Dr K.P.S. Dhama is an internationally renowned homoeopath who adopts a rational and analytical approach while treating any disease. He has cured several baffling ailments, which did not respond to traditional methods of treatment. Also, a large member of his articles and case reports have been published.

Dr (Mrs) Suman Dhama is a trained homoeopathic gynaecologist, and has vast experience in treating chronic cases. She is the author of a well-established book (in Hindi) on homoeopathy.

HOMOEOPATHY
The Complete Handbook

Dr. K.P.S. Dhama
&
Dr. (Mrs.) Suman Dhama

📖 UBSPD®
UBS Publishers' Distributors Pvt. Ltd.
New Delhi • Bangalore • Kolkata • Chennai • Patna • Bhopal • Ernakulam
Mumbai • Lucknow • Pune • Hyderabad • Bhubaneshwar • Coimbatore

UBS Publishers' Distributors Pvt. Ltd.

5 Ansari Road, New Delhi-110 002
Phones: 011-23273601-4, 23266646-47, 23274846, 23282281, 23273552
Fax: 23276593, 23274261• E-mail: ubspd@ubspd.com

10 First Main Road, Gandhi Nagar, Bangalore-560 009
Phones: 080-22253903, 22263901, 22263902, 22255153 • Fax: 22263904
E-mail: ubspd@bngm.ubspd.com, ubspdbng@airtelbroadband.in

8/1-B Chowringhee Lane, Kolkata-700 016
Phones: 033-22529473, 22521821, 22522910 • Fax: 22523027
E-mail: ubspdcal@cal.ubspd.com

60 Nelson Manickam Road, Aminjikarai, Chennai-600 029
Phones: 044-23746222, 23746351-2 • Fax: 23746287
E-mail: dbs@che.ubspd.com,ubspdche@che.ubspd.com

Ground Floor, Annapurna Complex, Naya Tola, Patna-800 004
Phones: 0612-2672856, 2673973, 2686170 • Fax: 2686169
E-mail: ubspdpat@pat.ubspd.com

Z-18, M.P. Nagar, Zone-I, Bhopal-462 011
Phones: 0755-4203183, 4203193, 2555228 • Fax: 2555285
E-mail: ubspdbhp@bhp.ubspd.com

No. 40/7940-41, Kollemparambil Chambers, Convent Road, Ernakulam-682 035
Phones: 0484-2353901, 2363905 • Fax: 2365511
E-mail: ubspdekm@ekm.ubspd.com

2nd Floor, Apeejay Chambers, 5 Wallace Street, Fort, Mumbai-400 001
Phones: 022-66376922, 66376923, 66102067, 66102069
Fax: 66376921 • E-mail: ubspdmum@mum.ubspd.com

9, Ashok Nagar, Near Pratibha Press, Gautam Buddha Marg, Latouche Road,
Lucknow-226 018 • Phones: 4025124, 4025134, 4025144, 6531753
Fax 4025144 • Email: ubspdlko@lko.ubspd.com

680 Budhwar Peth, 2nd floor, Near Appa Balwant Chowk, Pune-411 002
Phone: 020-24461653 • Fax: 020-24433976 • E-mail: ubspdpune@pun.ubspd.com

3rd & 4th Floors, Alekhya Jagadish Chambers, H.No.4-1-1058, Boggulkunta, Tilak Road,
Hyderabad-500 001 • Phones: 040-24754473, 24754474 • Telefax: 040-24754472
E-mail: ubspdhyd@hyd.ubspd.com

1st Floor, Plot No. 145, Cuttack Road, Bhubaneshwar-751 006
Phones: 0674-2314446, 2314447 • Fax: 0674-2314448
Email: ubspdbbh@bbh.ubspd.com

2nd & 3rd Floor, Sri Guru Towers, No. 1-7 Sathy Road, Cross III, Gandhipuram,
Coimbatore-641 012 • Phones: 0422-2499914, 2499916, 2499917
Fax: 0422-2499914 • Email: ubspdcbe@cbe.ubspd.com

Visit us at www.ubspd.com & www.gobookshopping.com

© Dr. K.P.S. Dhama and Dr. (Mrs.) Suman Dhama

First Published	1994	Sixteenth Reprint	2001
First Reprint	1995	Seventeenth Reprint	2002
Second Reprint	1995	Eighteenth Reprint	2002
Third Reprint	1995	Ninteenth Reprint	2003
Fourth Reprint	1996	Twentieth Reprint	2003
Fifth Reprint	1996	Twenty First Reprint	2004
Sixth Reprint	1996	Twenty Second Reprint	2004
Seventh Reprint	1997	Twenty Third Reprint	2005
Eighth Reprint	1997	Twenty Fourth Reprint	2005
Nineth Reprint	1998	Twenty Fifth Reprint	2006
Tenth Reprint	1998	Twenty Sixth Reprint	2006
Eleventh Reprint	1998	Twenty Seventh Reprint	2007
Twelfth Reprint	1999	Twenty Eighth Reprint	2008
Thirteenth Reprint	1999	Twenty Nineth Reprint	2009
Fourteenth Reprint	2000	Thirtieth Reprint	2009
Fifteenth Reprint	2000		

ISBN 978-81-86112-59-5

Cover Photo: Madan Mahatta

Printed at: Rajkamal Electric Press, Delhi

Preface

OUR PERSONALITY AND THE structure of our body are such that as soon as there appears any impurity or imbalance in them, its external signs start manifesting themselves in the form of various symptoms. If we can identify these symptoms in time and administer a homoeopathic medicine which shows similar symptoms, the malady can be cured. Such treatment does not clash with surgery, body exercises or yoga, or any other drugless system of treatment. It is said that a system of treatment, like homoeopathy, based on symptoms, attacking the malady from inside is generally not taken seriously. There can be only one answer to this situation: we, the homoeopaths, devote a great deal of our time and attention to the correct and precise analysis of symptoms and, based on that analysis, continue to administer our 'magic pills' undeterred.

An eminent allopath of England, Dr. Compton Burnett, was once himself afflicted with pleurisy. When allopathic treatment failed, he resorted to homoeopathic treatment and, after being cured, took to homoeopathic practice himself. He said if the homoeopathic method was kept secret the governments of the world would have been surprised by its curative powers and would be prepared to give anything to learn its secrets. How true is his statement! Homoeopathic medicines, if correctly prescribed, work like magic.

Illness or accident can strike at any time. In such a situation if we can administer quick medical treatment, many complications can be obviated. This book has been written to overcome such unexpected situations. The present work follows the shorter Hindi version after its unprecedented success and we are sure that this will be intelligible to an ordinary layperson who has a basic knowledge of English. This book will also be equally useful for quick consultation by the busy practitioner.

We have tried to present the subject matter in a way that will help the selection of medicines according to symptoms keeping in view the need to avoid unnecessary details. We have tried to be brief and to the point. If the readers wish to discuss the topics further, we are always prepared to do so provided a self-addressed and stamped envelope is sent.

Broadly speaking, the subject matter has been arranged ailment-wise in an alphabetical order, making it easy to locate medicines needed for individual ailments. Wherever necessary cross-references have also been given. For a better understanding of the subject and for easy practical application it would be necessary to go through the Introduction first.

We have benefited from the help and advice of many friends. The following names do merit special mention: Dr. Y.P. Chhibbar, Lt. Gen. R.P. Singh, and Shri S.J.S. Chhatwal. Shri Amit Nagi has prepared the final computerised manuscript with care and attention.

K.P.S.Dhama
Suman Dhama

Contents

✧ Contents ✧

❖ Contents ❖

✦ Contents ✦

✦ Contents ✦

Introduction to Homoeopathy

H OMOEOPATHY WAS INTRODUCED BY the famous German doctor, Samuel Hahnemann. It is a medical science that treats the ailments by medicines which have been tested on healthy persons and then validated. The question arises: Why on healthy persons? The answer will be clear after reading this introduction This makes the homoeopathic system foolproof and safe.

Dr. Hahnemann emphasized the futility of omnibus experiments or researches which tried to provide cures on the basis of the *overall disease* rather than focussing on *individual symptoms*. This is because human beings react differently from animals and also differently from each other. This phenomenon applies to both medicines and diseases. For example, *morphia* makes dogs vomit and renders them drowsy, whereas it excites cats; *aconite* kills sheep but does not affect horses and goats; *antimony* proves lethal to human beings and most animals except to hogs and elephants. The same logic can be extended to human beings. Therefore, each patient will have to be treated individually on the basis of his or her symptoms.

The basis of homoeopathy is a basic natural principle. In Latin this principle is stated as *similia similibus curentur* ("Let likes be treated by likes") – first propounded by Hippocrates. That is to say, that to cure any disease a drug must be found which is capable of producing similar symptoms when tested on healthy humans. Or in other words, a drug can only cure that which it can produce. The common person understands it as 'poison kills poison'. This principle is described in the Hindu texts as *vishasya vishmaushadham*. Everyone knows that iron cuts iron and heat symptoms can be cured by heat treatment.

According to science we cannot create anything; we can simply change the form. The things which exist today are because something was already there. A drug, in its **proving**, can evoke in each case only what was already there, latent in the prover – even as disease brings out only weak points and therefore does not affect two patients in exactly the same way. It requires many provers, of different types and different defective resistances, to bring out the complete picture of a drug pathogenesis.

It follows from this principle that the symptoms that are created in a healthy human body by taking a homoeopathic medicine will be cured by the same medicine if they are present during an ailment. For example, when a healthy person uses cannabis he/she suffers from hallucinations: one minute seems like an hour; nearby objects appear to be miles away; if the person laughs, he/she will go on doing so; if he/she starts to talk, will continue to talk; on passing urine there is cutting feeling and urine comes in drops; and the head starts aching. According to the homoeopathic principle, if in any ailment, these symptoms are present these will be cured by the homoeopathic medicine *Cannabis Indica* which is prepared from cannabis.

Thus in homoeopathy an ailment is treated according to its symptoms; the name of the ailment does not matter. To find out the symptoms of a medicine these are tested on healthy persons. This is known as *drug proving*.

> *Most of the substances that are used on the table as seasonings in foods will in the course of a generation or two be very useful medicines, because parents poison themselves with these substances as tea, coffee, pepper, and tobacco (though tobacco cannot be said to be on the table, yet it might as well be if it is used at all), and these poisonous effects in the parents cause in the children a predisposition to diseases, which are similar to the diseases produced by these substances.* **Kent**

Dr. M.L. Tyler describes the action-reaction as follows:

Every agent that acts on vitality (i.e., every medicine) more or less deranges the vital force, and causes, for a longer or shorter period, certain alterations in the health of the individual. This is termed *primary action*.

Although this primary action is a conjoint product of the medicinal and vital powers, it is principally due to the former.

To this primary action our vital force endeavours to apply energetic opposition: and this automatic, life-preserving reaction goes by the name of *secondary action,* or counteraction.

During the primary action of artificial morbific agents (medicines) on our healthy bodies, the vital force, as will be seen by the following examples, seems to behave in a passive, or receptive manner, as if compelled to receive impressions from without, acting on it and perverting its health. Then it appears to rally and to develop (a) an exactly opposite condition, if such be possible, the countereffect, proportionate to its own energy and to the intensity of the primary action. Or (b) where there is no condition exactly the opposite of the primary action, the vital force appears to "indifferentiate" itself, and, putting forth its superior strength, it extinguishes the morbid changes, thereby restoring normal health. This is the after-effect, or curative effect.

Examples of (a) are familiar to everybody. A hand bathed in hot water is at first much warmer than the other; but, taken out and dried well, it will, after a while, grow colder than the other hand (after-effect or secondary action). A person heated by violent exercise (primary action) is afterwards affected by chilliness and shivering (secondary action). To one heated the previous day by drinking a lot of wine (primary action), today every breath of air feels too cold (secondary action). Excessive vivacity after strong coffee (primary action) entails sluggishness and drowsiness for a long time afterwards (reaction – secondary action) if they are not removed for a short time by taking fresh supplies of coffee (palliative). After the profound, stupefied sleep caused by opium (primary action), the following night will be all the more sleepless (reaction – secondary action). After the constipation produced by opium (primary action) diarrhoea ensues (secondary action); and after purgation with medicines that irritate the bowels, constipation for several days ensues (secondary action).

In a like manner it always happens, after the primary action of a medicine which, in large doses, produces a great change in the health of a healthy person, that its exact opposite, provided there is such a thing, is produced in the secondary action by our vital force.

As following the action of minute homoeopathic doses in health, obvious secondary effects are perceived very little. For though such minute doses, closely observed, will be found to produce a perceptible primary effect, yet the living organism sets up only such countereffect as is absolutely required to re-establish normal conditions.

It must always be remembered that homoeopathy is essentially an individualistic treatment. It therefore never makes use of nor seeks specifics for disease. So it must not be thought that any remedy mentioned in this book will cover all the cases.

Thus we can draw the following conclusions:

1. Homoeopathy is based on basic natural principles.
2. Medicines can create ailments.
3. In order to find out full symptoms of a medicine it is tested on healthy persons.
4. For treating an ailment we have to administer a medicine which has the symptoms that are present in the ailment.

The mental and physical symptoms created in a healthy person by administering a medicine are catalogued in the homoeopathic *Materia Medica*.

HOW TO PREPARE HOMOEOPATHIC MEDICINES AND FROM WHAT

Homoeopathic medicines are prepared from plants (roots, bark, stem, buds, leaves. juices, gums, oils, etc., or whole plants), live substances (secretions of healthy organisms, poisons, etc.), body impurities, chemicals, synthetics, minerals, etc.. These medicines are available as mother tinctures, triturations or potencies.

The following media are used to prepare or to administer the medicines. These media do not have any medicinal quality of their own. These can be dry or in liquid form:

1. Sugar of milk – to prepare the trituration or to add medicine to.
2. Pharmaceutical grade cane sugar – for preparing globules or tablets.
3. Distilled water – to prepare and to administer medicines.
4. Alcohol – to prepare mother tinctures or potencies.
5. Glycerine – to preserve or to administer the medicines.
6. Vaseline – to prepare ointments.
7. Solvent ether – to test medicines.
8. Syrup simplex – to prepare syrups, etc..

Mother Tincture

Mother tinctures are generally prepared from plants which are soluble in alcohol. The alcohol percentage can be up to 90. Mother tincture is written as 'θ'.

Trituration

Substances that are not soluble in alcohol are ground with sugar of milk and triturations are prepared.

Potency

Mother tinctures and triturations contain the medicine in crude form. These are added to alcohol and are given successive strokes in a special way or are ground with sugar of milk in a mortar with a pestle to potentise them. For potentisation the mother tincture and alcohol, sugar of milk or distilled water can be in the ratio of 1 to 9 or 1 to 99. Medicines prepared from 1:9 are given the potentise name in 'X' along with the number, for example; 3X. This is a **decimal scale**. If the medicine is prepared as 1:99 (**centesimal scale**) we do not write anything along with the number: for example, Nux vomica 30.

HOW TO SELECT THE HOMOEOPATHIC MEDICINE

We have already mentioned that homoeopathy rests on a basic principle of nature. Allopathy or other Western systems do not pay any attention to the symptoms of the patient. The medicine is prescribed on the basis of the name of the ailment, whatever the symptoms.

Everyone knows that different patients suffering from the same ailment may show different symptoms. Different patients suffering from common cold may manifest the following different symptoms:

(a) Sudden cold; flowing nose; sneezing; aggravation of symptoms in a warm room; fear; restlessness; thirst; fever.

(b) Continuous sneezing because of cold; aggravation inside a warm room; too much watery, corroding flow; headache; cough; hoarseness. Eyes swollen and watering, not corroding; amelioration in open and cool place.

(c) Corroding flow from the nose; burning in eyes and nose; desire for sipping water at short intervals; restlessness and fear; weakness; sleeplessness because of headache; all symptoms are ameliorated by providing warmth.

(d) Flowing cold; constant flow of burning water from eyes; face hot, but the patient is cold and feels cold; aggravation of all the symptoms in the evenings and in warm room.

(e) Chill runs up and down the spine; tension and heaviness in head and on face; sneezing and post-nasal catarrh; feels sleepy; fever, which breaks without sweating and comes back; cold feeling accompanied by intense urination which lightens the head.

The above five patients are exhibiting different symptoms while suffering from common cold. They cannot be given the same medicine; their remedies will be as follows: (a) Aconite; (b) Allium cepa; (c) Arsenic alb.; (d) Euphrasia; and (e) Gelsemium.

If these five patients were go to an allopath they would have been given one and the same medicine. The allopath is not concerned with the increasing or decreasing of the flow, or with the type of the flow. He is simply concerned with cold which has one medicine. This medicine will not cure the cold but will suppress it. After some time, this suppressed cold can give rise to other more serious ailments.

The reason for giving a different medicine to every patient is that at the time of drug proving, different medicines produced different symptoms which shows that the homoeopathic medicine is selected on the basis of *similia similibus curentur*.

TREATMENT OF THE PATIENT NOT OF THE DISEASE

The reason behind every ailment is imbalance in the vital force. The equilibrium of the vital force maintains the body in a healthy state, this facilitates the flow of feelings and sensibilities. If for any reason this system of free communication is obstructed or derailed, the body becomes sick. This interruption of the line of communication is termed as shock; from an injury, from the death of a near relative or loved one, from drowning, from sudden cold, etc., a person is shocked. Shock lies at the root of all ailments.

Some people may maintain that illnesses have multifarious causes. It is correct that there may be numerous activating and contributing reasons to an ailment, but if they cannot cause a shock to the dynamic system, they cannot produce an illness.

It has been seen in some experiments that after administering anaesthesia a patient is not effected by even deadly poisons like potassium cyanide or prussic acid, though we all know that these can cause instantaneous death if administered to a healthy person even minimally. This shows that a deadly poison does not effect the anaesthetized person because in such a state the dynamic communication system itself does not work. So the question of its obstruction does not arise, hence the balance of the vital force is not disturbed and the person (dynamic plane or inner man) is not affected by the poison. The same thing happens when a person is in coma.

A human body lives as long as the vital force continues to function in it. This vital force is manifested in the mind, the dynamic system, etc., which are ethereal and not physical. As soon as the physical body is rendered devoid of the vital force, existence ends and the situation is defined as death.

Now the question is: *Why homoeopathy*? Crude or unpotentised drugs reduce our natural body defence system and lay the field open to ailments. A remedy, basically, performs the tasks of balancing the vital forces in the body so that the line of communication is maintained. As long as the vital force is undisturbed, the body remains healthy. If developments like gangrene kill the tissues, the vital force in that region is destroyed and the medicine will have no effect on that part but the homoeopathic medicines can re-establish the balance of vital force and throw out the dead tissues; and health is restored.

Every big or small accident produces some shock. It is necessary to observe the general rules of treating a shock (viz., to keep the victim warm, to use the hot water bottle, to cover with woollens, etc.). Homoeopathic medicine **Arnica 200**, a few doses given at short intervals, helps the victim to recover in a short time. Arnica is one of the basic medicines for shock.

If the victim becomes unconscious from a shock, *Arnica helps him or her in regaining consciousness*. Pain resulting from physical or mental injury is cured by Arnica. Inflammations at the time of dentition or pain, sprain, fracture, etc., respond well to Arnica.

DO NOT SUPPRESS AN ILLNESS

An illness is like garbage in your house. It has to be thrown out. Covering or pushing it aside will not make you secure against its harmful effects. Similarly, an ailment is a foreign element in the body and must be taken out. It is a folly to keep it covered and let it remain inside the body. Homoeopathy operates on the principle of removing the garbage and not putting it aside.

DOSAGE AND FREQUENCY OF MEDICINE

The medicine intake should be repeated in proportion to the acuteness of the illness: in an emergency, every 10 to 15 minutes, otherwise from two to four times a day is normally a safe principle. One has to remember that when the medicine starts showing its effect, the frequency should be reduced. Unnecessary repetition can produce the symptoms of the medicine in the patient.

In long-lasting ailments like influenza, typhoid or pneumonia one should keep on giving medicines three or four times a day for some time. The medicines work better on an empty stomach. Potentised medicine should be put in freshly cleaned mouth and allowed to dissolve. These medicines are available in tablets or in globules of different sizes. Generally globules No. 20 or 30 are used. In case of children two to three and in case of adults five to six globules make a dose. Tablets are generally of one grain in measure. In case of children one or two tablets and in case of adults five to six tablets are sufficient. In case of infants a few drops of a tablet dissolved in water will do. **Fifty millesimal** (fifty thousandth potency) are labelled as 0/1, 0/2, 0/3, and so on, or LM-1, LM-2, LM-3, etc. Generally they are prepared in distilled water. One teaspoon three or four times a day should be taken. We have not discussed this process in detail because it is not very common, but is very effective in chronic cases.

Mother tincture (denoted by 'θ') is administered in doses of from 1 or 2 to 10 to 15 drops, in water.

The vials or bottles containing medicine should be kept in some cool place, away from sunlight. They should be kept away from strong smells. You must buy medicines from some dependable place as these have to be in correct potency, etc. A wrong potency may not work and the ailment may become aggravated. You should not take anything up to half an hour before or after taking the medicine. Intake of onions, coffee, pickles, etc., is prohibited along with some medicines. Your doctor should inform you about this. If you feel an intense desire to eat something, take it. If something does not agree with you, shun it. Simple, bland and vegetarian diet helps during illness.

SYMBOLS/ABBREVIATIONS USED IN THE BOOK

☆	Effective in most cases
❑	Most commonly effective in other cases
●	Intercurrent/catalyst
❀	Based on our clinical experience
SOS	As and when required
( )	*(Consulting* Materia Medica *is necessary for any other clarification.) Figures in parentheses denote the number of maximum doses. When a particular potency is no more effective, the next higher potency is advisable.*

Warning: When pathological changes occur in the system, high potencies should not be used and the treatment should be under the guidance of an experienced physician only.

The users have to understand that such a work can never be a guarantee; the homoeopathic literature is just a long distance treatment and is no substitute for a face-to-face contact between the patient and the doctor.

ABDOMINAL PAIN
(See Colic Also)

Symptoms	Remedy	Frequency And Doses
☆ Violent pains; better hard pressure; umbilical region	Colocynth. 30	3 hourly
❑ Food lies like a stone in the stomach; stools hard, constipated; desire to lie quietly	Bryonia 30 or 200	2 hourly (3)
❑ Shooting pain; hysterical colic	Ignatia 30 or 200	3 hourly (3)
❑ Stitching pain; worse movements; colicky, before menses	Kali carb. 30 or 200	3 hourly (3)
❑ Pain spasmodic; cutting, soon after eating	Kali bich. 30	3 hourly
❑ With soreness above pelvis	Verat-vir. 30	3 hourly
❑ Pain after discharging flatus excessively; worse eating rich, fatty foods	Pulsatilla 30	3 hourly
❑ Radiating to other parts	Plumbum met. 30	3 hourly
❑ In upper abdomen; stools hard, constipated	Graphites 30	3 hourly
❑ In front portion of abdomen; tongue clean	Ipecac 30	3 hourly
❑ In lower abdomen	Viburnum op. 30	3 hourly
❑ In hypogastrium	Cimicifuga 30	3 hourly
☆ Pain suddenly shifts and appears in distant parts like in fingers and toes. Pain better bending backwards and stretching the body	Dioscorea 30	3 hourly
☆ After abdominal operation; indignation	Staphysagria 30 or 200	4 hourly
☆ After over eating; due to sedentary habits	Nux vomica 30	3 hourly

Symptoms	Remedy	Frequency And Doses
✰ Violent, spasmodic pain; better by hot drinks/applications	**Magnesia phos. 6X or 30**	2 hourly
	Bio-combination No.3	3 hourly

ABORTION
Miscarriage

To give birth to an embryo or foetus before it is viable is called miscarriage, it may be spontaneous due to fright, a fall or injury, etc., or induced (abortion). Some women are prone to miscarriage in specific months of pregnancy.

Threatened:

✰ From fright or excitement	**Aconite 200**	10 min. (3)
✰ Acute bleeding with continuous flow of bright red blood; colic; tongue clean	**Ipecac Q or 30**	1/2 hourly
✰ Abortion in any month (particularly 8th month). *The patient must take complete bed rest*	**Viburnum pr. Q or 30**	2 hourly
✰ For impending abortion; when bleeding starts	**Trillium p. Q,** 5-10 drops	1/2 hourly
❏ Threatened from a fall or shock, etc.	**Arnica 200**	10 min. (3)
❏ Threatened due to mental excitement	**Chamomilla 30 or 200**	2 hourly
❏ From over exertion or irritating emotions	**Helonias Q,** 5-10 drops	2 hourly
❏ With black, non-coagulable blood	**Crotalus h. 30 or 200,**	1/2 hourly (3)
❏ Due to weakness of uterus	**Caulophyllum 30**	3 hourly
❏ Abortion during 1st month	**Crocus sativa Q or 30**	3 hourly
❏ Tendency of abortion; specially in anaemic patients	**Aletris f. Q,** 5-10 drops	2 hourly
❏ When haemorrhage persists for some time	**Thlaspi bur-p. Q,** 5-10 drops	2 hourly
❏ After effects of abortion; pain in lower back and genitals, etc.	**Sabina 30**	6 hourly (6)
❏ To recover from weakness due to excessive bleeding	**China 30**	3 hourly

Symptoms	Remedy	Frequency And Doses

To Prevent Miscarriage (in tendency to):

The medicines can be given according to the symptoms at least one month previous to the expected time when abortion is expected (when miscarrige occurs in specific months).

Symptoms	Remedy	Frequency And Doses
❑ To prevent tendency of abortion when there is thyroid distrubance	**Thyroidinum 200**	*weekly (3)*
❑ In anaemic patients	**Ferrum met. 3X**	*3 hourly*
❑ Abortion due to hardening of cervix	**Aurum mur-nat. 3X**	*3 hourly*
❑ In fat and flabby women with profuse and early menstruation	**Calcarea carb. 200 or 1M**	*weekly (3)*
❑ In hysterical women with superiority complex	**Platina 1M**	*10 min. (3)*
❑ Abortion in early months; habitual in 2nd month	**Kali carb. 1M**	*weekly (3)*
❑ Habitual in 2nd, 3rd or 4th month	**Apis mel. 200**	*weekly (3)*
❑ During 3rd month with blackish bleeding	**Kreosotum 30 or 200**	*weekly (3)*
❑ During 3rd month; haemorrhage partly clotted; worse from least motion	**Sabina 200 or 1M**	*weekly (3)*
❑ Abortion - 5th to 7th month	**Sepia 30 or 200**	*weekly (3)*
❑ Abortion - 2nd and 7th month	**D.N.A. 1M**	*weekly (3)*
❑ Abortion after 7th month	**Opium 200 or 1M**	*weekly (3)*
❑ In women with weak and unhealthy uterus (history of profuse menses lasting for weeks together)	**Secale cor. 30 or 200**	*4 hourly*
● Intercurrent remedy; when there is tubercular family history	**Tuberculinum K. 200 or 1M**	*fortnightly (3)*
● Intercurrent remedy; when there is history of abortion	**Syphilinum 200 or 1M**	*fortnightly (3)*
Biochemic remedies	**Kali phos. 6X, Calcarea phos. 6X and Calcarea fluor. 6X**	*4 hourly*

If pain or bleeding starts, the patient should lie down in a comfortable position. In emergency hospitalisation is necessary.

To Induce Abortion (when menses are delayed for a few days only):

Gossypium Q, Pulsatilla Q, and *Secale cor. Q* in equal quantity can be tried in 40 drops doses, four times a day for 3-4 days (success is in 70% cases approximately).

ABSCESSES AND BOILS
Including Carbuncles, etc.

An ordinary inflammation may develop into a boil going on to become an abscess. All the three stages are covered here.

Symptoms	Remedy	Frequency And Doses
1st Stage		
(Inflammatory stage to suppurative stage)		
☆ In acute abscesses; blood boils, when pus develop with lightening rapidity (mammary, hepatic or glandular abscesses)	**Belladonna 30**	*2 hourly*
☆ Favours rapid formation of pus, useful for glandular abscesses with throbbing pain; worse from warmth of bed	**Mercurius sol. 30** (**Mercurius sol. 30** and **Belladonna 30** can be given alternately)	*3 hourly*
☆ In the beginning of suppuration; corroding, putrid, bloody pus formation with chill and sharp stitching pain; pus smells like old cheese. Though the patient is chilly but feels better in wet weather	**Hepar sulph. 30**	*4 hourly*
❑ In the beginning when the part is red with shining. Stitching pain; worse by slightest motion	**Bryonia 30**	*4 hourly*
❑ Swelling very red with shining and burning; fever with dry hot skin; worse in warm room, evening, and night	**Aconite 6 or 30**	*2 hourly*
❑ When Hepar sulph. fails and the pain is unbearable	**Chamomilla 30 or 200**	*3 hourly*
❑ To cut short the duration of suppuration. It often does the work of a knife. Abscesses on ends of fingers and phallenges	**Myristica seb. 1X or 3X**	*2 hourly*
❑ Small painful/sore boils in crops (summer boils)	**Arnica 30 or 200**	*4 hourly*
❀ To hasten suppuration	**Hepar sulph. 2X or 3X**	*2 hourly*
❀ To check suppuration	**Hepar sulph. 1M or 10M**	*10 min. (3)*

(**Hepar sulph.** in low potencies should not be given in tonsillitis in suppurative stage)

Symptoms	Remedy	Frequency And Doses

2nd Stage
(When the suppuration has taken place)

Symptoms	Remedy	Frequency And Doses
☆ When the suppuration continues and boil does not heal. To bring the suppurative process to maturity; chilly Patient; better in dry and warm weather	**Silicea 6X or 6**	*3 hourly*
❑ To form healthy granulation after Silicea	**Fluoric acid. 30**	*4 hourly*
☆ When Silicea fails and the suppuration continues; better in open air and worse in change of weather	**Calcarea sulph. 6X or 30**	*3 hourly*
☆ Copious, bloody, yellowish or greenish pus; worse after taking rich food, and warmth; better in cold, open air	**Pulsatilla 30**	*4 hourly*
❑ Abscesses in patient of tubercular diathesis	**Calcarea carb. 200**	*4 hourly (6)*
❑ When pus is thick and yellow without inflammation	**Calendula 30**	*3 hourly*
❑ Abscesses beneath skin; worse warm applications and warmth	**Lycopodium 30 or 200**	*4 hourly (6)*
❑ Useful for suppurating glands. Pus may be copious, corroding, thin and watery	**Rhus tox. 6 or 30**	*4 hourly*
❑ Pus thin and sticky. Eruptions in bends of limbs, groins, neck and behind ears	**Graphites 30 or 200**	*4 hourly*
❑ For recurring abscess conditions, fever, etc.. To clean the system and to prevent a recurrence	**Pyrogenium 200 or 1M**	*weekly (3)*
❑ For unhealthy offensive pus with a low condition and hepatic fever. Extreme burning sensation and restlessness	**Arsenic alb. 30 or 200**	*4 hourly*
❑ Carbuncles/boils with intense burning and high fever	**Anthracinum 200 or 1M**	*10 min. (3)*
❑ In low conditions of abscess; boils of bluish colour when the pus is thin, dark and	**Lachesis 30 or 200**	*10 min. (3)*

Symptoms	Remedy	Frequency And Doses
offensive in character. Burning pains; sensitive to touch		
❑ Painful and inflammed abscesses with tendency to gangrene; the neighbouring glands are swollen, hard and painful. Specific for abscesses under the armpit	**Tarentula c. 200 or 1M**	*weekly (3)*
❑ For bloody or greenish yellow pus; intense pain.	**Nitric ac. 200 or 1M**	*10 min. (3)*
❑ Boils or felons caused by needle pricks	**Ledum pal. 200 or 1M**	*10 min. (3)*
❑ To purify blood; when low fever persists due to infection	**Echinacea 1X or 30**	*4 hourly*
❑ Bad effects of burns. Pus may be bloody, greenish, greyish or yellowish; corroding, thin and watery	**Causticum 30 or 200**	*4 hourly*
❑ Ulcers which mature slowly. Burning pains; pus thin, watery and offensive may be bloody, brownish or yellowish. Tendency to gangrene. Better fanning	**Carbo veg. 30 or 200**	*3 hourly*
❑ Abscesses with excruciating pains; inflammation, chronic carbuncles, boils; abscesses in the joints especially left hip joint. Septic pus	**Stramonium 200 or 1M**	*10 min. (3)*
❑ Carbuncles on lumbar region with diabetes. Foul discharge of pus from several openings. Nausea and vomiting	**Carbolic acid 200**	*10 min. (3)*
❑ For boils, herpes zoster, ascariasis and blood poisoning; stools constipated	**Gunpowder 3X or 30**	*4 hourly*
❑ When the pus is blackish, thin, watery, putrid and offensive	**Kali phos. 6X or 30**	*3 hourly*
● For syphilitic and tubercular patients		
❑ Boils in axilla; glands swollen	**Kali iod. 200 or 1M**	*weekly (3)*
❑ For abscesses about the bones	**Carbo ani. 30 or 200**	*4 hourly (6)*

Symptoms	Remedy	Frequency And Doses
❑ Recurrent boils in external ear with past history of measles	**Phosphorus 200 or 1M**	*3 hourly (6)*
❑ Boils in the external ears; worse summer	**Morbillinum 200**	*10 min. (3)*
❑ Small, painful boils; pus greenish which mature slowly	**Picric acid. 30**	*4 hourly (6)*
	Secale cor. 30 or 200	*10 min. (3)*
● In chronic cases when the discharge of pus is profuse with emaciation and hepatic fever (intercurrent remedy)	**Sulphur 200**	*one dose*

Biochemic remedy

	Remedy	Frequency
	Calcarea sulph. 12X (to heal the tissues)	*4 hourly*

For External Use:

For dressing Calendula ext. Q and Echinacea ext. Q (lotion or ointment) is very useful. To relieve unbearable pain Arnica mont. Q and Cassia soph. Q as a paint are useful. To burst boils (paint the medicine on effected lesion) Pulsatilla Q, Dioscorea Q or Bryonia Q. To suppress boils Calcarea caust. 1X is very useful.

ACIDITY
Hyperacidity (Gastralgia)

An abnormal degree of acidity in the stomach which brings cramp, gnawing or contractive pains and burning, etc., in the stomach associated with anxiety, belching, headache and constipation, etc., is called hyperacidity.

Symptoms	Remedy	Frequency
☆ Excess of hydrochloric acid; burning in the food pipe, heart burn, nausea and chilly feeling	**Acid-sulph. 30**	*4 hourly*
☆ From nervous anticipation of coming events; desire for sweets	**Argentum nit. 30**	*4 hourly*
☆ Gastric complaints after taking rich fatty food; less or no thirst; better open air	**Pulsatilla 30**	*4 hourly*
❑ Hyperacidity; sour and bitter belchings	**Iris v. 30**	*4 hourly*
❑ Slow and imperfect digestion; offensive flatulence in upper part of abdomen; better after discharge of gas or eructations	**Carbo veg. 30**	*4 hourly*

Symptoms	Remedy	Frequency And Doses
❑ Gastric derangements due to sedentary habits or over-eating	**Nux vomica 30**	*4 hourly*
☆ Dyspepsia; better after eating	**Anacardium or. 30**	*4 hourly*
❑ Acidity with irritating eructations and frontal headache; worse night	**Robinia 30**	*4 hourly*
❑ Constant belching; tongue thickly white coated. Heartburn. Desire for acids, pickles, etc.	**Antim-crud. 30 or. 200**	*6 hourly*
❑ Digestion slow; no change after passing flatus or after belching. Flatulence affects middle part of the abdomen	**China 6 or 30**	*4 hourly*
❑ Abdomen bloated; easy satiety, gas affects lower part of the abdomen; worse in the evening – 4 to 8 p.m.	**Lycopodium 30**	*4 hourly*
☆ Pain and flatulence in stomach; smell of food causes nausea	**Colchicum 30**	*4 hourly (3)*
● Intercurrent remedy	**Psorinum 30**	*4 hourly (3)*
Biochemic remedy Specially for infants	**Natrum phos. 3 X or 6X**	*3 hourly*

ACNE
Pimples

An inflammatory follicular, papular and pustuler eruption involving the sebaceous apparatus on face, chest and back is called acne.

● Head remedy. Pimples worse during menses; worse after eating fats, sugar coffee and meat	**Psorinum 200 or 1M**	*weekly (3)*
☆ Pimples at the age of puberty with itching	**Asterias rub. 30**	*6 hourly*
☆ If *Asterias rub*. fails; pustular eruptions	**Kali brom. 30**	*6 hourly*
❑ Chronic cases; worse taking eggs and during winter season	**Streptococcin. 200 or 1M**	*weekly (3)*

Symptoms	Remedy	Frequency And Doses
❑ To clean the complexion	**Berberis aquifolium Q**, 7-8 drops	*4 hourly*
❑ Pimples; stools constipated like sheep's dung; worse from sea bathing	**Magnesia mur. 30**	*6 hourly*
❑ Acne of nose; better in damp weather	**Causticum 30**	*6 hourly*
❑ To cover tendency of pimples and to purify the blood	**Echinacea Q**, 5-10 drops	*4 hourly*
❑ Acne rosacea. Pimples are painful for some distance around; worse during menstruation	**Eugenia j.Q**, 5-10 drops	*4 hourly*
❑ Pimples hard like flee bites; chilblains	**Agaricus mus. 30 or 200**	*6 hourly*
❑ Skin moist; pimples; digestion slow; flatulence; better fanning	**Carbo veg. 30 or 200**	*6 hourly*
❑ Rose coloured pimples; pale, waxy skin; chilly persons	**Silicea 200 or 1M**	*weekly (3)*
● Acne in tubercular patients	**Tuberculinum k. 200 or 1M**	*weekly (3)*
❑ Acne hard; indurated base with pustule at apex; night sweats	**Arsenic iod. 3X or 6**	*4 hourly*
● When above remedies fail (intercurrent remedy)	**Sulphur 200 or 1M**	*weekly (3)*
Biochemic Remedy specially in young girls with menstrual disorders and general weakness	**Calcarea phos. 6X**	*4 hourly*

ADDICTIONS
To Reduce The Cravings

A wrong habit of taking of drugs or excessive use of alcohol, etc., harmful to the person.

❑ To opium	**Berberis vul. Q**, 5-10 drops	*4 hourly*
❑ To Morphia	**Avena sat. Q**, 10-20 drops	*4 hourly*

Symptoms	Remedy	Frequency And Doses
● Hereditary craving for alcohol	**Syphilinum 1M**	*weekly (6)*
Biochemic remedies		
To tone up the nervous system	**Kali phos. 6X** and **Natrum phos. 3X**	*4 hourly*

ADENOIDS

Hypertrophy of the lymphoid nodules in the posterior wall of the naso-pharynx resulting from chronic inflammation.

● To start the treatment; also as an intercurrent remedy	**Bacillinum 1M or 10M**	*fortnightly (3)*
☆ In fat and flabby children who takes cold at every change of weather; extremities cold	**Calcarea carb. 200 or 1M**	*weekly (6)*
☆ In children with recurring attacks of acute tonsillitis	**Baryta carb. 200 or 1M**	*weekly (6)*
☆ Fetid smell; thick, ropy, greenish - yellow discharge from nose; coryza with blockage of nose	**Kali bich. 30 or 200**	*4 hourly*
❑ With lymphoid hypertrophy; mucous yellowish in colour; post-nasal catarrh	**Hydrastis c. 30**	*4 hourly*
❑ Greenish, purulent expectoration; patient sensitive to cold	**Calcarea iod. 30 or 200**	*4 hourly*
❑ Patient sensitive to cold; sensation of heat and dryness in the throat; drinks water frequently; feels better after eating	**Cistus can. 30**	*4 hourly*
● Chronic catarrh; blockage of nose, offensive discharges; chilly patient	**Psorinum 200 or 1M**	*weekly (3)*
❑ Patient prone to cold; obstruction of nostrils; chronic tonsillitis. Breathes with open mouth	**Agraphis nut. 6 or 30**	*4 hourly*

Symptoms	Remedy	Frequency And Doses
Biochemic Remedies When adenoids cover post-nasal space and pharynx	**Calcarea fluor. 12X** and **Calcarea phos. 6X**	*4 hourly*

ALBUMINURIA

The presence of protein in urine, mainly the albumin is called albuminuria.

☆ Albuminous urine with burning and drawing pain in urethra	**Terebinth. Q**, 5-10 drops	*4 hourly*
☆ Urine turbid; offensive, contains ropy or bloody mucous; difficulty in passing urine	**Chimaphila umb. Q**, 5-10 drops	*4 hourly*
❑ Frequent; profuse, watery, milky urine; worse night	**Acid-phos. Q**, 5-10 drops	*4 hourly*
❑ Urine albuminous; alkaline, clear and profuse; contains phosphates	**Helonias Q**, 5-10 drops	*4 hourly*
● History of suppressed gonorrhoea. Painful, slow urination	**Medorrhinum 200 or 1M**	*10 min. (3)*
☆ Frequent urging; burning in urethra on beginning to urinate. Urine dark, scanty and bloody	**Mercurius sol. 200 or 1M**	*weekly (3)*
❑ Urine albuminous with great pain in urethra along with gout; during pregnancy	**Mercurius cor. 30**	*6 hourly*
❑ Frequent urging; scanty, dark, coffee coloured urine. Bladder distended	**Helleborus Q or 30**	*6 hourly*
☆ Urine turbid; brown with red sediments, haematuria; thirst for icy cold water	**Phosphorus 30 or 200**	*4 hourly (3)*
☆ Scanty; high coloured urine loaded with casts; burning and soreness while passing urine; loss of thirst; worse heat	**Apis mel. 30 or 200**	*4 hourly (3)*

Symptoms	Remedy	Frequency And Doses
❏ Urine dark; scanty or suppressed, bloody, brown, blackish; contains albumin; patient feels worse with smell of food	**Colchicum 30 or 200**	*4 hourly*
❏ When the urine contains blood and albumin; lightening like pain in locomotor ataxia, brain fag; nervousness and vertigo	**Zincum phos. 30**	*4 hourly*
☆ Urine albuminous, turbid and scanty; severe burning in urethra while passing urine	**Cantharis 30**	*4 hourly*
Biochemic remedy	**Kali phos. 6X**	*4 hourly*

ALCOHOL
Bad Effects Of

Symptoms	Remedy	Frequency And Doses
☆ For bad effects of excessive use of alcohol; tremors, delirium and gastric complaints, etc.; irritable and nervous patient	**Nux vomica 30 or 200**	4 hourly
☆ When patient can not digest even small quantity of food without taking alcohol	**Acid-sulph. 30**	*4 hourly*
❏ When patient becomes violent and talkative after prolonged use of alcohol	**Cannabis ind. 30 or 200**	*4 hourly*
❏ For patients who drink in excess and have many fears in mind. Delirium tremens	**Opium 200 or 1M**	*10 min. (3)*
❏ Patient becomes intoxicated after consuming small quantity of alcoholic drinks; especially old bachelors	**Conium mac. 200**	*6 hourly (6)*
❏ Usually constipated, stools hard; patient feels intoxicated with small quantity of alcoholic drinks	**Alumina 30 or 0/5 and above**	*4 hourly*
☆ For bad characters who are wicked and jealous by nature and talk nonsense even before drinking	**Lachesis 30 or 200**	*6 hourly*

Symptoms	Remedy	Frequency And Doses
❑ Delirium tremens - constant; loquacious	**Hyoscyamus 30 or 200**	*10 min. (3)*
☆ Delirium tremens - inflammatory; rush of blood towards head	**Belladonna 30**	*1/2 hourly*
☆ Delirium tremens-maniacal; hallucination, illusions and fear of dark	**Stramonium 200 or 1M**	*10 min. (3)*
❑ Mental depression and tremors; tries to injure himself	**Cimicifuga 30 or 200**	*1/2 hourly*
Biochemic remedy To tone up the nervous system	**Kali phos. 6X**	*4 hourly*

ALCOHOLISM
To Create Aversion

Symptoms	Remedy	Frequency And Doses
⚹ To create aversion to alcoholic drinks. Water causes coldness in the stomach; water must be mixed with liquors	**Acid-sulph. 30**	*4 hourly*
☆ For chronic drunkards with weak heart	**Strophanthus Q**, 10 drops	*4 hourly*
❑ To take away craving for alcohol	**Quercus g-s. Q**, 30-40 drops	*4 hourly*
❑ To produce disgust for liquor	**Angelica Q**, 10 drops	*4 hourly*
● Hereditary tendency (excessive desire) for alcoholic drinks	**Syphilinum 1M or 10M**	*weekly (12)*
✾ If Angelica Q fails	**Camphor Q**, 5 drops	*4 hourly (SOS)*
✾ Desire to take alcoholic drinks instead of water	**Arsenic alb. 30**	*3 hourly (SOS)*
❑ For weak and nervous persons who are addicted to alcohol	**Avena sat. Q**, 10-15 drops	*4 hourly*
Biochemic remedy	**Kali phos. 6X**	*4 hourly*

ALLERGIES

Hyper-sensitiveness to Certain Foods, Drinks and Medicines, etc.

To relieve allergic conditions in certain cases the same allergen can be given in minute amounts (potentised), so small that it be just short of producing symptoms. But in homoeopathy 'law of similia' is the only answer.

Symptoms (Allergen)	Remedy	Frequency And Doses
☆ Allergic to dust; smoke, strong perfumes	**Histamine 1M**	*weekly (3)*
❏ Allergic to bread; acidic food	**Nat-mur. 30 or 200**	*4 hourly*
❏ Allergic to beer; malt liquor	**Kali bich. 30**	*4 hourly*
❏ Allergic to dust (asthma)	**Pothos foe. 6 or 30**	*4 hourly*
❏ Allergic to warm boiled milk; fatty pork, (diarrhoea)	**Sepia 30 or 200**	*4 hourly*
❏ Allergic to milk	**Magnesia carb. 30 or 200**	*6 hourly*
❏ Allergic to cod liver oil	**Hepar sulph. 30**	*6 hourly*
❏ Allergic to aspirin; bad liquors, salt butter, bad eggs, poultry items	**Carbo veg. 30**	*4 hourly*
❏ Allergic to antibiotics	**Sulphur 30 or 200**	*6 hourly (3)*
❏ Allergic to castor oil	**Bryonia alb. 30**	*6 hourly*
❏ Allergic to coffee	**Nux vomica 30**	*4 hourly*
❏ Allergic to heat	**Apis mel. 30**	*4 hourly*
❏ Allergic to cold drinks; fruits, rotten food, iodine	**Arsenic alb. 30**	*4 hourly*
❏ Allergic to dampness	**Dulcamara 30 or 200**	*4 hourly*
❏ Allergic to smell of flowers (asthma)	**Ailanthus g. 6 or 30**	*4 hourly*
❏ Allergic to sweets; fatty meat, onion	**Thuja oc. 30 or 200**	*6 hourly (3)*
❏ Allergic to sugar	**Argentum nit. 30 or 200**	*6 hourly (3)*
❏ Allergic to rice	**Tellurium 30 or 200**	*6 hourly*
❏ Allergic to cabbage	**Petroleum 30 or 200**	*6 hourly*
❏ Allergic to cheese	**Nitri-spiritus dulcis Q or 30**	*6 hourly*

Symptoms	Remedy	Frequency And Doses
❑ Allergic to cold milk	**Kali iod. 200**	*6 hourly*
❑ Allergic to decayed vegetables	**Carbo animalis 30 or 200**	*6 hourly*
❑ Allergic to unripe fruits; prunes	**Rheum 200**	*6 hourly*
❑ Allergic to veal	**Kali nit. 200**	*6 hourly*
❑ Allergic to pastry; rich ice-cream, mixed variety food	**Pulsatilla 30**	*4 hourly*
❑ Allergic to lemonade	**Selenium 30 or 200**	*6 hourly*
❑ Allergic to indigestible food; tongue clean, constant nausea	**Ipecac 30 or 200**	*6 hourly*
❑ Allergic to melons	**Zingiber 30**	*4 hourly*
❑ Allergic to iodide of potassium	**Aurum met. 30 or 200**	*6 hourly*
❑ Allergic to sugar; bitter food	**Natrum phos. 6X or 30**	*4 hourly*
● Intercurrent remedy	**Psorinum 200 or 1M**	*fortnightly (3)*
❑ Allergic to vinegar; pickles, sour foods, acids	**Lachesis 200**	*weekly (3)*
❑ Allergic to strawberries	**Oxalic acid 30 or 200**	*weekly (3)*
❑ Allergic to oysters	**Lycopodium 200**	*weekly (3)*

ALLERGIC BRONCHITIS
(See Bronchitis and Allergies also)

Inflammation of the mucous membranes of the bronchial tubes due to altered reaction incited by an antigen or allergen is called Allergic Bronchitis.

❑ After preventive vaccines (***Triple antigen, polio oral vaccine*** or ***B.C.G.***)	**Drosera 1M** (never give in acute stage)	*fortnightly (3)*
❑ After vaccination against Small Pox	**Thuja oc. 200 or 1M**	*10 min. (3)*
❑ After vaccination against Diphtheria	**Diphtherinum 1M**	*10 min. (3)*
Biochemic remedies	**Ferrum phos. 6X** and **Kali mur. 6X**	*4 hourly*

ALLERGIC RHINITIS
(See Cold, Catarrh, Sinusitis and Cough also)

'Allergy' can be explained as an altered reaction capacity of an individual to any given substance to which normally individuals are not sensitive to the extent of producing symptoms. Hahnemann himself had envisaged these allergic reactions when he mentioned about 'Idio-syncracies', which he defines as peculiar corporeal constitutions which, although otherwise healthy possess a disposition to be brought into a more or less morbid state by certain things which seem to produce impression and no change in many other individuals.

Symptoms	Remedy	Frequency And Doses
☆ Allergic to dust; smoke, perfumes, and sprays, etc., usually of the naso pharynx which leads to sneezing and blockage of nose and then cough	Histamine 1M	weekly (3)
❑ Allergic to dust; coryza with profuse nasal discharge and sneezing in the evening, dull frontal headache; lachrymation with itching in eyes	Justicia adhatoda 30	4 hourly
☆ Profuse, watery coryza; itching in posterior chamber of nose	Solanum lycopersicum 30	4 hourly
Biochemic remedies	Natrum mur. 12X and Natrum sulph. 12X	3 hourly

AMOEBIASIS
(See Dysentery also)

☆ Tongue clean; stools slimy, greenish or like frothy molasses with gripping at naval	Ipecac 30 or 0/5 (and above)	4 hourly
☆ With despair, dejection and irritability; loss of weight	Emetine 30	4 hourly
❑ Stools greenish bloody and slimy; worse at night with pain and tenesmus in abdomen; never get done feeling	Mercurius sol. 30	4 hourly
❑ Fetid stools with flatus; great weakness after passing stool; involuntary stools, patient feels as if anus remained wide open	Phosphorus 30	4 hourly
Biochemic Remedy	Kali phos. 6X	

ANAEMIA

Symptoms	Remedy	Frequency And Doses
☆ Anaemia due to loss of vital fluids; blood loss, excessive menstruation, semen loss, dysentery, etc., with much weakness; extremities cold with dropsy	China 6 or 30	4 hourly
☆ Anaemia with breathlessness after slight exertion. Sudden fiery flushing of face with paleness of parts with dropsical swelling	Ferrum met. 3X or 6	4 hourly
❑ Anaemia due to over-indulgence in sex	Acid-phos. 30	4 hourly
❑ Anaemia caused by over-dosing of Iron. Menstrual disorders; absence or loss of thirst; better in open, cool air	Pulsatilla 30	4 hourly
❑ Anaemia with extreme prostration and anxiety; due to malarial and toxic influence. Irritability and restlessness; thirst excessive, sips water frequently	Arsenic alb. 30	4 hourly
☆ Anaemia after prolonged nervous tension	Phosphorus 200	3 hourly (3)
❑ Anaemia in fat and flabby persons who crave for indigestible things	Calcarea carb. 1M	weekly (3)
❑ Anaemia of business-man, studious persons, etc., due to sedentary life and more intake of stimulants like tea and alcoholic drinks, etc.	Nux vomica 30	4 hourly
❑ Anaemia with palpitation and breathlessness	Strophanthus Q, 5-10 drops	4 hourly
❑ Progressive and pernicious anaemia; brain-fag and sexual excitement	Picric acid. 30	4 hourly
❑ Anaemia with extreme weakness and throbbing all over the body; soft pulse; general depression; patient feels worse at 3 a.m.	Kali carb. 30 or 200	4 hourly (3)
● Anaemia with breathlessness; patient feels better lying flat and in warmth; desires warm clothings even in summer	Psorinum 200	weekly (3)

Symptoms	Remedy	Frequency And Doses
❑ For aplastic anaemia	**T.N.T. 200**	*weekly (3)*
❑ Anaemia after long continued malaria. Emaciation inspite of eating well; excessive thirst; depression; consolation aggravates. Desire to eat extra salt.	**Natrum mur. 6X or 30**	*4 hourly*
❑ Pernicious or chlorotic anaemia in young girls with waxy complexion	**Calcarea phos. 6X**	*4 hourly*
Biochemic remedies	**Ferrum phos. 1X or 3X** and **Calcarea phos. 6X**	*4 hourly*
	Bio-combination No.1	*4 hourly*

ANGER
Annoyance

❑ Anger when misunderstood; before convulsions	**Bufo rana. 200 or 1M**	*10 min. (3)*
❑ Anger worse from contradiction; when forced to answer	**Nux vomica 200 or 1M**	*10 min. (3)*
❑ Anger violent; strikes friends, attendants	**Tarentula h. 200 or 1M**	*weekly (3)*
❑ Anger easy; quarrelsome, obstinate and irritable person	**Kali carb. 200 or 1M**	*weekly (3)*
❑ Anger with trembling; irritable, hateful, vindictive and head strong person	**Acid-nit. 200 or 1M**	*weekly (3)*
❑ Anger on small matters; glandular affections; thyroid enlargement at puberty	**Calcarea iod. 200**	*10 min. (3)*
❑ Anger; violent fits; faints and falls down	**Moschus 200**	*10 min. (3)*
❑ Angereary; obstinate temperament; malignaucies	**Carcinocin 200 or 1M**	*weekly (3)*
❑ Anger easy; hard to please; quarrelsome	**Hepar sulph. 1M**	*weekly (3)*
❑ Anger easy; irritable and obstinate person; feels better in open, cold places	**Kali sulph. 200**	*10 min. (3)*

Symptoms	Remedy	Frequency And Doses
❏ Anger after Coition; obstinate; fat and flabby person	**Calcarea carb. 200 or 1M**	*weekly (3)*
❏ Anger during pregnancy	**Nux mosch. 200 or 1M**	*10 min. (3)*
❏ Anger; impulse violent; wants to kill	**Iodium 1M**	*weekly (3)*
❏ Anger, irritatable; abusive and cruel person	**Kali iod. 1M**	*weekly (3)*
❏ Anger; with changeable moods; repents afterwards	**Crocus sat. 200**	*10 min. (3)*
❏ Anger; bad temperament; angry without reasons; never smiles or enjoys	**Tuberculinum k.1M**	*weekly (3)*
❏ Wrong things make angry; oversensitive	**Staphysagria 1M**	*weekly (3)*
❏ Quarrels with colleagues and teachers though easily frightened; wants attention	**Phosphorus 200 or 1M**	*weekly (3)*
❏ Anger in children; desires some new things (like a toy, etc.) frequently and refuses it when given; changeable moods	**Chamomilla 200 or 1M**	*10 min. (3)*
❏ Indifferent to family members, children and loved ones; worse before menses	**Sepia 200**	*weekly (3)*

ANGINA PECTORIS

❏ Acute pain; suffocation and constriction in the chest (heart region)	**Cactus g. Q,** 10-15 drops	*15-20 min. (3)*
☆ Angina Pectoris with pain and numbness radiating to left arm and fingers; almost specific in acute stage	**Latrodectus m. 3X to 30**	*10 min. (3)*
❏ Pain chest and left arm; heart's action ceases suddenly; impending suffocation	**Cimicifuga 30**	*10 min. (3)*
❏ With violent beating of heart; depression and suicidal thoughts	**Aurum met. 200 or 1M**	*10 min. (3)*
☆ With feeling as if heart would cease to work; slow pulse; worse movements.	**Digitalis Q or 30**	*10 min. (3)*

Symptoms	Remedy	Frequency And Doses
❑ Angina with heart cramps	**Viburnum op.** **Q**, 5-10 drops	*1/2 hourly (3)*
❑ When patient can not lie on left side due to acute pain	**Spigelia 200**	*10 min. (3)*
❑ Angina due to weakness of heart	**Strophanthus** **Q**, 8-10 drops	*4 hourly (SOS)*
☆ When patient becomes unconscious due to intense pain and numbness of left arm	**Naja t. 30 or 200**	*15 min. (3)*
❑ Heart failure due to prolonged illness	**Ammonium carb. 30**	*1/2 hourly (3)*
☆ Angina with fainting; restlessness and weak pulse	**Acid-hydro. 30**	*10 min. (3)*
❑ Shooting pain of heart and arteries of left chest extending to left arm	**Lachesis 30**	*10 min. (3)*
❑ Angina with restlessness; burning sensation; excessive thirst and fear of death	**Arsenic alb. 30 or 200**	*10 min. (3)*
❑ Pain heart due to pressure of wind. Patient desires to be fanned; coldness and blueness of body	**Carbo veg. 30 or 200**	*10 min. (3)*
❑ Collapse with extreme coldness, blueness and weakness of body. Tobacco heart; one of the best heart stimulants	**Veratrum alb. 30 or 200**	*10 min. (3)*
❑ Palpitation with pain in heart; stitching pain in chest radiating to left shoulder and left hand; worse walking, after eating; hypertension; vertigo; darkness before eyes	**Terminalia arjuna** **Q or 6**	*1/2 hourly (SOS)*
❑ Heart tonic (to strengthen the heart)	**Cactus g. Q,** and **(Crataegus) Q,** 10-15 drops	*4 hourly*
❑ When pain extends from heart region to right shoulder or right clavicle or towards right knee	**Lac-can. 30 or 200**	*10 min. (3)*
Biochemic remedy	**Magnesia phos. 6X**	*1/2 hourly*

ANXIETY
WORRY
(See Fear Also)

Symptoms	Remedy	Frequency And Doses
☆ Sudden with restlessness and fear of death	**Aconite 30 or 200**	*1/2 hourly (3)*
☆ Prolonged with periodic and panic attacks	**Arsenic alb. 200**	*4 hourly (3)*
● With fainting spells; profuse sweating; worse in the morning	**Sulphur 30 or 200**	*3 hourly (3)*
☆ Makes patient walk fast; due to anticipation	**Argentum nit. 200**	*3 hourly (3)*
❑ Worse lying in bed and closing the eyes	**Carbo veg. 30 or 200**	*4 hourly (6)*
❑ Anxiety aggravated by upward or downward motion, going in an elevator; worse till 11 p.m.	**Borax 200 or 1M**	*3 hourly (3)*
❑ Anxious about business even when seriously ill	**Bryonia alb. 200**	*3 hourly (3)*
❑ Full of apprehensions in the evening	**Causticum 200**	*3 hourly (3)*
❑ Anxiety and fears in the evening with restlessness and palpitation	**Calcarea carb. 200 or 1M**	*3 hourly (3)*
❑ Anxiety worse while lying still. Sad music ameliorates the complaints	**Manganum acet. 200**	*3 hourly (3)*
☆ Anxiety due to fright, fear, exciting news; stage fright; worse while appearing for examination or interview, etc.	**Gelsemium 30 or 200**	*3 hourly (6)*
❑ Anxiety due to grief or shock in the sub-conscious mind	**Ignatia 200 or 1M**	*3 hourly (3)*
❑ Anxiety; better after eating	**Anacardium or. 30**	*4 hourly*
Biochemic remedy	**Kali phos. 6X**	*4 hourly*

APHTHAE
See Mouth Ulcers Also)

Small white spots often associated with small ulcerations on the mucous membrane of the mouth seen in thrush, sprue, or with Vincent's infection; though usually caused by a virus or fungus; they may occur after enteric use of the broad spectrum antibiotics, etc..

Symptoms	Remedy	Frequency And Doses
☆ Painful; whitish blister in the mouth; bleeds easily	Borax 30	3 hourly
☆ Painful blisters with foul smell from the mouth; excessive saliva; excessive thirst with moist mouth	Mercurius sol. 30	3 hourly
❑ Severe; painful blisters. Saliva acrid and offensive	Acid-nit. 30	4 hourly
❑ With fetid, sour smell from the mouth; sordes on teeth and gums; glands swollen	Acid-mur. 30	4 hourly
❑ Aphthae with swollen tongue and profuse salivation; gums bleed easily; pyorrhoea	Acid-sulph. 30	4 hourly
❑ Aphthae with burning blisters; marked prostration and restlessness; unquenchable thirst, sips water frequently	Arsenic alb. 30	4 hourly
❑ Severe aphthae with rawness and burning; gums swollen, spongy - bleeds easily; swelling of tongue. Patient feels worse after sleep	Lachesis 30	4 hourly
☆ Aphthae; stomatitis; tongue yellowish coated, large and flabby with imprints of teeth; constipation	Hydrastis can 30	4 hourly

Biochemic remedy

With watering from mouth	Natrum mur. 6X or 12 X	4 hourly

Natrum phos. 6X and *Kali mur. 6X*, 2 tablets each thrice daily gives wonderful results along with other indicated homoeopathic remedies.

For External Use:
i) *Borax mixed with Honey*
ii) *Hydrastis can. Q in One (1) part and Glycerine in Nine (9) parts (mixed together) gives good results.*
iii) *In severe cases Echinacea Q can be used for mouth wash (5 to 7 drops in half a glass of luke warm water).*

APOPLEXY
Lack of Sensation Due to Stroke

Symptoms	Remedy	Frequency And Doses
❑ Sudden onset due to draught of cold air	**Aconite nap. 200**	*3 hourly (3)*
❑ Complete unconsciousness; involuntary sighing. The look of the patient becomes idiotic	**Helleborus 200 or 1M**	*3 hourly (3)*
❑ Unconsciousness; rush of blood towards head	**Belladonna 200 or 1M**	*3 hourly (3)*
❑ Complete unconsciousness; cerebral apoplexy, jaws dropped	**Opium 1M or 10M**	*3 hourly (3)*
❑ Stupor with sudden sharp cries and startlings; unconsciousness	**Apis mel. 200 or 1M**	*3 hourly (3)*
❑ Mouth partly open and running of excessive salivation	**Baryta carb. 200 or 1M**	*3 hourly (3)*
❑ Apoplexy due to mechanical injury	**Arnica 200 or 1M**	*3 hourly (3)*
❑ Apoplexy due to suppressed anger	**Colocynth. 200 or 1M**	*3 hourly (3)*
❑ Apoplexy due to emotional disturbances; grief, shock, etc.	**Ignatia 1M or 10M**	*3 hourly (3)*
❑ With palpitation; cold and moist skin; convulsions of the facial muscles	**Laurocerasus 30**	*3 hourly*
● Intercurrent Remedy	**Sulphur 200**	*3 hourly (3)*
Biochemic remedy	**Kali phos 6X and Magnesia phos. 6X**	*4 hourly (4)*

For effective management of the case always try to find out the exact cause and treat accordingly.

APPENDICITIS

Inflammation of the vermiform appendix is called appendicitis.

☆ To start the treatment	**Baptisia CM**	*1 dose only*

Symptoms	Remedy	Frequency And Doses
☆ Severe pain in the ileocecal region; worse even with slight touch	**Iris tenax 1M**	*2 hourly (3)*
❏ Sudden severe pain; patient cannot bear even slightest pressure on effected lesion	**Belladonna 30 or 200**	*15 minutes (6)*
❏ Stitching pain; worse from slightest motion, even from breathing; better while lying quietly on painful - right side	**Bryonia Q**, 5-10 drops	*2 hourly*
❏ Pain worse during rest and better while moving	**Rhus tox. 30 or 200**	*2 hourly (6)*
❏ When sepsis starts; chill, diarrhoea, restlessness, anxiety and sudden sinking of strength; stitching pain with inflammation	**Arsenic alb. 200 or 1M**	*10 min. (3)*
❏ When pain is better by bending backwards. Bowels filled with gas; gripping and twisting pain	**Dioscorea 30 or 200**	*1/2 hourly (3)*
❏ Whole abdomen sensitive; stitching pain from the point of inflammation radiating to backward and downwards to the thigh; can not bear even touch of clothes on effected parts	**Lachesis 200**	*10 min. (3)*
❏ Pain severe and intolerable; even slightest exposure to cold or touch aggravates. Patient chilly	**Hepar sulph. 200 or 1M**	*15 min. (3)*
❏ Pain worse while lying on right side. Profuse sweat which does not relieve	**Mercurius sol. 200**	*15 min. (3)*
Biochemic remedies	**Ferrum phos. 6X,** **Kali mur. 6X** and **Magnesia phos. 6X,** in warm water	*1/2 hourly*

APPETITE
Excessive

Symptoms	Remedy	Frequency And Doses
☆ Due to worms; feels hungry even after eating food	**Cina 30 or 200**	*4 hourly*
☆ Worse especially at 11 a.m.; lack of food leads to headache	**Sulphur 200**	*10 min. (3)*
❑ With pain in the stomach; better after eating	**Lachesis 30**	*4 hourly*
❑ With Diarrhoea; hunger after passing stool	**Petroleum 30**	*4 hourly*
❑ After eating full meal; hurried feeling	**Argentum met. 30**	*4 hourly*
❑ Feeling of emptiness even after eating full meal; fat and flabby patient	**Calcarea carb. 200**	*weekly (3)*
❑ Easily satisfied but feels hungry even at night and eats at odd hours	**Lycopodium 30 or 200**	*4 hourly*
❑ Ravenous appetite though emaciating; stomach feels as if swimming in water	**Abrotanum 30**	*4 hourly*
❑ Feels better during and after eating; loosing weight even though eating good food	**Iodium 30**	*4 hourly*
❑ Excessive hunger; hardly satisfied; nausea in the morning before eating	**Sepia 30**	*4 hourly*
❑ Feels hungry even when stomach is full; desires stimulants	**Staphysagria 30**	*4 hourly*
❑ Hungry with intense thirst; sensitive to music	**Tarentula h. 30**	*4 hourly*
❑ Feels hungry but no appetite	**Rhus tox. 30**	4 hourly
❑ Hungry with hic-cough; prefers hot food and drinks	**Chelidonium Q or 6**	*4 hourly*
Biochemic remedies	**Kali phos. 6X** and **Natrum phos. 6X**	*3 hourly*

APPETITE
Loss of

Symptoms	Remedy	Frequency And Doses
☆ Head remedy; craving for wine & coffee	**Lecithin. 3X**	*4 hourly*
❑ Loss of appetite after acute illness	**Gentiana lut. Q**, 5-10 drops	*4 hourly*
❑ Tongue thickly whitish coated; foul eructation; wind passes downwards	**Antim-crud. 30**	*4 hourly*
❑ Loss of appetite with desire to eat	**Mezereum 30**	*4 hourly*
❑ Complete loss of appetite in morning but craving for food during noon and at night	**Abies nig. 30**	*4 hourly*
❑ Hungry without appetite; bad effects of tea; digestion slow	**China off. 30**	*4 hourly*
❑ Loss of appetite when totally exhausted after prolonged work; fat and chilly patient	**Calcarea carb. 30**	*4 hourly*
❑ Loss of appetite due to indigestion; bitter taste; tongue thickly coated at back	**Nux vomica 30**	*4 hourly*
❑ Easily satisfied; appetite decreases after few mouth full of food	**Lycopodium 30**	*4 hourly*
❑ Complete loss of appetite for ordinary food. Craving for indigestible, acidic and variety foods	**Ignatia 30**	*4 hourly*
❑ With loss of thirst and desire for open, cool air	**Pulsatilla 30**	*4 hourly*
❑ Fluctuates greatly with aversion to food; nausea and vomiting of undigested food	**Ferrum phos. 6X or 6**	*4 hourly*
☆ General tonic	**Alfalfa Q**, 5-10 drops	*4 hourly*
● Intercurrent remedy	**Sulphur 30**	*3 hourly (3)*

ARTHRITIS
Including Gout, Arthritis Deformans and Rheumatism

❑ Pain knee joints; worse by movements; better initial movements, continuous pain in joints worse while rising from seat; pain in heels; worse by movements	**Cassia sophera 30**	*4 hourly*

Symptoms	Remedy	Frequency And Doses
☆ Acute attack of gout of joints of the feet. Pain with bright red swelling	**Aconite nap. 200**	*2 hourly*
❑ Pain with inflammation; worse by movements	**Bryonia alb. 200 or 1M**	*6 hourly*
☆ Complaints worse after rest and exposure to cold; better by movements	**Rhus tox. 200 or 1M**	*4 hourly*
❑ Complaints worse during menstruation; beginning at the time of menopause; more in hands and feet	**Caulophyllum 30**	*4 hourly*
● When the origin of complaints is gonorrhoeal; worse during day time	**Medorrhinum 1M**	*fortnightly (3)*
● When the origin of complaints is tubercular	**Tuberculinum k. 1M**	*fortnightly (3)*
☆ Complaints of small joints with red or pale swelling; tenderness and shifting pains; worse by motion. Main remedy for gout during cold weather	**Colchicum 30**	*4 hourly*
☆ When Rhus tox. cease to work; pain is worse in cold damp weather and better by movements	**Calcarea carb. 200 or 1M**	*6 hourly (6)*
☆ Nodosities in the joints with gastric complaints. At last nodules become painless (Rheumatoid arthritis). Tongue whitish thickly coated.	**Antim-crud. 30 or 200**	*6 hourly*
❑ Complaints of ankles and feet; stiffness	**Drosera 200**	*fortnightly (3)*
❑ Complaints of long bones; contraction of ligaments	**Causticum 30 or 200**	*4 hourly*
❑ Pain worse at night; in wet weather; Rheumatism of large muscles	**Cimicifuga 30**	*4 hourly*
❑ Rheumatism; worse in damp cold weather. Gout. Pain in limbs and hip joints	**Natrum sulph. 30 or 200**	*4 hourly*
❑ Pain travels downwards affecting the large part of a limb and passes through quickly along the course of nerve	**Kalmia lat. 30 or 200**	*6 hourly*
❑ Pains worse during rest, night, and warmth; better by cold, open air and movements	**Pulsatilla 30 or 200**	*4 hourly*

Symptoms	Remedy	Frequency And Doses
❏ Pain - violent; bruised or as if sprained; can not bear touch; feels somebody coming near him may hit the affected part	**Arnica mont. 200**	*4 hourly*
❏ Gout of great toe and joints with swelling; soreness and drawing pain on stepping; worse in warmth, pressure and by motion. Pain travels upwards; better cold compresses	**Ledum pal. 200**	*4 hourly*
❏ Gouty nodosities of joints; tearing pain extremities and contraction of the muscles	**Guaiacum 30**	*4 hourly*
❏ Chronic nodosities of the joints; hands twisted, out of shape due to deposits of water of soda	**Ammonium phos. 6 or 30**	*4 hourly*
❏ Gouty complaints with offensive urine	**Acid-benz. 6 or 30**	*4 hourly*
❏ When there is red sand in urine in gouty patients	**Lycopodium 30**	*4 hourly*
❏ Severe pain with enlargement of the joints; worse during rest and when storm approaches	**Rhododendron 200 or 1M**	*10 min. (3)*
☆ Almost a specific for gout (to drain out uric acid and urates)	**Urtica u. Q**, *8-10 drops* in hot water	*4 hourly*
❏ Arthritic deformans (chronic rheumatoid, particularly of fingers)	**Picric acid. 30**	*4 hourly*
☆ Rheumatic pains or arthritis after checked diarrhoea	**Abrotanum 30 or 200**	*4 hourly (6)*
☆ Specific for pain with numbness. Pain so severe that patient says he would prefer death than the pain	**Chamomilla 200 or 1M**	*1/2 hours (3)*
❏ Pain appear diagonally as right arm and left leg with sensation of cold, numbness and tingling	**Agaricus mus. 30 or 200**	*4 hourly*
❏ In weak persons; burning pain with chilliness; feels better by heat, while eating, and worse in cold open air	**Capsicum 30 or 200**	*4 hourly*

Symptoms	Remedy	Frequency And Doses
● Unbearable pain; rigidity and stiffness. Superiority/inferiority complex	**Platina 1M**	*weekly (3)*
❏ Pain flies like electric shock; due to exposure to damp cold weather. Better warmth and rest	**Phytolacca 30 or 200**	*4 hourly*
❏ Rheumatic pain; worse after washing clothes, doing laundry work	**Sepia 30 or 200**	*4 hourly*
❏ Pain in long bones; may be due to injury or rheumatism	**Ruta g. 200**	*6 hourly*
❏ Pain worse on slightest touch specifically after loss of vital fluids like excessive bleeding, diarrhoea, vomiting, etc..	**China off. 6 or 30**	3 hourly
❏ Pain in the small joints of extremities with swelling. Backache; worse in morning before rising	**Staphysagria 30 or 200**	4 hourly
❏ Pain heels; better by putting most of the weight on them	**Berb-vul. Q**, 8-10 drops	4 hourly
❏ Shifting pain in all parts of the body; worse by motion	**Stellaria Q**, 8-10 drops in warm water	*4 hourly*
❏ Rheumatic pain without swelling; pain joints; worse at night	**Iodium 30**	*4 hourly*
● Osteo-arthritis of large joints with degeneration. Pain, swelling, stiffness and tenderness of joints; worse by motion (cracking joints) and cold; better by warmth	**O.A. Nosode,** 1M or 1002	*weekly (6)*
❏ Chronic muscular rheumatism of back and neck. Intense pain along the sciatic nerve. Numbness alternates with pain	**Gnaphalium 30 or 200**	*4 hourly*
❏ Muscular atrophy; rigidity and stiffness	**Strychninum 3X or 6X**	*4 hourly*
● Rheumatism accompanied with skin ailments and itching; can not walk erect	**Sulphur 200**	*10 min. (3)*
❏ Rheumatism of the knee joint; with round worms	**Natrum phos. 6X or 30**	*4 hourly*

Symptoms	Remedy	Frequency And Doses
❑ For defective bony growth; better by warmth and worse by cold	Calcarea fluor. 12X or 30	4 hourly
Biochemic remedy	Magnesia phos. 6X	4 hourly
	Biocombination No.19	4 hourly

ASCITES
Dropsy of the Abdomen

Ascites is a watery effusion in the cavity of the peritonium, which causes much swelling of the abdomen. The symptoms often are in the form of fever, restlessness at night, faulty digestion, foul smell from the mouth, nausea or vomiting, constipation, scanty, high coloured urine, pain lower back and liver region.

The ailment is usually due to complication of other ailments like rheumatism, anasarca, heart or liver disorders, albuminuria, menstrual disorders, etc.. The treatment should be according to the symptoms.

Symptoms	Remedy	Frequency And Doses
❑ When the disease is an out come of excitability; urine dark and scanty; stools loose - jelly like	Helleborus 30 or 200	4 hourly
❑ Debility, prostration and restlessness; thirst - unquenchable, sips little water frequently	Arsenic alb. 30 or 200	4 hourly
☆ Ascites due to loss of vital fluids; short, dry cough with or without expectoration; paleness of skin; chilliness; small, feeble and slow pulse	China off. 6 or 30	4 hourly
❑ Pain and disagreeable sensations are experienced in the region of the kidneys	Zincum met. 6 or 30	4 hourly
☆ Ascites after eruptive fever with loss of thirst and scanty urine. Skin pale, transparent and puffy. Worse by heat and better by cold	Apis mel. 30 or 200	4 hourly
❑ Dropsy due to chronic albuminuria or liver disorders, etc. or due to faulty nutrition	Lac defloratum 30 or 200	6 hourly
❑ Due to urinary complaints; brick-dust sediments in urine; retention of urine	Thlaspi bur-p. Q, 5-10 drops	4 hourly

Symptoms	Remedy	Frequency And Doses
❑ With• great thirst but scanty urination. Complaints after long continued fevers like typhoid, etc.. Cold and cold drinks aggravate	Apocynum can. Q, 5-10 drops	4 hourly
☆ Patient can not tolerate even the touch of clothings on the abdomen; lies on back lifting clothes from the abdomen	Lachesis 30 or 200	3 hourly (6)
Biochemic remedy	Kali phos. 6X	3 hourly

ASPHYXIA
Apparent Death

We know that individuals sometimes to all appearances suddenly expire, when infact there is but a mere suspension of animation; and in as much as absolute and sudden death frequently occurs when it might be mistaken for a suspension of the kind. In all such cases where there is least uncertainty to exercise the greatest care - we should not do any thing that may cause death and we should not interfere until certain of putrefaction.

Apparent death may be a result of:

1. From hunger
2. From falling or an injury
3. From lightening
4. From drowning
5. From suffocation due to inhaling noxious vapours, chemicals, etc.
6. From cold or being frozen
7. From long continued or sudden ailments
8. From sunstroke, etc.

1. From hunger:

When an individual has been without food since long and animation has become suspended inconsequence, warm milk should be given repeatedly, in the beginning it may be given drop by drop and gradually increased to a tea spoonful; after short interval a small quantity of wine and beef tea or **Avena sat. Q** 10-15 drops in warm water; when animation has been restored and the patient has had a sound sleep, small quantity of food may be given. The food may be given at short intervals (but little at a time) and the patient should return to his normal mode of living slowly.

2. From falling or an injury:

When the result is after a fall or injury the patient should be carefully placed upon a bed in a quiet place with his head keeping high and he should be given **Arnica mont. 200** (few doses) repeatedly every half an hour or so. **Arnica** can be given orally or it can be rubbed on the skin also.

3. From lightening:

When the result is due to lightening the patient should be kept in open air and cold water should be showered upon his face, neck and chest; warm friction should be applied if the body is cold. Artificial respiration should be given if required.

4. From drowning:

When the result is because of drowning the patient should be stripped and rubbed, and the body should be wrapped in warm clothes and should be kept in a warm place. Throat, mouth and nostrils should be cleaned. Warmth should be applied to the spine, hot water bottle, etc. may be used. The soles and the feet of the patient should be rubbed constantly. Artificial respiration should be given. *Lachesis 30 or 200* or any other indicated remedy can be given frequently.

5. From suffocation due to inhaling noxious vapours, chemicals, etc.:

When the result is from inhaling poisonous gases, carbon-di-oxide, etc., the patient should be kept in open and artificial respiration should be given immediately. *Carbo-veg. 30 or 200* should be given repeatedly. Sometimes in cases of coal gas poisoning the face of the patient looks pinkish and thus he looks in best of health, which at times mislead and is very dangerous.

In cases of complete unconsciousness *Opium 200* or 1M should be used. If the body of the patient is cold then the patient should be surrounded with warm clothes. Hot water, etc. may be used.

6. From cold or being frozen:

When animation becomes suspended in consequence of exposure to cold the patient should be gently removed to a place of shelter or cool room as a moderate degree of heat might prove an obstacle to restoration so he should not be exposed to a draught of air.

The patient may be covered with snow keeping his mouth and nostrils free in such a position that the melted snow may run off easily. The same process can be renewed. If snow is not available then a bath in icy cold water can be substituted. The body should be immersed for a short time only and then should be covered with wet clothes covering with dry blankets. As the animation returns, the patient should be handled carefully.

Carbo veg. 200, Arsenic alb. 200 or *Veratrum alb. 200* can be given according to the symptoms, half hourly.

7. From long continued or sudden ailments

Treat according to the symptoms (see different ailments).

8. From sunstroke, etc.:

If the result is due to sunstroke (prolonged exposure to the sun) the patient should be kept in a dark, shady and quiet place and the clothes should be loosened. A wet cloth (wet in hot water) should be wrapped around the head changing it frequently and the whole body should be sponged with warm water simultaneously. *Glonoine 6 or 30* (few doses) should be given repeatedly. *Glonoine* can be given orally or it can be rubbed on the skin. Saline water, glucose or electrol powder should be given frequently in small quantities at a time.

ASTHMA
Bronchial Asthma

The inflammation of bronchial tract due to the congestion by cough or due to some allergen and allergic condition, increase in the percentage of eosinophilia, etc., are the pathological conditions. Constant breathing trouble, dyspnoea, dry cough with wheezing sound are chief complaints of bronchial asthma.

Symptoms	Remedy	Frequency And Doses
☆ Dyspnoea aggravates during winter; worse from exposure to dust, change of weather, cold drinks, exertion, inhaling smoke and in the morning. Hoarseness of voice. Cough with pain in chest	**Cassia sophera Q or 30**	*4 hourly*
❑ Dry cough; worse rest; dyspnoea at 4 a.m.	**Penicillinum 200**	*4 hourly*
☆ During acute attack when there is anxiety, fear and dyspnoea	**Aconite. Q and Ipecac Q**, 5-10 drops *alternate*	*1/2 hourly*
● In children with spasm, secretion of mucous and infection (as an intercurrent remedy)	**Bacillinum 1M**	*fortnightly (6)*
● In adults with spasm, secretion of mucous and infection (as an intercurrent remedy)	**Tub-koch. 1M**	*fortnightly (6)*
● In sycotic patients; worse during daytime; better knee-chest position and sea side	**Medorrhinum 200 or 1M**	*fortnightly (3)*
● For patients coming for homoeopathic treatment after taking steroids, etc., bad effects of vaccination; chilly patient	**Thuja 200 or 1M**	*weekly (3)*
☆ For chilly patients; worse after taking cold drinks or being angry; anxiety, restlessness and unquenchable thirst	**Arsenic alb. 30**	*2 hourly*
❑ In children with history of worms	**Cina 10M or 50M**	*weekly (3)*
● Bronchial asthma with high eosinophil count; thyroid disturbance	**Thyroidin. 1M**	*weekly (3)*
☆ Better while lying on the back with his arms and legs spread apart	**Psorinum 200 or 1M**	*weekly (3)*
☆ Worse on falling asleep and after sleep, worse taking sour food or vinegar, etc.	**Lachesis 30 or 200**	*3 hourly (3)*

Symptoms	Remedy	Frequency And Doses
❑ Excessive dyspnoea, cough and much mucous secretion; emphysema	Antim ars. 6 or 30	3 hourly (6)
● Dyspnoea in middle of night and early morning; wants windows open	Sulpur 200 or 1M	weekly (3)
❑ Respiratory trouble due to foundry or traffic pollution	Acid sulphurosum 30 or 200	4 hourly
❑ Patient can breathe properly only while standing	Cannabis sativa 200 or 1M	4 hourly (6)
❑ Asthma of stone cutters, silk/cotton mill workers (should be used with great care)	Silicea 30 or 200	4 hourly (S.O.S.)
❑ Smell of flowers causes asthma	Ailanthus-g. 30	4 hourly
☆ Desires fanning during acute attack though body may be cold	Carbo-veg. 30	1/2 hourly
❑ Difficult and hurried breathing; feels as if every breath will be the last; loss of thrist	Apis mel. 30	4 hourly
❑ Attacks during rainy season and dampness with looseness of bowels at each attack	Natrum sulph. 6 or 30	4 hourly
❑ Due to nervousness; spasm and constriction of chest; better drinking water	Cuprum met. 30 or 200	4 hourly
❑ Due to anger; suffocative tightness of chest	Chamomilla 200 or 1M	4 hourly
❑ Worse in dry, cold weather and better in damp weather	Hepar sulph. 30 or 200	4 hourly
☆ Patient can not breathe properly while lying in bed	Grindelia Q, and Blatta or. Q, 5-10 drops	alternate 2 hourly
● Asthma worse at night; when well selected remedies fail	Syphilinum 1M	weekly (3)
❑ Due to suppressed emotions; grief (Psychosomatic); little expectoration; worse inhaling smoke	Ignatia 1M or 10M	4 hourly (3)
❑ Amelioration while passing stools; worse inhaling dust	Pothos foe. 6 or 30	4 hourly

Symptoms	Remedy	Frequency And Doses
❑ Difficulty in getting air into the lungs. Better at sea; worse after coming on land; asthma of seafaring men	**Bromium 30 or 200**	*4 hourly*
☆ Want of breath on least motion; to stimulate respiratory centres to increase oxygen in the blood	**Aspidosperma Q,** 5-10 drops	*2 hourly*
❑ Due to strong odours; of gastric origin; dyspnoea and constriction of chest	**Sanguinaria 30 or 200**	*4 hourly*
☆ Collapse due to acute attack; paralysis of lungs; cyanosis	**Acid-hydro. 30 or 200**	*1/2 hourly (3)*
❑ Catarrhal asthma; desire for open air; uterine disorders	**Sabina 30 or 200**	*4 hourly*
❑ Dry, splenic asthma; dyspnoea and stitches in chest	**Scilla mar. 30**	*4 hourly*
❑ Hysterical asthma; cough; worse warmth of bed	**Nux moch. 30 or 200**	*4 hourly*
❑ Nervous, spasmodic asthma; chocking on falling asleep	**Valeriana Q or 30**	*4 hourly*

Histamine and *Eosinophilinum 200 or 1M* in potencies are also very useful when eosinophil count is high.

AVERSIONS

❑ To smiling faces	**Ambra-gr. 200 or 1M**	*4 hourly (6)*
❑ To certain persons	**Ammon-mur. 200**	*4 hourly (6)*
❑ Aversion to her own children. Aversion to women in homosexuals	**Platina 1M**	*weekly (3)*
❑ Aversion to friends during pregnancy	**Conium mac. 200**	*weekly (3)*
❑ Aversion to parents and wife	**Flouric acid. 1M**	*weekly (3)*
❑ Aversion to apples	**Antim-tart. 200 or 1M**	*weekly (3)*
❑ Aversion to bananas and plums	**Baryta carb. 200 or 1M**	*weekly (3)*

Symptoms	Remedy	Frequency And Doses
❑ Aversion to beef, brandy and dry food	**Merc. Sol. 200 or 1M**	*weekly (3)*
❑ Aversion to beer	**Nux vomica 200**	*weekly (3)*
❑ Aversion to brandy; cabbage	**Carbo veg. 200**	*weekly (3)*
❑ Aversion to bread, butter, hot food, melons	**Natrum mur. 200 or 1M**	*weekly (3)*
❑ Aversion to butter milk and craving for sweets	**Cina 200 or 1M**	*weekly (3)*
❑ Aversion to cereals; boiled milk, onion, oranges, pastry, spices, puddings and warm drinks	**Phosphorus 200 or 1M**	*weekly (3)*
❑ Aversion to cheese and craving for sweets	**Argentum nit. 200 or 1M**	*weekly (3)*
❑ Aversion to chicken	**Bacillinum 200 or 1M**	*weekly (3)*
❑ Aversion to chocolate; cocoa, spices	**Tarentula h. 200 or 1M**	*weekly (3)*
❑ Aversion to coffee; gruel, milk	**Calcarea carb. 200 or 1M**	*weekly (3)*
❑ Aversion to cold drinks	**Arsenic alb. 200 or 1M**	*weekly (3)*
❑ Aversion to cold water; garlic, onion, wine	**Sabadilla 200 or 1M**	*weekly (3)*
❑ Aversion to cooked food	**Lycopodium 200 or 1M**	*weekly (3)*
❑ Aversion to eggs	**Ferrum met. 200 or 1M**	*weekly (3)*
❑ Aversion to fat; fruits, ham, hot drinks, pastry, spices	**Pulsatilla 200 or 1M**	*weekly (3)*
❑ Aversion to fish; hot drinks, salt, soup, sweets	**Graphites 200 or 1M**	*weekly (3)*
❑ Aversion to honey; milk	**Natrum carb. 200 or 1M**	*weekly (3)*
❑ Aversion to ice-cream	**Radium brom. 200 or 1M**	*weekly (3)*
❑ Aversion to melons; pastry	**Silicea 200 or 1M**	*weekly (3)*
❑ Aversion to pickles	**Abies can. 200 or 1M**	*weekly (3)*
❑ Aversion to soup	**Rhus tox. 200 or 1M**	*weekly (3)*
❑ Aversion to sweets; starchy food, strawberries	**Sulphur 200 or 1M**	*weekly (3)*
❑ Aversion to vegetables	**Magnesia carb. 200 or 1M**	*weekly (3)*

Symptoms	Remedy	Frequency And Doses
❑ Sudden backache due to exposure to dry, cold wind	**Aconite 200**	*3 hourly*
☆ Due to exposure to cold; over exertion, sprains etc.; worse initial movements better continued movements	**Rhus tox. 200 or 1M**	*3 hourly*
☆ With stiffness; worse movements and cold; better lying quietly	**Bryonia 200 or 1M**	*6 hourly*
❑ Backache due to injury or over strain; bruised pains	**Arnica 200 or 1M**	*3 hourly*
❑ Pricking pain, weakness and sweating; complaints worse 3-4 a.m.	**Kali carb. 200**	*10 min. (3)*
❑ In fat and flabby patients; worse while bathing and exposure to cold	**Calcarea carb. 200 or 1M**	*10 min. (3)*
❑ Pain lower back; better sleep and rest; patient desires cold, open air	**Pulsatilla 30 or 200**	*4 hourly*
❑ Backache better by belching. Chilly patient. Aversion to family members	**Sepia 200 or 1M**	*10 min. (3)*
☆ In chilly, constipated patients who lead sedentary life; irritable by nature; pain worse cold, motion, particularly turning in bed patient has to sit up and then turn in bed	**Nux vomica 30 or 200**	*4 hourly*
❑ Pain lower back due to constipation and piles. Better only while standing	**Aesculus h. 30 or 200**	*6 hourly*
❑ Backache worse damp cold and bending for long hours	**Dulcamara 200 or 1M**	*10 min. (3)*

Symptoms	Remedy	Frequency And Doses
● Severe pain in lower back and coccyx. Cannot walk erect. Pain better damp and cold; worse night. Burning of soles	**Sulphur 30 or 200**	*10 min. (3)*
❑ Rheumatic pains back, neck, lumbar - sacral regions - down thighs;stiffness and contraction; spine quite sensitive; pain in scapula and right shoulder	**Cimicifuga 30**	*3 hourly*
❑ Worse while sitting; better motion; itching and frozen feeling of toes and feet	**Chelidonium 30**	*4 hourly*
❑ Worse night; better movements and daytime; sweating do not relieve the pain	**Mercurius sol. 30 or 200**	*6 hourly*
● Pain lumbo-sacral region which extends to lower extremities; worse during day; better sea-shore and lying on abdomen	**Medorrhinum 200 or 1M**	*weekly (3)*
☆ Pain back and more in small of the back which at last settles on the upper part of thigh and buttock. Patient limps and at last pain becomes so severe that patient is unable to walk and stand; better pressure and heat	**Colocynthis 200 or 1M**	*10 min. (3)*
❑ Pain worse at rest and during storm; better warmth and eating	**Rhododendron 200 or 1M**	*10 min.(3)*
❑ Pain deep into the bones after Malarial fever with excessive thirst and chill	**Eupatorium perf. 30 or 200**	*3 hourly*
❑ Backache is better by hard pressure. Patient puts a hard thing under the back like a book or wooden plank while sitting or lying in bed	**Natrum mur. 30 or 200**	*4 hourly*
❑ Backache due to excessive indulgence in sex	**Symphytum 30**	*4 hourly*
☆ Backache due to nerve injury	**Hypericum 30 or 200**	*4 hourly (6)*
❑ Violent pain in upper three dorsal vertebrae extending through scapulae; pains descending, lumbar pain of nervous origin	**Kalmia lat. 30 or 200**	*3 hourly*

Symptoms	Remedy	Frequency And Doses
Biochemic remedies		
Pain in nape of neck and cervical region, weakness and pain in back	**Calcarea phos. 6X**	*3 hourly*
Backache worse rest; extending to sacrum; better by heat	**Calcarea fluor. 6X or 12X**	*3 hourly*
Backache better heat; worse cold	**Magnesia phos. 6X**	*3 hourly*

BAD BREATH

❑ Putrid discharges and fetid breath	**Acid-carb. 30**	*4 hourly*
❑ With metallic taste and excessive salivation	**Mercurius sol. 30**	*4 hourly*
● Intercurrent remedy	**Prorinum 200**	*weekly (3)*
Biochemic remedy	**Kali phos. 6X**	*4 hourly*

BARBER'S ITCH
(See Other Skin Ailments Also)

❑ Cracks with bleeding; skin sensitive, dry and rough	**Petroleum 30**	*4 hourly*
☆ Eruptions papular. Patient feels the hair erect	**Sulphur iod. 3X or 30**	*4 hourly*
☆ Obstinate cases with excessive burning and itching with swelling and redness of effected lesion	**Radium brom. 30**	*4 hourly*
☆ Burning and itching with vesicular eruptions; worse wet, rainy season and cold.	**Rhus tox. 30 or 200**	*4 hourly (3)*
❑ With sticky discharge; little injury suppurates; unaffected part of skin hard	**Graphites 30 or 200**	*4 hourly (3)*
❑ Eruptions scaly. Abscess under the eruptions; worse warmth and warm applications	**Lycopodium 30 or 200**	*4 hourly (3)*

Symptoms	Remedy	Frequency And Doses
☆ Ring - shaped eruptions; much itching and offensive odour from affected parts	**Tellurium 6 or 30**	*3 hourly*
❑ When cracks re-appear after suppuression and oozing starts; bluish, purplish appearance of effected lesion	**Lachesis 30 or 200**	*10 min. (3)*
❑ Worse after shaving. Exudation forms into a hard, lemon - coloured crust	**Cicuta v. 30**	*4 hourly*
● When the complaints are worse after washing the face or bathing	**Sulphur 30 or 200**	*10 min. (3)*
● When there is pain along with itching	**Psorinum 200**	*10 min. (3)*

BED-SORES

☆ In cases of typhoid fever or long continued ailments	**Baptisia Q or 6**	*3 hourly*
☆ In the beginning when there is bruised feeling in the bed - sores	**Arnica 30 or 200**	*4 hourly*
❑ When bed - sores are very painful even touch is intolerable; patient oversensitive	**Hepar sulph. 30 or 200**	*10 min. (3)*
❑ In chronic cases; when thin, bloody, offensive pus oozes constantly	**Silicea 12X or 30**	*4 hourly*
☆ With blue edges; worse touch. Oozing of decomposed blood	**Lachesis 30 or 200**	*4 hourly (6)*
❑ When affected parts become gangrenous	**Crotalus h. 30 or 200**	*4 hourly (6)*
❑ Due to blood poisoning; septic conditions, gangrenous bed sores (*Echinacea* lotion can be used externally)	**Echinacea Q or 30**	*4 hourly*
● In chronic cases when bed-sores turn into gangrene	**Sulphur 30 or 200**	*10 min. (3)*
● Intercurrent remedy for tubercular patients	**Tuberculinum k. 200**	*weekly (3)*
Biochemic remedy	**Calcarea sulph. 6X**	*4 hourly*

For External Use:

Calendula lotion should be used for general cleaning and calendula ointment for dressing.

BED WETTING
Enuresis

Symptoms	Remedy	Frequency And Doses
❑ Bed-wetting immediately after sleep; patient chilly	**Sepia 200**	*10 min. (3)*
☆ Unconsciously; during Ist part of night	**Causticum 30 or 200**	*4 hourly (3)*
❑ In nervous patients when Causticum fails	**Gelsemium 30**	*4 hourly*
❑ In fat and flabby children; perspires easily, prone to catch cold	**Calcarea carb. 200 or 1M**	*weekly (3)*
☆ Bed wetting; worse after measles; hot patient; changeable disposition; thirstlessness and desire for open air	**Pulsatilla 30 or 200**	*4 hourly (6)*
☆ Urine of low specific gravity, strong smelling; wet the bed several times during sleep	**Acid-benz. 3 or 6**	*4 hourly*
☆ Wetting the bed in deep sleep with dreams of urinating at proper places; caries of teeth	**Kreosote 30 or 200**	*4 hourly (6)*
❑ Habitual bed wetting with dreams or nightmares	**Equisetum 30**	*4 hourly*
● Wetting the bed during full moon. When well selected remedy fails. Psoric patient	**Psorinum 200 or 1M**	*weekly (3)*
❑ Patient wakes up after wetting the bed in dream	**Lac caninum 200**	*weekly (3)*
❑ Due to strangury (urine dribbles drop by drop with tenesmus and pain)	**Magnetis pol-austral. 200**	*weekly (3)*
❑ Involuntary urination during sleep; fear of being alone, apprehensive	**Lycopodium 30 or 200**	*10 min. (3)*
❑ Bed wetting due to worms	**Cina 30 or 200**	*4 hourly*
Biochemic remedies	**Calcarea phos 6X, Kali phos 6X** and **Natrum phos 6X**	*4 hourly*

Symptoms	Remedy	Frequency And Doses

BEREAVEMENT

Symptoms	Remedy	Frequency And Doses
❑ Severe shock due to sudden death of loved ones; restlessness, anxiety and fear	Aconite 200	10 min. (3)
❑ Prolonged mournings; can not overcome the loss of the loved ones	Ignatia 1M or 10M	6 hourly (3)
❑ When the grief is in the conscious mind; patient weeps; does not like sympathy	Natrum mur. 200 or 1M	6 hourly (3)
❑ For chronic grief and indignation	Staph. gria 200 or 1M	weekly (3)
Biochemic remedy	Kali phos 6X	4 hourly

BEAUTY TIPS
Plastic Medicines To Improve Complexion/Glow

Symptoms	Remedy	Frequency And Doses
● For dry and rough skin. Aversion to take bath; scratching of the effected lesions	Sulphur 30 or 200	weekly (3)
● Pain after scratching with rough and dry skin. Patient likes cold climate	Psorinum 200 or 1M	weekly (3)
● Dark circles around eyes due to shock or grief	Natrum mur. 200 or 1M	weekly (3)
☆ Eyes sunken and face pale due to loss of vital fluids	China 6 or 30	4 hourly
❑ Saddle like brownish complexion of nose and cheeks. Yellow spots on chest. Sallow look	Sepia 200	weekly (3)
☆ Dark circles around eyes due to nervous weakness or prolonged nervous tension	Phosphorus 200	weekly (3)
❑ For blackish spots; dry, rough, scaly skin; burning sensation. Restlessness	Arsenic alb. 30	4 hourly
❑ Bluish, purple spots; face pale, jaundiced. Patient can not tolerate pressure of even clothes around throat, abdomen and waist	Lachesis 30 or 200	6 hourly (3)

Symptoms	Remedy	Frequency And Doses
❑ Complexion yellow due to anaemia	**Ferrum met. 3X**	*4 hourly*
❑ Face deathly pale with blue rings around the eyes	**Bismuth 200**	*weekly (3)*
❑ Warts, epithelioma; freckles and blotches; brownish spots	**Thuja oc. 200**	*weekly (6)*
☆ Face pimply, dry, rough, scaly skin; to clean the complexion	**Berberis aq.Q**, 4-5 drops	*4 hourly*
❑ To dissolve scar tissue	**Thiosinaminum 3X**	*4 hourly*
☆ Old burn or injury marks; bleeds easily; warts	**Causticum 30 or 200**	*6 hourly*
Biochemic remedy For birth marks; scar marks, hard skin	**Calcarea fluor. 12X**	*4 hourly*

BIRTH MARKS
(See Beauty Tips)

Though it is not possible to cure any unwanted birth mark etc., but there are certain medicines in homoeopathy (constitutional and symptomatic) which help considerably.

BITES
Of Animals, Insects, Etc.

Any of the following medicines according to the symptoms can be given for bites till specific medical treatment, if required is given.

❑ Bee bite (Urtica u. lotion can be used externally)	**Apis mel. 30**	*3 hourly*
❑ Wasp bite	**Arnica 200**	*1/2 hourly (3)*
❑ Mosquito bites	**Staphysagria 30**	*3 hourly*

Symptoms	Remedy	Frequency And Doses
❑ Serpent/snake/venomous bite. **Hoang-nan Q** or **Golondrina Q** can be given in 10 drops doses 15 minutes (6). (**Lycopus Q** is also helpful) (**Cedron 200** *1/2 hourly* is also helpful)	**Belladonna 200** and **Mercurius sol. 200**,	*alternate 10 min. (6)*
❑ Flee bite	**Pulex irritans 30**	*2 hourly*
❑ Gnat bite	**Cantharis 200**	*15 min. (3)*
❑ Dog bite; bite of rabid animals	**Lyssin 200**	*10 min. (3) externally Echinacea lotion*
❑ Rat or scorpion bite	**Ledum pal. 200**	*1/2 hourly (3)*

BLADDER AND URETHRA
Affections Of
(See Cystitis Also)

☆ Burning pains; urine comes drop by drop	**Cantharis 30**	*3 hourly*
☆ Burning pain; worse at rest; better walking in open air	**Terebinth. Q.** 7-8 drops,	*4 hourly*
❑ Burning pain in the urethra while passing urine; thirst excessive - drinks quite often but little at a time	**Arsenic alb. 30**	*4 hourly*
❑ Paralysis of bladder; dribbling of urine while coughing or sneezing	**Causticum 30 or 200**	*4 hourly (3)*
❑ Bladder weak - no expulsive power	**Opium 30 or 200**	*4 hourly (3)*
❑ Constant desire to urinate; urine milky, scanty and hot	**Lilium tig. 30 or 200**	*4 hourly (3)*
❑ Bladder feels full; constant feeling of as if contents would fall out	**Sepia 30 or 200**	*4 hourly (3)*
❑ Inflammation of bladder with much difficulty in passing urine	**Conium mac. 200**	*10 min. (3)*

Symptoms	Remedy	Frequency And Doses
❑ Pain in the bladder with rigidity of cervical muscles. Back stiff; pain better by lying on back	**Strychnin. 3X or 30**	*4 hourly*
❑ Prolapse of bladder	**Pyrus americana 30**	*4 hourly*
❑ Haematuria while no pathological condition can be found; weakness of bladder	**Belladonna 30**	*4 hourly*
❑ Haemorrhage from the bladder	**Rhus aromatica 30**	*4 hourly*
❑ Stone in the bladder - with sharp pain in loins	**Calcarea renalis 30 and Hydrangea Q**	*3 hourly alternately*
Biochemic remedy Pain due to haemorrhage from urethra or bladder	**Ferrum phos. 3X**	*4 hourly*

BLEEDING
Gums

Symptoms	Remedy	Frequency And Doses
☆ Soreness of gums; bleeding after extraction of teeth	**Arnica 200 or 1 M**	*1/2 hourly (3)*
☆ Gums swollen and sensitive to hot and cold; worse night; unhealthy gums, excessive saliva	**Mercurius sol. 30**	*4 hourly*
☆ Easy and passive bleeding, blood does not coagulate easily	**Phosphorus 30 or 200**	*6 hourly (3)*
❑ Excessive bleeding from gums. Flatulence; hot and sour belching	**Salicylic acid. 30**	*4 hourly*
❑ Oozing of decomposed, thin blood. Gums swollen, spongy, sensitive to touch, bleed easily; worse morning	**Lachesis 30 or 200**	*6 hourly (3)*
❑ Gums retracted and bleed easily; pyorrhoea	**Carbo veg. 3X or 6**	*3 hourly*
Biochemic remedy	**Ferrum phos. 3X**	*4 hourly*

BLEEDING PILES
Haemorrhoids

Symptoms	Remedy	Frequency And Doses
● Head remedy - Haemorrhage and constipation	**Sulphur 1M**	*weekly (3)*
☆ For bleeding piles; only till bleeding persists	**Dolichos Q**, 4-5 drops,	*6 hourly*
☆ If Dolichos Q do not act; blood bright red	**Millefolium Q**, 5-10 drops or 200	*4 hourly*
❑ Blood bright red; the proven Indian drug	**Ficus relig. Q**, 5-10 drops	*4 hourly*
☆ Blood dark clotted (venous); soreness; haemorrhoids and pulsation in the rectum	**Hamamellis Q**, 5-10 drops or 30	*4 hourly*
☆ When bleeding is in a small stream with every stool	**Phosphorus 200**	*10 min. (3)*
☆ With constipation or alternate diarrhoea; loss of appetite; specially during pregnancy; painful bleeding piles	**Collinsonia 30 or 200**	*4 hourly*
❑ Ancient Indian medicine for bleeding piles	**Blumea od. Q**, 5-10 drops	*4 hourly*
❑ Painful bleeding haemorrhoids; severe cutting pain after passing stools lasting for hours	**Nitric-acid. 200 or 1M**	*10 min. (3)*
❑ With burning pain; itching, smarting and stinging in anus while passing stools	**Capsicum 30**	*4 hourly*
❑ Haemorrhoids-blind and bleeding; worse during climacteric	**Aesculus hipp. 30 or 200**	*4 hourly*
Biochemic remedy	**Ferrum phos 3X**	*4 hourly*

BLEEDING
Vagina

Symptoms	Remedy	Frequency And Doses
❑ Bleeding follows (next day) after coitus	**Kreosote 30 or 200**	*10 min. (3)*
❑ Bleeding from vagina after breast feeding; chilly patient	**Silicea 6X or 30**	*4 hourly*
Biochemic remedies	**Ferrum phos. 3X** and **Natrum mur. 6X**	*4 hourly*

Symptoms	Remedy	Frequency And Doses

BLEPHARITIS
Inflammation of Eye-Lids

❏ In syphilitic cases; sensitive to touch, heat or cold	**Mercurius cor. 200**	*10 min. (3)*
☆ Inflammation; between eye-lids and eye brows specially upper eye-lids	**Kali carb. 200**	*10 min. (3)*
● Inflammation with throbbing pain; suppurative stage; sensitive to touch and cold; better warmth	**Hepar sulph. 3X** to abort pus or **1M** to suppress if possible (should be used with great care)	
☆ Oedematous swelling; lower eye-lid; worse heat; loss of thirst	**Apis mel. 30 or 200**	*4 hourly (3)*
❏ Swelling on margins of eye-lids with loss of eye lashes	**Petroleum 30**	*4 hourly*
❏ Oedematous swelling; under eye-lids; thirst for icy cold water/drinks	**Phosphorus 30 or 200**	*10 min. (3)*
❏ Swelling of eye-lids with profuse lachrymation; worse cold and better by warmth; restlessness	**Rhus tox. 30**	*4 hourly*
❏ With hardness due to styes or cyst on eye lids	**Staphysagria 30 or 200**	*6 hourly (3)*
❏ Swelling on eye-lids due to tumours; malignancy etc.	**Conium 200 or 1M**	*10 min. (3)*
❏ Swelling; burning and redness of eye-lids due to fistulous lachrymation; chilly patient	**Silicea 12X or 30**	*4 hourly*
Biochemic remedy	**Ferrum phos. 6X** and **Kali mur. 6X**	*4 hourly*

BLINDNESS

❏ Sudden; when the reason is not known	**Aconite 200 or 1M**	*10 min. (3)*
❏ Nervous blindness; color blindness	**Santoninum 6**	*4 hourly*

Symptoms	Remedy	Frequency And Doses
❑ Night blindness	**Ranunculus bulb. 30**	*4 hourly*
❑ Day blindness	**Bothrops 30**	*4 hourly*
❑ In anaemic; weak, hysterical patient	**Ferrum met. 30**	*4 hourly*
❑ Due to lightening; fear, nervous tension etc.	**Phosphorus 30 or 200**	*4 hourly (3)*
❑ Night blindness; sees only one half of the object	**Lycopodium 30 or 200**	*6 hourly (3)*
☆ Night blindness; increasing myopia	**Physostigma 30**	*4 hourly*
❑ Blindness of leprosy patients	**Hura brazil. 30**	*6 hourly*
Biochemic remedies	**Calcarea phos. 6X** and **Kali phos. 6X**	*4 hourly*

BLISTERS
Skin

Symptoms	Remedy	Frequency And Doses
❑ Due to insect bites; loss of thirst	**Apis mel. 30**	*4 hourly*
❑ Due to excessive walking; exposure to fire, sun burn etc.	**Cantharis 30**	*4 hourly*
❑ On fingers; large, filled with dark serum	**Ailanthus g. 30**	*4 hourly*
❑ Blisters crusty; in typhoid fever	**Acid-phos. 30**	*4 hourly*
❑ Blisters in typhoid fever (sordes)	**Baptisia 6 or 30**	*4 hourly*
❑ Blisters with much itching and redness surrounding it	**Rhus tox. 30**	*4 hourly*
❑ Blisters with white pus inside; sensitive to touch	**Hepar sulph. 30**	*4 hourly*
❑ Fever blisters especially around lips	**Natrum mur. 6X or 30**	*4 hourly*
Biochemic remedy	**Silicea 6X or 12X**	*4 hourly*

Symptoms	Remedy	Frequency And Doses

BLOID PRESSURE HIGH
(See Hypertension)

BLOOD PRESSURE (LOW)
(See Hypotension)

BODY ODOUR
(See Bad Breath Also)

❑ Due to sweating etc. especially forehead	**Calcarea carb. 200**	*4 hourly (3)*
❑ Offensive odour of body like old cheese with sensitive skin	**Hepar sulph. 30**	*4 hourly*
❑ With excessive odorous, viscid perspiration which stains the clothes yellow but sweating do not relieve the complaints	**Mercurius sol. 30**	*4 hourly*
● With unhealthy looking skin; aversion to take bath	**Sulphur 30 or 200**	*4 hourly (3)*
☆ Offensive sweat on feet, hands, and axillae; chilly patient	**Silicea 30 or 200**	*4 hourly*
● Intercurrent remedy	**Psorinum 200**	*weekly (3)*

BONE AFFECTIONS
Including Injuries and Caries

☆ To aid all kinds of bone injuries	**Ruta g. 30**	*4 hourly*
☆ For fractured or broken bone	**Symphytum 3X or 6**	*4 hourly*
❑ Caries; due to suppression of foot sweat	**Acid salicylic 30**	*4 hourly*
❑ Caries of cervical bones	**Aurum met. 200**	*weekly (3)*
❑ Caries of the spinal cord	**Calcarea carb. 200 or 1M**	*weekly (3)*
❑ Tuberculosis of bone	**Drosera 200 or 1M**	*fortnightly (3)*

Symptoms	Remedy	Frequency And Doses
Biochemic remedies		
For fractures and caries of bones etc.	**Calcarea phos. 6X** and	
For caries of bones; offensive and profuse sweat of forehead and feet	**Silicea 12X**	*4 hourly*

BRAIN
Affections Of

❑ Anaemia of brain	**Tabacum 30 or 200**
❑ Inflammation of brain	**Arum triph. 30 or 200**
❑ Injury of brain or after effects of injury	**Natrum sulph. 200 or above**
❑ Paralysis of brain; brain fag	**Zincum met. 30 or 200**
❑ Tumors of brain	**Plumbum met. 30 or 200**
❑ Inflammation of brain due to injury	**Ruta g. 30 or 200**
❑ Brain fag due to excessive mental work	**Kali phos. 6X or 30**
❑ Dread of making any mental effort; chilly patient	**Silicea 12X or 30**
❑ Atrophy of brain after nervous tension or fright	**Phosphorus 30 or 200**
❑ Affections of brain occuring in infants during - Nux Mosch. attack of cholera.	**Nux Mosch. 30 or 200**

BREAST - AFFECTIONS OF
(See Mammary Glands)

BRONCHIECTASIS
(See Bronchitis and Asthma Also)

Dilation of a bronchus or of the bronchial tubes is called Bronchiectasis.

❑ Cough; worse change of position. Caries of teeth	**Kreosote 30**	*4 hourly*

Symptoms	Remedy	Frequency And Doses
❑ Feels better in knee - chest position; worse during day; better see side	**Medorrhinum 200 or 1M**	*fortnightly (3)*
❑ Cough often ends in a sneeze; expectoration difficult; tough and profuse mucous	**Senega Q**, 5-7 drops	*4 hourly*
❑ Emphysema with excessive dyspnoea and cough; difficult expectoration and excessive mucous secretions	**Antim ars. 6 or 30**	*4 hourly*
❑ Cyanosis; venously congested lungs; dry, spasmodic, suffocative cough	**Acid Hydrocyanic 30**	*2 hourly (3)*
Biochemic remedy	**Silicea 6X or 12X**	*4 hourly*

BRONCHITIS
Acute
(See Cough Also)

Inflammation of the mucous membrane of the bronchial tubes is called Bronchitis.

1st Stage

☆ In healthy persons; due to sudden exposure to dry cold air; anxiety and chilly feeling, high fever, pulse fast; fear and restlessness	**Aconite 30 or 200**	*2 hourly*
☆ Eyes red, face shiny red, high fever; respiration short, rapid and difficult; dry cough and hoarseness; skin hot and dry but moist on covered parts	**Belladonna 30**	*2 hourly*
❑ Fever; inflammatory bronchial catarrh, soreness in chest and exhaustive cough; sweating does not relieve; mouth moist with saliva	**Mercurius sol. 30**	4 hourly
☆ Dry cough which hurts the head with fever. Thirst excessive for large quantities of cold water at long intervals. Worse movements	**Bryonia 30 or 200**	*3 hourly*
● In weak patients with high fever	**Ferrum phos. 6X or 30**	*3 hourly*

Symptoms	Remedy	Frequency And Doses

○ If there is no improvement with above medicines then give one dose of **Sulphur 30 or 200** and wait for one or two days and again give the medicine according to the symptoms. **Tuberculinum-bov. 1M** should be given once a month for 6 months to the patients who are prone to Bronchitis

	Biochemic remedy	**Ferrum phos. 6X** and **Kali mur. 6X**	*4 hourly*

IInd Stage

	Symptoms	Remedy	Frequency
☆	When cough begins to loosen; complaints worse cold, even uncovering of body parts aggravate. Coughing chokes	**Hepar sulph. 30**	*4 hourly*
☆	Much rattling in the chest due to mucous in the bronchial tubes; tongue clean; dyspnoea and nausea	**Ipecac 30**	*4 hourly*
☆	Wheezing; rattling chest, loose cough, but no phlegm comes out even after prolonged coughing. Tongue whitish coated	**Antimonium tart. 200**	*10 min. (3)*

IIIrd Stage

	Symptoms	Remedy	Frequency
☆	When mucous becomes yellow; patient feels better in open air; loss of thirst	**Pulsatilla 30**	*4 hourly*
❑	When no phlegm comes out; if any, it is blood streaked; pulse rapid and patient becomes very weak	**Ammonium carb. 30**	*4 hourly*

BRONCHITIS
Chronic

	Symptoms	Remedy	Frequency
●	For persons who are constantly catching cold with chronic suffocative cough	**Bacillinum 200 or 1M**	*weekly (3)*
☆	Wheezing and oppression in the chest. Breathing stops when falling asleep;	**Grindelia Q or 6**	*½ hourly (3)*

Symptoms	Remedy	Frequency And Doses
wakes up with a start and gasps for breath. Must sit up to breathe; can not breath when lying down		
❑ Chronic Bronchitis. Pain in distant parts of body on coughing	**Capsicum 30**	4 hourly
❑ Cough worse after midnight; dry and painful which makes the patient to hold his chest; worse on talking	**Drosera 200**	one dose only
❑ When breathing is rapid and hard; wheezing with excessive dyspnoea; expectoration very difficult	**Antimonium ars. 6 or 30**	4 hourly (6)
❑ Hard, croupy cough with inability to raise the sputum	**Antimonium iod.30**	4 hourly
✩ Cough with soreness in chest; better drinking cold water. Involuntary escape of urine while coughing	**Causticum 30**	4 hourly
❑ Must cough for a long time before he can raise the mucous because it is strong and sticky; involuntary escape of urine	**Squilla 30**	4 hourly
✩ Extreme restlessness with prostration. Thirst for small quantities of water at short intervals. Cough dry worse after drinking; and midnight must sit up. Chilly patient	**Arsenic alb. 30**	4 hourly
✩ When body turns blue and cold; patient wants to be fanned	**Carbo veg. 30**	4 hourly
❑ Copious expectoration with dilatation of bronchial tubes	**Sabal ser. Q or 6**	4 hourly
❑ Painful spasmodic cough and dyspnoea; worse night	**Naphthaline 30**	4 hourly
❑ Breathlessness after attack of bronchitis	**Chloralum 30**	4 hourly

Symptoms	Remedy	Frequency And Doses

BURNS

❏ Head remedy - For burns of any kind — **Cantharis 30** — *4 hourly*

❏ Sun burns; rush of blood towards head, flushed face — **Belladonna 30** — *4 hourly*

❏ Radium, X- ray burns — **Phosphorus 200 or Cadmium iod 30** — *4 hourly (3)*

❏ When there is fear of death and anxiety due to burns. Burnt area is hot and swollen with fever — **Aconite 30 or 200** — *15 min. (6)*

● If the part mortifies (leading towards gangrene) — **Silicea 30 or Sulphur 30** — *3 hourly (3)*

❏ If pus forms; effected part becomes very sensitive — **Hepar Sulph. 200** — *10 min. (3)*

❏ Burns due to pouring of hot water or hot oil; when blisters has not formed — **Urtica urens. 30** — *2 hourly*

For External Use:

Cantharis lotion. If wounds form then apply Calendula lotion.

CANCER
(Of Different Organs)

The medicines which have special affinity on particular organs have been given here. If the totality of symptoms of the patient as a whole tallies with a particular medicine then it can be given accordingly. The repetition should be with great care only.

Symptoms	Remedy	Frequency And Doses
❏ Cancer of stomach with constant vomiting of black fluid	Cadmium sulph. 30	3 hourly
❏ Cancer of pancreas or of bones, especially the lower jaw and tibia	Phosphorus 30 or 200	3 hourly
❏ Cancer of bone, periosteum, especially the joints	Symphytum 6 or 30	3 hourly
❏ Cancerous ulcer; especially when out-come is after suppression of Malaria	Chininum sulph. 30 or 200	3 hourly
❏ Cancer of stomach, of axilla, oesophagus; painful cracks in corner of the mouth	Condurango 30 or 200	3 hourly
❏ Cancer of bladder, breast; disposition to pimples at adolescence	Asterias rubens 30 or 200	3 hourly
❏ Cancer of caecum, pylorus, duodenum; painful contraction with duodenal distention	Ornithogalum Q or 6	3 hourly
❏ Cancer of cervix; bleeds easily; sensation of boiling water along the back	Ustilago Q or 6	3 hourly
❏ Cancer of face; ill-effects of vaccination. Rapid exhaustion and emaciation	Thuja oc. 30 or 200	3 hourly
❏ Cancer of lungs; sleep always disturbed by lewd dreams	Cobaltum. 30	3 hourly
❏ Cancer of glands of the neck; patient sensitive to cold. Sensation of coldness in various parts	Cistus can. 30	3 hourly
❏ Cancer of testicles	Cadmium phos. 30	3 hourly
❏ Cancer of vagina; prostate; can not control the urine; urine dribbles constantly while lying	Kreosote 30	3 hourly

Symptoms	Remedy	Frequency And Doses
● Cancerous history in the family or past history of cancer in the patient	**Carcinocin 200 or 1M**	*fortnightly (3)*
☆ Cancerous diathesis; over irritability	**Strychninum 200 or 1M**	*fortnightly (3)*
❑ To expel the poison from the effected lesion	**Silicea 12X or 30**	*4 hourly*
❑ When carbuncle turns towards gangrene; marked burning and restlessness	**Arsenic-alb. 30**	*4 hourly*
❑ Cancer affecting lower bowel with prolapsus	**Ruta grav. 6 or 30**	*4 hourly*

For External Use: **Hypericum lotion.**

CHANGE OF LIFE
(See Menopause)

CARIES OF TEETH

☆ Decay of teeth in children as soon as they appear; bed wetting	**Kreosote 30**	*4 hourly*
☆ Decay of teeth; pain and soreness	**Plantago 30**	*4 hourly*
☆ Decay of teeth; bleeding gums, sensitive to hot or cold	**Merc-sol. 30**	*4 hourly*
● Intercurrent remedy	**Syphilinum 200 or 1M**	*weekly (3)*
Biochemic remedyies	**Calcarea fluor. 12X, Calcarea phos. 6X and Silicea 12X**	*4 hourly*

For External Use: **Plantago Q or Kreosote Q.**

CAUSATION – AILMENTS DUE TO
(See Different Ailments and Occupational Ailments, Etc., Also)

❑ Ailments due to carrying heavy weight in labourers, etc.	**Ruta gr. 30 or 200**	*6 hourly*

Symptoms	Remedy	Frequency And Doses
❑ Effect of cold drinks; (when over heated; takes cold drinks or water and suffers)	Bellis p. 30	*4 hourly*
❑ Due to fasting	Dioscorea 30	*4 hourly*

CERVICAL SPONDYLOSIS
(See Slipped Disc, Etc., Also)

☆ Vertigo; worse closing eyes due to degeneration of spinal cord	Theridion 30	*4 hourly*
☆ With muscular weakness; perspiration of hands, specially in bachelors	Conium mac. 200 or 1M	*3 hourly (3)*
☆ With numbness; worse night	Kali iod. 200 or 1M	*3 hourly (3)*
☆ Head remedy; tearing pain with weakness	Acid-phos. 30	*4 hourly*
● Intercurrent remedy	Psorinum 200 or 1M	*weekly (3)*
☆ Pain nape of neck; better movements, worse by rest, cold and damp, after drinking icy cold water	Rhus tox. 200 or 1M	*4 hourly*
Biochemic remedies	Calcarea fluor. 12X and Calcarea phos. 6X	*4 hourly*

CHICKEN-POX

✪ Preventive medicine	Variolinum 200	*10 min. (3)*
❑ High fever with anxiety and shiny red face	Aconite 30 or 200	*2 hourly*
❑ Fever without thirst, though throat is dry; desire for open, cold air	Pulsatilla 30	*4 hourly*
❑ Fever with headache and shiny red face; rush of blood towards head	Belladonna 30	*3 hourly*
❑ Itching in eruptions; tip of tongue red; restlessness	Rhus tox. 30	*4 hourly*
❑ When fever is over and eruptions starts drying up	Merc sol. 30	*4 hourly (3)*
Biochemic Remedies	Kali mur. 6X and Ferrum phos. 6X	*alternate 2 hourly*

CHILBLAINS

Symptoms	Remedy	Frequency And Doses
☆ Painful; worse in cold weather, winter	**Agaricus m. 30**	*4 hourly*
☆ When there are cracks which bleed easily; worse winter and cold climate	**Petroleum 30**	*4 hourly*
❑ With itching; worse by warmth; better in cold, open air	**Pulsatilla 30**	*4 hourly*
☆ With redness and swelling of the skin; itching and burning; restlessness	**Rhus tox. 30**	*4 hourly*
Biochemic remedies	**Calcarea phos. 6X** and **Calcarea fluor. 12X**	*4 hourly*

For External Use:

Rhus ven. Q and Glycerine in 1: 9.

CHILDREN DISEASES
(See Different Ailments)

❑ Mongol child; mentally and physically retarded; irritable; lack of concentration	**D.N.A. 1M or 1002**	*fortnightly (6)*

Constitutional remedies are helpful for all sorts of complications of children.

CHOLERA

Cholera is an acute infectious disease caused by the Bacillus Vibrio Cholerae. The spread of disease is through water or contaminated food. In the beginning there is diarrhoea which becomes watery and profuse very soon. There is sudden loss of fluids. Acute vomiting , weak pulse, blood pressure falls down, urine becomes scanty. If not managed properly patient may die due to loss of fluid.

❑ Prophylactic remedy	**Cuprum met. 200** and **Verat-alb. 200**, alternate weekly throughout an epidemic	

Symptoms	Remedy	Frequency And Doses
☆ Head remedy - when body becomes cold with internal chill	**Camphor Q or 30**	*1/2 hourly*
❑ Desire for cold drinks - violent colic, especially around naval. Patient feels as if anus remains wide open after passing stools	**Phosphorus 30 or 200**	*1/2 hourly*
☆ Stools - white, like rice water; cold sweating and uncontrollable retching with drawing and cramps in fingers	**Verat-alb. 30**	*1/2 hourly*
☆ When deathly nausea and cold sweat persist	**Tabacum 30**	*1/2 hourly*
☆ Body cold and bluish. Spasmodic diarrhoea, spasm starts from lower extremities and spread to upper extremities, muscles of abdomen and chest	**Cuprum met. 30**	*1/2 hourly*
☆ Large, yellow, greenish, offensive stools	**Podophyllum 30**	*1/2 hourly*
☆ Burning sensation all over the body; restlessness, difficulty in breathing. Rapid onset of collapse. Thirst for small quantities of water at frequent intervals	**Arsenic alb. 30**	*1/2 hourly*
❑ When vomiting stops but diarrhoea continues; extremities icy cold but patient doesn't want to cover them. More retching than vomiting	**Secale cor. 30**	*1/2 hourly*
☆ When body becomes cold; respiration weak and laboured; patient desires to be fanned	**Carbo veg. 30**	*1/2 hourly*
❑ When cholera symptoms are associated with loud, violent and deathly hiccough	**Cicuta v. 30**	*1/2 hourly*
❑ When Cholera is followed by croup	**Spongia 30**	*1/2 hourly*
Biochemic remedies	**Magnesia phos. 6X, Ferrum phos. 12X, Kali mur. 6X, Natrum sulph. 12X, Kali phos. 6X** and **Natrum mur. 12X**	*1/2 hourly*

During acute stage when vital force goes down the above medicines should be given at short intervals according to the symptoms in higher potencies (200 and above).

CHOLERA INFANTUM

Symptoms	Remedy	Frequency And Doses
❑ Complaints with cough, stools golden yellow; patient craves for icy cold drinks	**Phosphorus 30**	*1/2 hourly*
☆ When there is marked sour smell in the stools	**Rheum 30**	*1/2 hourly*
☆ When there is frequent thirst for small quantity of water. Vomiting with frequent and watery stools; restlessness	**Arsenic alb. 30**	*1/2 hourly*

Other Useful Remedies:

Aethusa 30, Antim-crud. 30, Calcarea phos. 6X or 30, Chamomilla 30, China 30, Opium 30 or 200, Phosphorus 30, Podophyllum 30, etc..

CHOREA
Involuntary Movements of Muscles
(See Nervousness Also)

❑ With pain and numbness	**Asafoetida 30**	*6 hourly*
❑ Angular; better during sleep	**Argentum nit. 30 or 200**	*6 hourly*
❑ Jerking of arms and legs	**Mygale 200**	*weekly (3)*
☆ Due to disturbed emotions; specially of facial muscles; worse after inhaling smoke	**Ignatia 200**	*6 hourly*
❑ Movements of head backward and forward; fear of dark	**Stramonium 200 or 1M**	*6 hourly*
❑ Tremors of hands; profuse sweating which do not relieve the complaints	**Mercurius sol. 30 or 200**	*6 hourly*
❑ In chilly, weak, worn-out patients; worse by cold	**Zincum phos. 30**	*6 hourly*
☆ Loss of control; movements of extremities; worse during sleep; contraction of muscles	**Causticum 30 or 200**	*6 hourly*
Biochemic remedies	**Kali phos. 6X and Magnesia phos. 6X**	*4 hourly*

COITION - Male
(See Erections Impotency, Spermatorrhoea, Etc., Also)

Symptoms	Remedy	Frequency And Doses
❑ Aversion to coitus due to impotency; constipated patients; who are prone to be obese	**Graphites 200 or 1M**	*weekly (3)*
✫ Desire lost or diminished. Complete loss of erection	**Lycopodium 200 or 1M**	*weekly (3)*
● Intercurrent remedy	**Psorinum 200**	*weekly (3)*

Only constitutional treatment gives the desired results in sex related ailments.

COLD, CATARRH AND CORYZA

Ist Stage

✫ Icy coldness of whole body; internal and external both. To give heat to the system	**Camphor 6 or 30**	*1/2 hourly*
✫ Cold due to sudden exposure to dry cold wind; chilly feeling, headache, watering of eyes and sneezing; anxiety and fear; feverish feeling	**Aconite 30 or 200**	*2 hourly*
✫ Running of nose during day and blockage at night with chilly feeling	**Nux vomica 30**	*3 hourly*
✫ Cold with sneezing and profuse discharge from eyes and nose; worse in warmth and indoor; better in open air	**Allium cepa. 30**	*3 hourly*
❑ Dryness of nose with headache; worse from motion; thirst more; lips parched and dry; stools constipated	**Bryonia 30 or 200**	*3 hourly*
❑ Sneezing; watering of nose and eyes; throat sore with constant desire to swallow saliva; foul smell from mouth; feverish with sweat which do not relieve. Worse at night	**Mercurius sol. 30**	*3 hourly*

Symptoms	Remedy	Frequency And Doses
☆ Watering and burning of eyes with streaming nose; acrid discharges	**Euphrasia 30**	3 hourly
☆ Chilly feeling though face is hot; restlessness and un-quenchable thirst, drinks often but little at a time; better hot drinks	**Arsenic alb. 30**	3 hourly
☆ Acrid discharge from nose which corrodes the upper lip. Nose filled with phlegm; breathes through the mouth	**Arum triph. 30**	3 hourly
☆ Cold; running of nose and sneezing; redness and pain forehead; watering eyes	**Sabadilla 30**	4 hourly
❏ Cold; pain throat; red face, rush of blood towards head	**Belladonna 30**	4 hourly
☆ Aching pain, dullness, chilliness in back; sneezing, bland and thick discharge from nose; feverish; better passing urine	**Gelsemium 30**	3 hourly
☆ Coryza with sneezing and aching in bones of extremities with soreness of flesh	**Eup-perf. 30**	3 hourly
❏ Cold; better from cold bathing	**Calcarea sulph. 30**	4 hourly
❏ Dripping of nose while eating	**Trombidium 30 or 200**	6 hourly
❏ Dripping of nose while going to sleep	**Thuja oc. 30 or 200**	6 hourly
❏ Dry coryza; sniffles of infants, blockage of nose	**Sambucus nig. 30**	4 hourly
Biochemic remedies	**Calcarea phos. 6X** and **Ferrum phos. 6X**	*alternate 3 hourly*

IInd stage

❏ Discharge from nose; yellowish or greenish; stringy	**Kali bich. 30**	4 hourly
❏ Greenish yellow mucous from nose; loss of taste and thirst; better open air	**Pulsatilla 30**	4 hourly
❏ Thick yellow discharge from nose; post nasal catarrh; constipation	**Hydrastis c. 30**	4 hourly

Symptoms	Remedy	Frequency And Doses
❏ Watering from nose like a tap; thirst more; stools constipated; cold aggravates till noon and ameliorates after noon	**Natrum mur. 30** (in acute stage **Bryonia 30**)	*4 hourly*
❏ In fat and flabby patient; worse after bathing; chilly patient	**Calcarea carb. 200**	*6 hourly*
❏ Watery discharge from nose in the beginning and finally it becomes thick, yellow. Pain in the throat on swallowing as if full of splinters; sensitive to cold	**Hepar sulph. 30**	*4 hourly*
● Cold worse early morning; chronic, dry catarrh; aversion to take bath	**Sulphur 200**	*weekly (3)*
● Chronic catarrh; dry coryza, with blockage of nose; worse change of weather and cold.	**Psorinum 200**	*weekly (3)*
● Chronic cases with tubercular history	**Tuberculinum k. 200 or 1M**	*fortnightly (6)*
● Obstinate chronic cases, when indicated remedy fails	**Bacillinum 1M**	*weekly (3)*

Biochemic remedies

Symptoms	Remedy	Frequency And Doses
— Yellowish phlegm; worse by warmth	**Kali sulph. 6X**	*4 hourly*
— Head cold with thick yellow green discharge	**Calcarea fluor. 6X or 12X**	*4 hourly*
— For acute or chronic catarrh	**Calcarea phos. 6X and Natrum mur. 12X**	*4 hourly*

COLIC
(See Abdominal Pain Also)

Symptoms	Remedy	Frequency And Doses
❏ Due to food poisoning; un-quenchable thirst sips at frequent intervals; anxiety and restlessness	**Arsenic-alb. 30**	*2 hourly*
☆ Due to acidity and ulcers; patient desires constant fanning, fresh air	**Carbo veg. 30**	*4 hourly*

Symptoms	Remedy	Frequency And Doses
☆ Agonising, cutting pains; better bending double	Colocynth. 30	4 hourly
❑ After over - eating; especially spicy - rich food or milk, etc.	Nux vomica. 30	3 hourly
☆ During cholera with cold sweating	Veratrum alb. 30	2 hourly
❑ Pain in abdomen due to worms	Cina 200 or 1M	6 hourly
❑ Due to flatulence; better bending backwards	Dioscorea v. 30	4 hourly
❑ While eating; burning pain around the navel	Calcarea renal. 30	4 hourly
❑ After abdominal operation.	Staphysagria 30	4 hourly
❑ When pain comes and goes suddenly	Belladonna 30	4 hourly
❑ After taking rich fatty food with loss of thirst; desire for cold, open air	Pulsatilla 30	4 hourly
☆ When pains are intolerable; especially in pregnant woman; worse after anger	Chamomilla 200	2 hourly
❑ Severe; spasmodic pain; violent and intermittent	Cuprum met. 30	4 hourly
Biochemic remedy	Magnesia phos. 6X	2 hourly

COLITIS
(See Dysentery Also)

Symptoms	Remedy	Frequency And Doses
☆ Symptoms worse after anger; bitter taste. Severe cutting pain in abdomen causing patient to bend over double	Colocynth. 30	3 hourly
☆ Greenish watery stools, gushing out with great force; abdomen distended	Magnesia carb. 30	4 hourly
❑ Yellowish watery stools with flatulence; worse after eating, taking icy cold water or preserved fruits; digestion slow	China 6 or 30	4 hourly

Symptoms	Remedy	Frequency And Doses
❑ Offensive, loose stools. Patient can not tolerate even touch of clothes on abdomen; worse during spring and after sleep	**Lachesis 30 or 200**	*4 hourly (3)*
❑ Ulcerative or simple colitis; after indignation (such as rape or other inhuman acts; etc.)	**Staphysagria 200 or 1M**	*fortnightly (3)*
❑ Stools contain white shreddy particles; distention of abdomen; pain over liver region; oversensitive to smell of foods	**Colchicum 30**	*4 hourly*
Biochemic remedy	**Magnesia phos. 6X**	*3 hourly*

COLLAPSE
(See Fainting and Unconsciousness Also)

To fall into a state of profound physical depression is called collapse.

(Seek medical aid immediately - the following medicines can be given according to the symptoms till proper medical aid is given). Try to find out the basic cause and treat accordingly.

☆ When there is internal as well as external coldness; after sudden exposure to cold; during cholera	**Camphor. Q or 30**	*15 min. (6)*
☆ Though the body is cold but patient desires fanning	**Carbo veg. 30 or 200**	*1/2 hourly*
❑ Sudden; due to fear or exposure to dry cold air	**Aconite 200 or 1M**	*1/2 hourly*
❑ Due to concussion (injury)	**Arnica 200 or 1M**	*1/2 hourly (3)*
❑ Due to exhaustive discharges, such as loss of blood, excessive vomiting, diarrhoea or semen loss, etc.	**China 30**	*1/2 hourly*
❑ In epileptic fits	**Cuprum met. 30 or 200**	*1/2 hourly*
❑ Due to sun stroke	**Glonoine 30 or 200**	*1/2 hourly*
☆ With cold sweating	**Veratrum alb. 30 or 200**	*1/2 hourly*
Biochemic remedies	**Kali phos 6X, Magnesia phos. 6X** and **Natrum mur. 12X** in like warm water	*1/2 hourly*

Symptoms	Remedy	Frequency And Doses

Other Useful Remedies:

Arsenic alb., Phosphorus, Conium mac., Hydrocyanic acid., Opium, Colocynth, etc..

CONJUNCTIVITIS
(See Trachoma Also)

Inflammation of the conjunctiva (the mucous membrane covering the anterior surface of the eyeball) is called conjunctivitis.

Symptoms	Remedy	Frequency And Doses
☆ Sudden watering from the eyes with inflammation after exposure to cold	**Aconite 30 or 200**	*3 hourly*
☆ Eyes fiery red with pain and inflammation; face red	**Belladonna 30**	*4 hourly*
☆ Acrid, watery discharge from eyes; patient can not bear bright light	**Euphrasia 30**	*3 hourly*
☆ Headache; profuse, purulent discharge from eyes which makes vision hazy, should be cleared immediately; acute granular swelling	**Argentum nit. 30**	*4 hourly*
❑ Eye-lids swollen, red; worse by heat	**Apis mel. 30**	*4 hourly*
☆ Greenish yellow discharge from eyes; worse by heat and better in open, cold air	**Pulsatilla 30**	*4 hourly*
☆ Acrid lachrymation; severe burning, soreness of the eyes, sensation of foreign body in the eyes. Eye-lids get gummed	**Mercurius Cor. 30**	*4 hourly*
❑ Stringy, whitish discharge from the eyes	**Kali bich. 30**	*4 hourly*
❑ Redness and inflammation of the eyes; eyes can be open with great force only	**Rhus tox. 30**	*4 hourly*
● Itching and burning of eyes; worse by washing	**Sulphur 30 or 200**	*4 hourly (3)*
Biochemic remedies	**Kali mur. 6X** and **Ferrum phos. 6X**	*alternate 2 hourly*

For External Use: *Euphrasia eye drops*

Symptoms	Remedy	Frequency And Doses

CONSTIPATION

❏ Chronic constipation; much flatus, distention of abdomen	**Coca Q**, 10 drops in luke warm water	*6 hourly*
☆ Due to fast, sedentary life; ineffectual urging, passing stools many times in a day	**Nux vom. 30 or 200**	*6 hourly*
☆ Hard stools, due to dryness and non peristaltic action of the intestinal tract. Desire for dry food	**Alumina O/7 or above** (50 millesimal potency)	*6 hourly*
❏ Stools hard; dry as if burnt, seems too large. No desire to pass stools; thirst increased, drinks large quantity of water at a time at long intervals	**Bryonia 30 or 200**	*6 hourly*
☆ Tonic for proper bowel movements	**Cascara sag. Q**, 10-15 drops	*4 hourly*
❏ Feels better normal when constipated; fat, flabby and chilly patient	**Calcarea carb. 200**	*4 hourly (3)*
❏ Patient can pass stools only in standing position	**Causticum 30 or 200**	*6 hourly*
❏ Constipation with sinking feeling in stomach; tongue flabby, white and slimy	**Hydrastis can. Q or 6**	*4 hourly*
☆ In chilly patient who lacks vital energy; stools goes back into the rectum when partially expelled	**Silicea 12X or 30**	*4 hourly*
Biochemic remedy	**Bio-combination No.4**	*4 hourly*

Other Useful Remedies:

Selenium, Sulphur, Graphites, Opium, Mag-carb., etc.

CONTACT DERMATITIS

Contact dermatitis means dermatitis due to allergy to a locally applied agent.

Useful remedy for acute stage is *Apis mel. 30* and for chronicity *Graphites*, *Natrum mur.*, *Sulphur* and *Thuja-oc.*, etc..

Symptoms	Remedy	Frequency And Doses

CONVULSIONS
Fits

❏ Convulsions after seeing water; especially in cases of hydrophobia	**Lyssin 200 or 1M**	*10 min. (3)*
❏ Convulsions due to whooping cough	**Cuprum met. 30 or 200**	*3 hourly*
❏ Convulsions due to worms in children	**Cina 200 or 1M**	*6 hourly*
❏ Convulsions with hot, red skin, flushed face and glaring eyes; during teething period	**Belladonna 30**	*4 hourly*
❏ Violent convulsions; with violent distortions; fear of dark	**Stramonium 30**	*3 hourly*
❏ Violent distortions; back bent backward like an arch	**Cicuta v. 30 or 200**	*3 hourly*
Biochemic remedies	**Kali phos. 6X, Magnesia phos. 6X** and **Natrum phos. 6X**	*4 hourly*

In acute attack above medicines can be given at short intervals.

CORNS

☆ Painful; specially on the soles; tongue thickly whitish coated	**Antim-crud. 200 or 1M**	*6 hourly (6)*
☆ Corns due to pressure of shoes; painful	**Sulphur 200**	*weekly (3)*
❏ Corns with soreness and tearing pain	**Lycopodium 200**	*weekly (3)*
❏ Corns of toes; re-appears after cutting	**Hydrastis can. 30**	*4 hourly*
❏ Corns with deep cracks; stools hard, constipated	**Graphites 30**	*4 hourly*
Biochemic remedy Soft, inflamed and sore corns	**Silicea 12X or 30X**	*4 hourly*

For External Use: *Thuja oc. Q.*

Symptoms	Remedy	Frequency And Doses

CORONARY THROMBOSIS

A clot in blood vessel or in one of the cavities of the heart, formed life from constituents of blood; it may be occlusive or attached to the vessel or heart wall obstructing the lumen.

(Seek medical aid immediately and in the mean while any of the following medicines according to the symptoms can be given).

Symptoms	Remedy	Frequency And Doses
❏ Tightness and contraction in the chest; bruised pains	**Arnica 200**	*1/2 hourly (3)*
❏ Constriction of the heart region as if the heart squeezed by a tight band	**Cactus g. Q** or **30**	*1/2 hourly (6)*
❏ With numbness of the left arm and left sided paralysis. Can't bear tight clothings around neck or waist	**Lachesis 200**	*1/2 hourly (3)*
❏ Coronary thrombosis due to bad effects of anger	**Colocynth. 200**	1/2 hourly (3)
Biochemic remedies	**Magnesia phos. 6X, Ferrum phos. 6X** and **Kali mur. 6X**	*1/2 hourly*

Other Useful Remedies:

Ammon-carb., Apis mel., Baryta carb., Belladonna, Bothrops lan., Calcarea ars., Kali mur., Lilium tig., Lycopodium, Hyoscyamus, Medorrhinum, Mercurius sol., Opium, Phosphorus, Secale cor., Sulphur, etc., are also useful remedies.

(For myocardial infarction or coronary thrombosis see thrombosis also).

COUGH
(See Hoarseness, Wheezing, etc., Also)

Symptoms	Remedy	Frequency And Doses
❏ Cough with sensation of dust in the throat	**Chelidonium 6 or 30**	*4 hourly*
❏ Dry, violent cough due to exposure to dry cold wind; anxiety and fear in mind	**Aconite 30 or 200**	*4 hourly*
❏ Listening of music brings on cough	**Ambra gr. 30**	*4 hourly*
❏ Coughing causes pain in distant parts	**Capsicum 30**	*4 hourly*
❏ Looseness of brain while coughing	**Carbo ani. 30 or 200**	*4 hourly*
❏ Dry cough during sleep; worse after anger	**Chamomilla 30 or 200**	*4 hourly*

Symptoms	Remedy	Frequency And Doses
❏ Every paroxysm of pain excites nervous cough	**Hura b. 30**	*4 hourly*
❏ Every time patient stands still while walking he coughs; worse inhaling smoke; feels sleepy after every spell of coughing	**Ignatia 30 or 200**	*4 hourly*
❏ Cough worse while going down in comparison of going up; worse 4-8 p.m.	**Lycopodium 30 or 200**	*4 hourly*
❏ Cough better while lying down	**Manganum acet. 30**	*4 hourly*
❏ Cough at night and diarrhoea during day	**Petroleum 30**	*4 hourly*
☆ Cough worse inspiration and only during day	**Rumex c. 30**	*4 hourly*
❏ Cough always ends into sneezing	**Senega 30**	*4 hourly*
❏ Cough followed by hic cough	**Trillium p. 6 or 30**	*4 hourly*
☆ Dry, painful cough with headache; worse by movements and moaning. Thirst excessive; stools constipated	**Bryonia 30 or 200**	*4 hourly*
☆ Cough with hoarseness and loss of voice; desire to drink icy cold water	**Phosphorus 30 or 200**	*4 hourly*
☆ With sticky, ropy phlegm; chronic sinusitis; pain in the ears while coughing	**Kali bich. 30**	*4 hourly*
☆ Cough worse between 2-4 a.m.	**Kali carb. 30 or 200**	*4 hourly*
☆ Cough worse in warm room; better open air; thirstlessness with dry mouth	**Pulsatilla 30**	*4 hourly*
☆ Dry cough; sibilant (hissing) sounds like a saw driven through a pine board	**Spongia 30**	*4 hourly*
☆ Urine escapes while coughing; better in damp cold; dry cough	**Causticum 30 or 200**	*4 hourly*
☆ Cough worse after first sleep (1-2 hours after sleep)	**Aralia r. Q or 30**	*4 hourly*
☆ Cough with constant nausea and wheezing; tongue clean	**Ipecac 30**	*4 hourly*

Symptoms	Remedy	Frequency And Doses
☆ Rattling of chest; it is difficult to raise the phlegm; tongue whitish coated; cough and yawning alternate	**Antimonium tart. 30**	*1/2 hourly (3)*
❏ Dry cough at night with chocking; face turns red on coughing with congestion of head	**Belladonna 30**	*4 hourly*
☆ Cough after exposure to cold wind; sensation of foreign body in the throat with pain while swallowing; Patient over-sensitive to cold, touch, etc.	**Hepar sulph. 30**	*4 hourly*
● Symptoms constantly change and well selected remedies fail to act; cold is taken from the slightest exposure	**Tuberculinum b. 200**	*weekly (3)*
❏ Cough with itching in larynx, spasmodic with gaggling and vomiting of mucous; after any inflammatory disease like measles, etc.	**Carbo veg. 30**	*4 hourly*
● Cough dry, hard; worse at night; better during day and moving about slowly	**Syphilinum 200 or 1M**	*weekly (3)*
❏ Phlegm yellowish and sweetish in taste; weakness and emptiness in chest	**Stannum met. 30**	*4 hourly*
❏ Children loose their breath while coughing; face becomes bluish and purplish, gasping for breath. Cough rapid and short like gun fire	**Corallium r. 30**	*4 hourly*
❏ Cough following measles or suppression of intermittent fever	**Eupatorium perf. 30**	*4 hourly*
❏ Cough with thick ropy mucous; worse in warm room and taking warm drinks. It comes on while in cold water but relieved by cold drinks and washing face with cold water	**Coccus cacti 30**	*4 hourly*
❏ Cough, dry with desire for hot, salty drinks	**Lac caninum 30 or 200**	*4 hourly*
❏ Cough better while smoking - short of breath after each attack; cough while or after weeping	**Tarentula h. 30 or 200**	*4 hourly*

Symptoms	Remedy	Frequency And Doses
❑ Catarrhal cough; involuntary spurting of urine; sneezing	**Scilla mar. 30**	*4 hourly*
❑ Cough dry; worse from air into larynx, tobacco smoke, fog and while talking	**Mentha pip. 30**	*4 hourly*
❑ Cough explosive; persistent, recurring after influenza	**Strychninum 30**	*4 hourly*
❑ Cough during pregnancy; spasmodic	**Viburnum op. 30**	*4 hourly*
❑ Dry cough; has to stoop to cough; no expectoration with cough	**Kali-mur 6X or 30**	*4 hourly*
❑ Much rattling of mucous, loose cough; worse after bathing and morning	**Sulphur 200**	*weekly (3)*
Biochemic remedy	**Bio-combination No.6**	*4 hourly*

CRAMPS
Writer's Cramp, Etc.

Symptoms	Remedy	Frequency And Doses
☆ Cramps in cold water in swimmers. Cramps in calf muscles at night by stretching the legs in bed	**Rhus tox. 30 or 200**	*4 hourly*
❑ Cramps of abdomen	**Aesculus glab. 30**	*4 hourly*
❑ Writers cramp; pain in parts of hand where bones lie near surface; worse cold	**Cyclamen 30**	*4 hourly*
❑ Cramps due to fatigue; bruised feeling as if beaten	**Arnica 30 or 200**	*3 hourly*
❑ With icy coldness of limbs and body, as in cholera, etc.	**Camphor. Q or 6**	*1/2 hourly*
❑ Cramps of calf muscles, soles and palms, beginning from fingers and toes; spasmodic	**Cuprum met. 30**	*4 hourly*
❑ Cramp like drawing, in upper gluteals when standing; cold sweating	**Verat-alb. 30**	*4 hourly*

Symptoms	Remedy	Frequency And Doses

CRAVINGS
Desires for Eatables, Etc.

❏ To chew clean cloth; raw food	**Alumina 200** or above	*6 hourly (3)*
❏ Craving for fat; lime, slate, pencils, chalk and clay, etc.	**Acid-nit. 30 or 200**	*6 hourly (3)*
❏ For salt (extra salt in food)	**Natrum mur. 200 or 1M**	*6 hourly (3)*
❏ For eggs	**Calcarea carb. 200 or 1M**	*6 hourly (3)*
❏ For sweets	**Argentum nit. 30 or 200**	*6 hourly (3)*
❏ For pickles and sour food	**Sepia 200 or 1M**	*6 hourly (3)*
❏ For lemonade	**Pulsatilla 30 or 200**	*6 hourly (3)*
❏ For banana	**Theridion 30 or 200**	*6 hourly (3)*
❏ For icy cold drinks	**Phosphorus 200**	*6 hourly (3)*
❏ For milk	**Rhus fox 200**	*weekly (3)*

CROUP

Croup becomes dangerous disease if not attended well in time. It consists of a peculiar inflammation of the lining membrane of the wind pipe, ending in the secretion of a thick, viscid, opaque membrane, like boiled white of an egg when the symptoms fully develop. The symptoms may come as a common cold after exposure to cold or damp atmospheric changes, cold wind, etc., with cough, sneezing, hoarseness and fever. Shortly the cough becomes deep with hoarseness with a deep ringing sound as if the breath were passing through a metallic tube.

❏ Sudden attack; worse after exposure to dry cold winds (*1st day of treatment*)	**Aconite 200**	*15 min. (3)*
❏ Sudden attack, (*2nd day of treatment*)	**Spongia 200**	*4 hourly (3)*
❏ When the cough is loose, much rattling, (*3rd day of treatment*)	**Hepar sulph. 200**	*4 hourly (3)*

Symptoms	Remedy	Frequency And Doses
○ The best result is obtained by giving **Aconite 200**, 1 dose Ist. then after 3 hrs. 1 dose of **Hepar sulph. 200** then after 4 hrs. one dose of **Spongia 200** and after that **Hepar sulph. 200** and **Spongia 200** alternate, 4 hourly (2 doses each)		
❏ When there is much rattling in chest; tongue white coated, expectoration difficult	**Antimonium tart. 200**	*10 min. (3)*
❏ Rattling in chest; tongue clean	**Ipecac 30**	*4 hourly*
❏ Recurrent attacks, when there is membrane formation; stringy phlegm	**Kali bich. 30 or 200**	*4 hourly*
❏ Spasmodic cough	**Cuprum met. 30**	*4 hourly*
Biochemic remedies (In acute stage)	**Ferrum phos. 6X, Magnesia phos. 6X** and **Kali mur. 6X**	*3 hourly*

CYSTITIS
Inflammation of Bladder

Symptoms	Remedy	Frequency And Doses
☆ Head remedy; intense burning in urinary passage, urine comes drop by drop	**Cantharis 30**	*4 hourly*
☆ Frequent urination; last drop burns, urine mixed with blood, passes only a few drops at a time; loss of thirst	**Apis mel. 30**	*4 hourly*
❏ Constant urging with great straining; pain travels down to thigh while making effort to pass urine	**Pareira brava. Q or 6**	*4 hourly*
☆ Thick, muddy urine mixed with blood and albumin; constant tenesmus	**Terebinth. Q**, 5-10 drops	*4 hourly*
● Intercurrent remedy	**Medorrhinum 200 or 1M**	*weekly (3)*

Symptoms	Remedy	Frequency And Doses
Biochemic remedies	Ferrum phos. 6X, Kali mur. 6X and Kali phos. 6X	4 hourly

---

CYSTS
Eye-lids
(See Stye Also)

❑	Cysts on eye-lids	**Kali iod. 30 or 200**	6 hourly
☆	Recurrent; after styes	**Staphysagria 200**	6 hourly
	Biochemic remedy	**Calcarea fluor. 12X or 30**	4 hourly

DANDRUFF

Symptoms	Remedy	Frequency And Doses
☆ Dandruff with itching of scalp and headache; worse bathing with hot water	**Lycopodium 30 or 200**	*4 hourly (3)*
❑ When the whole scalp is covered with dandruff and hair falls in large bunches	**Phosphorus 30 or 200**	*4 hourly (3)*
● Dandruff with itching of scalp; hair dry, crispy	**Medorrhinum 200 or 1M**	*fortnightly (3)*
❑ Dandruff with intolerable itching; scalp sensitive, dry scales	**Arsenic alb. 30**	*4 hourly*
● Dandruff white; scaly; hair dry, falls out; worse damp, humid atmosphere	**Thuja oc. 200 or 1M**	*weekly (6)*
☆ Dandruff worse margins of scalp; oily, greasy skin and scalp	**Natrum mur. 12X or 30**	*4 hourly*
● Intercurrent remedy; hair dry, rough, lustreless, scalp foul smelling; itching intolerable	**Psorinum 200 or 1M**	*fortnightly (3)*
❑ Dandruff profuse, scaly, profuse sweat on occiput	**Sanicula 30**	*4 hourly*
☆ Dandruff in circular patches, like ringworms; itching not relieved by scratching	**Sepia 30 or 200**	*4 hourly (3)*
❑ Yellowish, copious dandruff; ringworm; eczema on scalp; worse by heat	**Kali sulph. 6X or 30**	*4 hourly*
❑ Whitish, copious dandruff	**Kali mur. 6X or 30**	*4 hourly*

Other Useful Remedies:

Calcarea carb., Cantharis, Graphites, Mezereum, Staphysagria, Sulphur, etc..

Symptoms	Remedy	Frequency And Doses

DEAFNESS
Loss of Hearing

Symptoms	Remedy	Frequency And Doses
☆ Sudden; due to exposure to dry cold winds	Aconite 200 or 1M	4 hourly
❑ To the sounds of voice only	Chenopodium anth. 30 or 200	4 hourly
❑ Deafness only to the sound of human voice	Phosphorus 30 or 200	4 hourly
❑ Obstruction deafness in noisy places; can hear better while riding in a car/bus, etc.	Graphites 30 or 200	6 hourly
☆ With blockage of eustachian tubes	Mercurius dul. 30 or 200	6 hourly
❑ Due to suppression of discharges or eczema	Lobelia inf. 30 or 200	6 hourly
❑ After scarlet fever; patient oversensitive to cold, touch, etc.	Hepar sulph. 30 or 200 (alternate with Belladonna 200)	6 hourly
❑ Feels as if ears are stuffed; feels as if some thing were being forced outward; better cold and open air	Pulsatilla 30 or 200	6 hourly
☆ Due to paralysis of auditory nerve	Causticum 30 or 200	6 hourly
❑ Due to shock or nervous disturbances	Magnesia carb. 30 or 200	4 hourly
❑ With cold and clammy feet; sensitive to change of weather; chilly patient	Calcarea carb. 200 or 1M	weekly (3)
● Intercurrent remedy	Sulphur 200 or 1M	weekly (3)
Biochemic remedies	Ferrum phos. 6X, Kali mur. 6X and Silicea 30X	4 hourly

DENGUE FEVER

Symptoms	Remedy	Frequency And Doses
☆ With extreme pain deep into the bones; better sweating	Eupator-perf. 30	3 hourly
☆ With muscular pains and restlessness; better by motion	Rhus tox. 30 or 200	3 hourly

Symptoms	Remedy	Frequency And Doses
❏ Bilious, remittent fever; thirst before and during chill and heat; better after vomiting	**Nyctanthes a. Q or 30**	*3 hourly*
☆ Chilliness up and down the back; muscular soreness and exhaustion; dull, heavy head	**Gelsemium 30**	*3 hourly*
☆ Bursting, splitting headache; body-ache; thirst excessive; stools constipated; worse by motion	**Bryonia 30 or 200**	*3 hourly*
❏ High fever; restlessness with exhaustion, thirst unquenchable, sips water frequently	**Arsenic alb. 30**	*3 hourly*
Biochemic remedy	**Bio-combination No.11**	*4 hour y*

DENTITION
Affections Of
(Teething)

At the time of teething general irritation, loss of appetite, diarrhoea, fever, sleeplessness and weight loss, etc., are the usual complaints of a child. In homoeopathy there are certain remedies which are very useful for teething complaints.

☆ Fever with restlessness and sleeplessness; child cries because of teething pain	**Aconite 6 or 30**	*4 hourly*
☆ Convulsions during teething period; followed by sleep; face red with high fever	**Belladonna 30**	*3 hourly*
☆ In fatty children, teething slow; profuse sweat on head; chilly patient	**Calcarea carb. 200**	*weekly (3)*
☆ Diarrhoea; watery, greenish slimy stools; general irritability, child wants to be carried all the time; worse at night	**Chamomilla 30 or 200**	*4 hourly (6)*
☆ Diarrhoea; profuse stools; child presses the gums or puts something hard in the mouth to press	**Podophyllum 30**	*4 hourly*
Biochemic remedies	**Calcarea phos. 6X or Bio combination No. 21**	*4 hourly*
Paralysis during teething period	**Kali phos. 6X** and **Magnesia phos. 6X**	*3 hourly*

Symptoms	Remedy	Frequency And Doses

DIABETES MELLITUS
(See Sugar in Urine Also)

Symptoms	Remedy	Frequency And Doses
☆ Very efficacious remedy for blood sugar	**Syzygium j. Q,** 8-10 drops	*4 hourly*
❑ Diabetes mellitus with emaciation	**Uranium nit. 3X**	*4 hourly*
❑ When diabetes mellitus is due to nervous weakness; apathetic condition; general weakness; specially in men	**Acid-phos. Q or 6**	*4 hourly*
❑ Complaints with excessive thirst; wasting disease; melancholy; constipation; in sad persons	**Natrum mur. 12X or 30**	*4 hourly*
● Intercurrent remedy	**Medorrhinum 200 or 1M**	*fortnightly (3)*
☆ General debility; thirst for large quantity of water; profuse and frequent urination; recurrent boils with much itching; diabetic itching	**Cephalandra ind. Q,** 5-10 drops	*4 hourly*
☆ Dryness of mouth, thirst increased; frequent urination at night; urine-profuse; weakness after passing urine; general debility; pruritus vulvae without eruptions	**Gymnema syl. Q,** 5-10 drops	*4 hourly*
❑ Dryness of mouth without thirst. Feels thirsty for large quantity of cold water at night; involuntary urination. Weakness in legs; better rest and pressure	**Sulphonamide 30**	*4 hourly*
Biochemic remedy	**Natrum sulph. 12X or 30**	*4 hourly*
—	**Bio-combination No.7**	*4 hourly*

DIARRHOEA
(Loose Motions, Gastroenteritis, Etc.)

Constitutional treatment is very useful in chronic cases.

Symptoms	Remedy	Frequency And Doses
❑ Diarrhoea with intestinal spasm; stools with nauseating odour; feels hungry with hollowness in stomach. Thirst for large quantities of cold drinks, aversion to sweets	**Chloromycetin 30**	*4 hourly*

Symptoms	Remedy	Frequency And Doses
☆ Sudden diarrhoea with anxiety and restlessness; pain abdomen due to sudden exposure to dry cold winds	**Aconite 30 or 200**	*1/2 hourly*
❏ Diarrhoea comes by riding in cars or other modes of automobiles; worse lack of sleep	**Cocculus ind. 30**	*4 hourly*
☆ Stools come out with force like a shot, as water from a hydrant; better drinking warm water	**Croton tig. 30 or 200**	*3 hourly*
❏ Chilliness in the rectum before passing stools; worse 4-8 p.m.	**Lycopodium 30 or 200**	*4 hourly*
❏ Shivering while passing stools; smells sour	**Rheum 30**	*4 hourly*
❏ Diarrhoea during day and cough at night; after suppression of skin ailments	**Petroleum 30**	*4 hourly*
❏ Though diarrhoea persists for a long time but it does not debilitate	**Acid-phos. 6 or 30**	*4 hourly*
❏ Diarrhoea due to cancer (especially rectum)	**Carduus m. Q, or 30**	*4 hourly*
❏ Diarrhoea after taking boiled milk	**Sepia 30 or 200**	*4 hourly (3)*
❏ Diarrhoea after eating fish	**Chin-ars. 30**	*4 hourly*
☆ After taking melons or drinking dirty water (as from ponds, nallahs, etc.)	**Zingiber 30**	*4 hourly*
☆ Eating rich, spicy food in excess; stools ineffectual; can not tolerate milk	**Nux vomica 30**	*4 hourly*
❏ After eating fatty rich food; pastry, non-veg, variety food, etc.; colour and consistency of stools changing constantly; worse at night; thirst-lessness with dry mouth	**Pulsatilla 30**	*4 hourly*
☆ Passing watery stools; without pain with excessive weakness; thirst more; sweating all over the body; desire for constant fresh air; abdomen bloated	**China off. 30**	*4 hourly*
☆ Diarrhoea during teething period; marked irritability; worse after anger	**Chamomilla 30 or 200**	*4 hourly (6)*

Symptoms	Remedy	Frequency And Doses
☆ Unable to control stools; even attempt to pass flatus is accompanied by a spurt of faeces; stools found in bed	**Aloe soc. 30**	*4 hourly*
❑ Diarrhoea with intense colic; better by pressure, doubling up; worse after anger	**Colocynth. 30**	*4 hourly*
☆ With great restlessness; thirst excessive, drinks little water at a time but very frequently; food poisoning; worse taking icy or preserved foods	**Arsenic alb. 30**	*3 hourly*
❑ In fat and flabby persons; chronic diarrhoea with ravenous appetite, craving for indigestible things like chalk, coal, pencil, etc.	**Calcarea carb. 200**	*4 hourly (6)*
❑ Greenish stools; milk passes undigested in nursing children	**Magnesia carb. 30**	*4 hourly*
● Morning diarrhoea; driven from bed in the morning due to great pressure	**Sulphur 30 or 200**	*4 hourly*
☆ Diarrhoea due to excitement and anxiety about coming events, apprehensions, etc.	**Gelsemium 30**	*4 hourly*
❑ Severe diarrhoea; pain abdomen and lower extremities; marked coldness of body; stools thin and whitish	**Veratrum alb. 30**	*4 hourly*
● Diarrhoea; worse during night	**Syphilinum 200**	*weekly (3)*
Biochemic Remedy	**Bio-combination No.8**	*3 hourly*

DIRECTION OF SYMPTOMS

❑ Diagonally	**Agaricus m., Bothrops**
❑ Diagonally; upper left, lower right	**Antimonium tart., Stramonium**
❑ Diagonally; upper right, lower left	**Ambra gr., Bromium, Medorrhinum, Phosphorus, Sulphuric acid.,**

Symptoms	Remedy	Frequency And Doses
❑ Downward	**Borax, Cactus g., Kalmia lat., Lycopodium, Sanicula**	
❑ Outwards	**Kali carb., Sulphur**	
❑ Upwards	**Conium mac., Benzin., Eupatorium perf., Ledum pal.**	
❑ Left side, then right side	**Lachesis**	
❑ Lower half of body	**Bacillinum**	
❑ Symptoms change sides	**Lac-can.**	

DREAMS

The important remedies which are helpful for curing many ailments when a particular dream is noticed repeatedly have been given here.

❑ Of pools of blood	**Solanum tub. 200 or 1M**	*weekly (3)*
❑ Of falling from height; heavy he is; of misfortune	**Thuja oc. 200 or 1M**	*weekly (3)*
❑ Black animals; beasts, gold, pleasant	**Pulsatilla 200 or 1M**	*weekly (3)*
❑ Another person lying in bed with him/her	**Petroleum 200 or 1M**	*weekly (3)*
❑ That he was blind; a lion	**Physostigma 200 or 1M**	*weekly (3)*
❑ Business of; roaming over fields	**Rhus tox. 200 or 1M**	*weekly (3)*
❑ Disappointments; hunger, intellectual mental exertion	**Ignatia 200 or 1M**	*weekly (3)*
❑ Fearful; followed by a dog, earthquake, past events, fights, pursued by, thieves	**Silicea 200 or 1M**	*weekly (3)*
❑ Excelling in mental work; fire	**Anacardium or. 200 or 1M**	*weekly (3)*
❑ Feasting; joyful	**Asafoetida 200 or 1M**	*weekly (3)*
❑ Fleeing of	**Zincum met. 200 or 1M**	*weekly (3)*
❑ Flying	**Apis mel. 200 or 1M**	*weekly (3)*
❑ Knives	**Lachesis 200 or 1M**	*weekly (3)*

Symptoms	Remedy	Frequency And Doses
❑ Marriage; pleasant	**Opium 200 or 1M**	weekly (3)
❑ Nightmare; unpleasent	**Sulphur 200 or 1M**	weekly (3)
❑ Pleasant	**Calcarea carb. 200 or 1M**	weekly (3)
❑ Quarrels	**Nux vomica 200 or 1M**	weekly (3)
❑ Robbers; thieves, thirsty of being	**Natrum mur. 200 or 1M**	weekly (3)
❑ Snakes; being bitten by	**Bovista 200**	weekly (3)
❑ Thunder - storms; threats	**Arsenic alb. 200**	weekly (3)
❑ Unsuccessful effort to talk	**Magnesia carb. 200**	weekly (3)
❑ Water	**Ammon-mur. 200**	weekly (3)

DRYNESS OF MOUTH

Symptoms	Remedy	Frequency And Doses
❑ Dryness of mouth; as if burnt	**Medorrhinum 200**	weekly (3)
❑ Dryness of mouth; like burnt leather	**Hyoscyamus 30 or 200**	4 hourly
❑ Dryness of mouth and tongue	**Kali bich. 30**	4 hourly
❑ Extreme dryness of mouth; of mucous membranes of mouth, nose and throat	**Wyethia 30**	4 hourly
❑ With excessive thirst; for large quantities of water at long intervals; stools constipated	**Bryonia alb. 30 or 200**	4 hourly
❑ With excessive thirst; for small quantities at short intervals; restlessness	**Arsenic alb. 30 or 200**	4 hourly
❑ Dryness of mouth without thirst; tongue sticks to the roof of the mouth due to dryness	**Nux mosch. 30 or 200**	4 hourly
❑ In diabetic patients	**Acid-phos. 6 or 30**	4 hourly
❑ Dryness of mouth, without thirst	**Pulsatilla 30 or 200**	4 hourly

DYSPEPSIA
(See Flatulence Also)

Indigestion or upset stomach with gastric complaints.

Symptoms	Remedy	Frequency And Doses
☆ Nausea worse in the morning; greenish yellow vomiting with great weakness; canine hunger, desire for sweets; flatulence with heaviness of abdomen worse after eating; bitter taste; indigestion from fried foods; hyperacidity with sour eructations	Atista indica 30	4 hourly
☆ Pain epigastric region with flatulence; tongue yellowish brown with imprints of teeth on edges	Penicillinum 30	4 hourly
❑ With cramps and distention of abdomen soon after eating	Gratiola 30	4 hourly
❑ When dyspepsia is caused by eating sugar and fats	Faecalis al. 30	4 hourly
☆ With dull gastric pain; sour eructations and nausea, loss of appetite, tongue large, flabby and slimy	Hydrastis can. 6 or 30	4 hourly
❑ Dyspepsia after taking calomel	Podophyllum 30	4 hourly
❑ Dyspepsia of alcoholics	Natrum sulph. 12X or 30	4 hourly
Biochemic remedy Due to nervousness	Kali phos. 6X or 30	4 hourly

DYSENTERY
(See Colitis Also)

❑ Amoebic dysentery; thirst for small quantities of water at short intervals	Arsenic alb. 30	4 hourly
☆ Amoebic dysentery; with nausea and clean tongue	Ipecac 0/5 or higher (50 millesimal)	4 hourly
● Amoebic dysentery (intercurrent remedy)	Thuja oc. 200 or 1M	fortnightly (6)

Symptoms	Remedy	Frequency And Doses
❏ Tearing down pain thighs and legs while passing stools	**Rhus tox. 6 or 30**	*4 hourly*
☆ Bacillary dysentery; blood in stools with tenesmus and never get done feeling	**Mercurius cor. 6 or 30**	*4 hourly*
● Bacillary dysentery (intercurrent remedy)	**Streptococcin. 200 or 1M**	*fortnightly (6)*
❏ Indigestion with sour eructations; anorexia, profuse salivation, bitter taste of mouth; tongue, coated brown; flatulence with distension of abdomen; stool loose mixed with mucus; urge for stool after eating; worse at night	**Terminalia chebula 30**	*4 hourly*
☆ Stools with mucous; worse at night	**Mercurius sol. 30**	*4 hourly*
❏ Chronic dysentery with discharge of pus and blood	**Staphylococcin. 200 or 1M**	*fortnightly (3)*
❏ Dysentery in camp life and in immigrants	**Septicimin. 30 or 200**	*3 hourly (6)*
☆ With large quantities of mucous; gurgling, pain rectum after passing stools, passing stools unnoticed	**Aloe soc. 30**	*4 hourly*
❏ Every drink of cold water causes chill and is followed by a hurried stool	**Capsicum 30 or 0/5 or above**	*4 hourly*
● Chronic dysentery when indicated remedies fail; worse in the morning	**Sulphur 200**	*4 hourly (3)*
☆ With violent cutting pains as from knives; passing almost pure blood instead of normal stools; sensation of anus wide open	**Phosphorus 30 or 200**	*4 hourly (3)*
❏ Stools loose; watery, yellowish, mixed with mucous and blood	**Aegle folia. Q or 6**	*4 hourly*
Biochemic remedy	**Bio-combination No.9**	*3 hourly*

DYSMENORRHOEA
(See Menstruation Affections Of)

EAR-ACHE
Otalgia

Symptoms	Remedy	Frequency And Doses
☆ Sudden; due to exposure to dry cold wind	**Aconite 30 or 200**	*2 hourly*
❑ Throbbing pain with redness of face; hot feeling; rush of blood towards head	**Belladonna 30**	*2 hourly*
☆ Intolerable pain; worse by warmth, at night and after anger	**Chamomilla 30 or 200**	*2 hourly*
☆ Severe pain in eustachian tubes; with acute cold ; worse indoors and warmth	**Allium cepa 30 or 200**	*2 hourly*
❑ Due to pressure in ears from collection of wax	**Spigelia 30 or 200**	*10 min. (3)*
❑ Due to sinusitis; stringy phelgm	**Kali bich. 30**	*4 hourly*
❑ Due to boil in the ear; perforation, discharge of fetid pus; worse by cold	**Hepar sulph. 200**	*10 min. (3)*
☆ With thick, yellowish discharge; better at cold place and cold open air	**Pulsatilla 30 or 200**	*3 hourly*
Biochemic remedies	**Kali mur. 6X** and **Ferrum phos. 6X**	*alternate 2 hourly*

For External Use: *Mullein oil - ear drops.*

Other Useful Remedies:

Colocynth., Sulphur, Syphilinum,, Pyrogenium, etc..

Symptoms	Remedy	Frequency And Doses

ECZEMA

Symptoms	Remedy	Frequency And Doses
✩ Acute; eruptions with tendency to scale formation	**Rhus tox. 30 or 200**	3 hourly (3)
✩ Weeping; with cracks, sticky discharge; stools constipated	**Graphites 30 or 200**	4 hourly (3)
✩ At the borders of hair; raw, red and inflammed; worse eating salt or at seashore	**Natrum mur. 30 or 200**	4 hourly (3)
❑ Due to Staphylococcus or Streptococcus infection	**Sulphuric acid. 30**	4 hourly (3)
✩ With yellowish pus; worse by heat; better by cold, open air	**Pulsatilla 30 or 200**	4 hourly (3)
● Dry and scaly eruptions; worse on scalp and face; worse by warmth of bed. Thin, fetid, excoriating discharge; looks dirty	**Psorinum 200**	10 min. (3)
❑ Eczema of beard; watery, oozing with itching; worse by washing	**Arsenic iod. 30**	3 hourly (3)
❑ With thick crusts; of head, ears, face and body; scratching changes location of itching	**Staphysagria 30 or 200**	3 hourly (3)
❑ With digestive, liver or urinary disorders; skin becomes thick and indurated	**Lycopodium 30 or 200**	4 hourly (3)
❑ Of fingers and toes eruptions like variola; with loss of nails	**Borax 30 or 200**	4 hourly (3)
❑ At hair margins; eruptions like variola	**Hydrastis can. 30**	4 hourly (3)
❑ Without itching; exudation forms into a hard, lemon coloured crust	**Cicuta v. 30 or 200**	4 hourly (3)
● Chronic; with irritation; worse by warmth of bed at night	**Sulphur 30 or 200**	4 hourly (3)
❑ With redness; irritability and anxiety; unquenchable thirst	**Arsenic alb. 30 or 200**	4 hourly (3)

Symptoms	Remedy	Frequency And Doses
❑ Weeping; in the bend of elbows and knees; foul breath	Mercurius sol. 30 or 200	4 hourly (3)
❑ After Mercurius sol.; pustular; sensitive patient; better by warmth; worse by cold	Hepar sulph. 30 or 200	4 hourly (3)
❑ Eczema on the palms; blisters; burning and intense itching	Ranun-bulb. 30	4 hourly (3)

✪ Repeat the medicine with great care in skin ailments to avoid aggravation or use 50 millesimal potencies repeatedly.

Biochemic remedies	Kali mur. 12X, Kali sulph. 6X, Natrum mur. 12X and Natrum phos. 6X	4 hourly

---

EMACIATION
(See Marasmus And Weakness Also)

Extreme loss of flesh due to chronic constitutional derangements, etc..

❑ Late learning to walk and talk; emaciation mostly in the neck	Natrum mur. 30 or 200	fortnightly (3)
❑ Emaciation lower limbs, and spreads upwards	Abrotanum 30 or 200	fortnightly (3)
❑ Loosing flesh though eats well	Iodium 30 or 200	fortnightly (3)
Biochemic remedies	Calcarea phos. 6X and Natrum mur. 6X	

Constitutional treatment is very helpful. Proper attention should be paid for diet also.

ENCEPHALITIS
Inflammation of the Brain

The inflammation of the brain occurs due to various reasons; as trauma, various kinds of infections, viral infections or allergic reactions, etc.. The constitutional or indicated remedy according to the symptoms is helpful.

In severe cases hospitalization should be preferred.

Symptoms	Remedy	Frequency And Doses

Aconite, Cuprum met., Eupatorium perf., Belladonna, Nux vomica, Hyoscyamus, Opium, Stramonium, Verat-vir., Zincum met., Helleborus, etc., are the main remedies in homoeopathy for this ailment.

Complete rest in a dark, airy and quiet room; and light diet (easily digestible and nutritious) is necessary.

EOSINOPHILIA

The increase in number of eosinophil cells of blood is called eosinophilia. It can be due to many reasons such as bronchial asthma, skin diseases, filariasis, allergic hay fever, pernicious anaemia, tropical eosinophilia, etc..

Symptoms	Remedy	Frequency And Doses
● Expectoration scanty and difficult; patient can not tolerate least opposition. Thyroid disturbances	**Thyroidin. 200 or 1M**	*weekly (3)*
❑ Dyspnoea, suffocation; worse pressure of anything around throat; during and after sleep; worse taking vinegar and sour foods	**Lachesis 0/5 and above**	*6 hourly*
● Intercurrent remedy	**Thuja oc. 200 or 1M**	*weekly (3)*
❑ Digestive disorders with allergic manifestations	**Histamine 200 or 1M**	*weekly (3)*
❑ Dyspnoea during damp weather; every fresh cold brings out complaints; worse after eating rice, banana, etc.	**Natrum sulph. 200 or 1M**	*weekly (3)*
❑ A well tried homoeopathic medicine; is very useful in acute or chronic cases	**Cassia soph. Q or 30**	*4 hourly*
❑ Dyspnoea with wheezing; worse by cold in any form; patient oversensitive to cold, touch, etc.	**Hepar sulph. 30 or 200**	*6 hourly*
Biochemic remedies	**Natrum mur.,12X** and **Natrum sulph. 12X**	*alternate 2 hourly*

Other Useful Remedies:

Silicea, Arsenic alb., Ipecac, Bacillinum, Tuberculinum, Phosphorus, Medorrhinum and Syphilinum, etc.. Milk contains the internal secretion of the thyroid gland so it should be avoided.

Symptoms	Remedy	Frequency And Doses

EPILEPSY

A nervous disease with loss of consciousness and with tonic and clonic convulsions.

❑ Worse before menstruation	**Oenanthe cro. 30**	*4 hourly*
☆ During moon phases; spasmodic affections, cramps, convulsions, etc., beginning in fingers and toes	**Cuprum met. 30 or 200**	*4 hourly*
❑ During sleep at night	**Bufo rana 30 or 200**	*4 hourly (6)*
❑ Due to fright; loud screaming or unconscious state	**Opium 200 or 1M**	*6 hourly (3)*
❑ Due to worms; itching of nose and anus	**Cina 200 or 1M**	*weekly (3)*
❑ Due to suppression of eruptions	**Agaricus m. 30 or 200**	*4 hourly*
❑ Due to unfortunate love; shock or grief	**Ignatia 200 or 1M**	*4 hourly*
❑ Due to head injury	**Natrum sulph. 200 or 1M**	*fortnightly (3)*
❑ Due to menstrual disorders	**Cedron 200**	*weekly (3)*
❑ With swelling of stomach; thumbs turn inwards during attack; worse touch or jar	**Cicuta v. 30**	*4 hourly*
Biochemic remedy	**Kali mur. 6X, Kali phos. 6X** and **Magnesia phos. 6X**	*4 hourly*

In acute attack, above medicines can be given at short intervals.

EPISTAXIS
Bleeding From Nose

☆ Head remedy. Bleeding worse by slightest motion (especially beneficial for young-esters)	**Bryonia Q,** 5-6 drops	*3 hourly*
☆ Bleeding easy and passive; worse blowing the nose; blood do not coagulate easily; thirst for icy cold drinks/water	**Phosphorus 200**	*weekly (3)*
☆ Blood bright red; nausea; tongue clean	**Ipecac 6 or 30**	*1/2 hourly (3)*

Symptoms	Remedy	Frequency And Doses
❏ Blood dark in colour; do not coagulate easily; worse while washing face or hands	**Ammonium carb. 30**	*4 hourly*
❏ With redness of face; rush of blood towards head	**Belladonna 30 or 200**	*1/2 hourly*
❏ Persistent bleeding (repeated); burning pains and irritability	**Arsenic alb. 30**	*6 hourly*
☆ Epistaxis at menopause	**Lachesis 30 or 200**	*4 hourly (3)*
❏ Blood dark and clotted; bleeding so profuse that it causes fainting and ringing in ears; patient wants to be fanned	**China 30**	*1/2 hourly*
❏ Due to relaxation of capillaries; puffiness of the body; worse at night and morning	**Bovista 30**	*4 hourly*
⊙ Epistaxis with bright red blood; aggravates from heat of sun; after coughing	**Cynadon dactylon Q or 6**	*3 hourly*
Biochemic remedy	**Ferrum phos. 3X**	*4 hourly*

For External Use:

Any one of Ficus relig. Q, Trillium p. Q, Hamamelis Q or Millefolium Q, 10-15 drops should be poured on an ice soaked cotton plug and apply on and in the nostrils.

ERECTIONS – *Affections of*
(See Other Male Ailments Also)

❏ Erections day and night; at night; incomplete during coition, though desire is strong; violent erections	**Phosphorus 30 or 200**	*4 hourly (3)*
❏ Erections in the morning	**Ammon-carb. 200**	*6 hourly*
❏ Erections while standing; painful, after coition	**Acid-phos. 30**	*4 hourly*
❏ Erections with shivering and great desire; delayed; wanting	**Baryta carb. 200**	*weekly (3)*

Symptoms	Remedy	Frequency And Doses
❑ Erections after night pollution	Nitric-acid. 200	weekly (3)
☆ Erections during sleep; excessive; strong; violent	Fluor-acid. 200	weekly (3)
❑ Erections with urging to urinate	Rhus tox. 30 or 200	4 hourly
❑ Erections on walking; painful during coition	Hepar sulph. 30 or 200	6 hourly
❑ Erections after coition	Sepia 200 or 1M	weekly (3)
❑ Erections painful; night, excessive; during sleeplessness; strong; violent	Cantharis 30 or 200	4 hourly (3)
❑ Erections with retention of urine	Colocynth. 200 or 1M	weekly (3)
❑ Erections during erotic thoughts; strong violent with headache	Picric-acid. 30	4 hourly
❑ Frequent erections; with loss of prostatic fluid	Pulsatilla 30 or 200	4 hourly
☆ Erections incomplete; during coition; desire lost or diminished	Lycopodium 200 or 1M	weekly (3)
❑ Erections incomplete during coition; delayed; stools constipated	Graphites 200 or 1M	weekly (3)
❑ Erections violent in the morning; penis becomes relaxed during coition	Nux vomica 30 or 200	4 hourly
❑ Erections fail when coition is attempted	Argentum nit. 200 or 1M	weekly (3)
❑ Erections painful; over excitement	Cannabis sat. 200 or 1M	weekly (3)
❑ With coldness of scrotum	Capsicum 200 or 1M	weekly (3)
❑ Erections while sitting	Cannabis indica 200 or 1M	weekly (3)
❑ Erections after sleep; intense excitement of sexual organs	Lachesis. 200 or 1M	weekly (3)
❑ Erections without sexual desire while passing stools	Thuja oc. 200 or 1M	weekly (3)
❑ Strong erections while undressing in a cold room	Lyssin 200 or 1M	weekly (3)

Symptoms	Remedy	Frequency And Doses
❑ Violent erections; arrogant patient; contempt for others	**Platinum 1M**	*weekly (3)*
☆ Erections wanting; parts cold, relaxed; desire lost	**Agnus cast. 30 or 200**	*6 hourly*
❑ Erections wanting; erections when half - asleep only	**Caladiums 30 or 200**	*6 hourly*
❑ Erections wanting; in fat, flabby and chilly patients	**Calcarea carb. 200 or 1M**	*weekly (3)*

ERUCTATIONS

☆ Foul; tasting the food taken; tongue thickly whitish coated as if painted	**Antim-crud. 30 or 200**	*4 hourly (3)*
☆ Due to hyperacidity; rancid, sour, putrid eructations; better discharge of gas and in fresh open air	**Carbo veg. 30 or 200**	*4 hourly (3)*
❑ After taking rich fatty foods; green vegetables, fruits, cakes, pastries, and non-veg food; loss of thirst with dry mouth	**Pulsatilla 30 or 200**	*4 hourly (3)*
❑ Difficult; causing faintness; worse taking sweets	**Argent-nit. 30 or 200**	*4 hourly (3)*
❑ With bad taste and breath	**Acid-carb. 30**	*4 hourly*
● Empty eructations; worse drinking milk; intercurrent remedy	**Sulphur 30 or 200**	*4 hourly (3)*
❑ With pain in stomach after eating	**Abies nig. 30**	*4 hourly*

ERYSIPELAS

Erysipelas is an acute streptococcal infection of the skin. Its main symptoms are fever, chill, headache, vomiting and hot skin. The symptoms of infection appear with oedema in the subcutaneous tissues.

Symptoms	Remedy	Frequency And Doses
❏ Eruptions with sore and bruised feeling all over the body; the bed feels too hard	**Arnica mont. 30 or 200**	*4 hourly*
❏ Sudden onset due to exposure to dry cold wind; high fever, restlessness and fear of death	**Aconite 30 or 200**	*2 hourly*
❏ Symptoms with oedema, pale and shiny skin; stinging and burning pains; sack like swelling of eye-lids; better from cold; worse from heat	**Apis mel. 30 or 200**	*4 hourly*
❏ Vesicular eruptions; burning with chill and fever; restlessness; eruptions on face with burning. Worse damp and cold; better by motion	**Rhus tox. 30 or 200**	*4 hourly*
❏ Intense itching; scratching intolerable; feels as if insects are creeping on the face. Cough and eruptions alternate	**Croton tig. 30 or 200**	*6 hourly*
❏ When the eruptions turn into malignancy or gangrene. Secretion acrid; burning in eruptions; better by heat. Anxiety, restlessness and prostration	**Arsenic alb. 30 or 200**	*4 hourly*
❏ Eruptions smooth, bright red, with throbbing pain; skin intensly hot and dry	**Belladonna 30**	*3 hourly*
☆ Eruptions on face with blisters and severe burning; even small touch aggravates burning sensation	**Cantharis 30**	*3 hourly*
❏ Complaints with offensive breath and sweat; bitter or salty salivation	**Mercurius sol. 30**	*4 hourly*
☆ Post vaccination erysipelas. Profuse sweat only on uncovered parts	**Thuja oc. 200**	*4 hourly (3)*
❏ Symptoms accompanied by delirium; narrow, well defined, red streak right through the middle of tongue.	**Verat-v. 30**	*4 hourly*
❏ When eruptions disappear suddenly. Cramps, spasmodic convulsions sets in	**Cuprum met. 30**	*4 hourly*
❏ When eruptions turn into malignancy and healing does not take place; large quantity of pus in eruptions	**Hippozaeninum 30**	*4 hourly*

Symptoms	Remedy	Frequency And Doses
❏ Purple, mottled and puffy eruptions; worse after sleep. Loquacious, suspicious and jealous patient. Can't tolerate even mild touch on throat	**Lachesis 30 or 200**	*4 hourly (3)*
☆ Recurring erysipelas on face. Skin separated from muscles by a fetid fluid. Symptoms develop with unusual rapidity	**Crotalus h. 30 or 200**	*4 hourly (3)*
❏ Eruptions with a feeling as if a mice is creeping under the skin	**Secale cor 30 or 200**	*4 hourly (3)*
❏ Gangrenous erysipelas; better by cold	**Baptisia 6 or 30**	*4 hourly*
❏ Great sensitiveness to the slightest touch, draught of air, noise. Instability and anger more prominent	**Hepar sulph. 30**	*4 hourly*
❏ In patients who are mild but irritable; weeps easily, craves for sympathy and open air. Thirstlessness. Worse from heat	**Pulsatilla 30**	*4 hourly*
● When well selected remedies fail. Burning sensation, worse from heat. Patient hungry especially at 10-11 a.m.. Worse contact of water, washing, etc.	**Sulphur 200**	*10 min. (3)*
❏ Eruptions with transparent glutinous fluid; and fever at night. Stools hard and constipated	**Graphites 30**	*4 hourly (3)*
Biochemic remedies	**Ferrum phos. 6X, Kali phos. 6X** and **Kali sulph. 6X**	*3 hourly*

EXPOSURE *Affections Of*
(See Catarrh, Cold, Etc., Also)

❏ To dry cold weather	**Aconite 30 or 200**	*1/2 hourly*
❏ With high fever after hair cut	**Belladonna 30**	*1/2 hourly*
❏ To wet air	**Dulcamara 30 or 200**	*10 min. (3)*
❏ As a tonic	**Avena sat. Q,** 10-15 drops	*2 hourly*
Biochemic remedy	**Ferrum phos. 6X** in warm water	*1/2 hourly*

Symptoms	Remedy	Frequency And Doses

EYE *Affections of*
(See Other Related Chapters Also)

Symptoms	Remedy	Frequency And Doses
❑ Stitches in eyes; sharp, sticking pains; syphilitic iritis; bleeding from eyes while blowing nose	Nitric acid. 30 or 200	4 hourly (3)
❑ Eyes stick while sneezing	Gambogia 30	4 hourly
❑ Atrophy of retina	Carbo-sulph. 30	4 hourly
❑ Detachment of retina	Naphthaline 30	4 hourly
❑ Sudden electric spark like flushes before eyes; sensation as if bright stars are dancing in front of the eyes	Crocus sat. 30	4 hourly (3)
❑ Congestion of retina due to heart disease	Cactus g. 30	4 hourly
❑ Eyes red hot; apoplexy of retina	Glonoine 30	4 hourly
❑ Bleeding from eyes; bruised pain	Arnica 30 or 200	4 hourly (3)
❑ Oedema; burning with acrid lachrymation	Arsenic alb. 30	4 hourly
❑ Congestion of eyes	Ailanthus g. 30	4 hourly
❑ Cannot stand light; bland lachrymation	Allium cepa 30	4 hourly
❑ Stitching pain in eyes; worse by motion	Bryonia 30 or 200	4 hourly
❑ Aching pain in eyes	Capsicum 30	4 hourly
❑ Pain over left eye; eyes yellow (due to jaundice)	Chelidonium 6 or 30	4 hourly
❑ Neuralgia in and over right eye	Sanguinaria c. 30 or 200	4 hourly
❑ Post orbital neuralgia; due to vaccinations	Thuja oc. 200 or 1M	4 hourly (3)
❑ Dark spots before eyes; feels as if veil or gauze is before eyes	Sulphur 30 or 200	4 hourly (3)
❑ Eyes sickly round; twitching of eyes; retinitis; worms infestations	Cina 30 or 200	4 hourly
❑ Blueness around eyes; diplopia, sensitive to light	Crotalus h. 30 or 200	4 hourly (3)

Symptoms	Remedy	Frequency And Doses
❏ Eyes agglutinated; pustular inflammation, photophobia	**Rhus tox. 30 or 200**	*4 hourly*
❏ Eyes dim and fatigued from too much reading or doing fine work; spasms of eye-lids	**Ruta g. 6 or 30**	*4 hourly*
❏ Itching of eyes; thick, profuse, yellow, bland discharges; lids inflamed; worse by heat	**Pulsatilla 30**	*4 hourly*
❏ Eyes seems as if pulled outwards; weakness in eyes; epithelioma of eye-lids	**Conium mac. 200**	*weekly (3)*
❏ Styes; inflammation of external canthi; eczema of eye-lids	**Graphites 30 or 200**	*4 hourly (3)*
❏ Smoky appearance before eyes; eye-lids heavy, dim-sighted	**Gelsemium 30**	*4 hourly*
❏ Eyes feels too large; glaucoma; optic neuritis	**Plumbum met. 30**	*4 hourly*
❏ Watery, bloody fluid from eyes; fiery, sparkling, staring look; burning in eyes	**Cantharis 30**	*4 hourly*
❏ Cold feeling behind eyes	**Calcarea phos. 12X or 30**	*4 hourly*
❏ Swelling of conjunctival membrane; purulent ophthalmia; catarrhal ulceration	**Argentum nit. 30 or 200**	*4 hourly (3)*
❏ Burning of eyes with aversion to light; sore canthi	**Ammon-carb. 30**	*4 hourly*
❏ Coldness; crawling in eyes; objects look smaller than they are	**Platinum 200 or 1M**	*weekly (3)*
❏ Loss of sight due to haemorrhages	**China off. 6 or 30**	*4 hourly*
❏ Opacity; spots and ulcers on cornea; chronic dilatation of pupils	**Calcarea carb. 200**	*weekly (3)*
❏ Trachoma; lids swollen, red, oedematous; lachrymation hot	**Apis mel. 30 or 200**	*4 hourly (3)*
❏ Recurrent styes; pain in inner canthi	**Staphysagria 30**	*4 hourly*
❏ Swelling of right lachrymal gland	**Silicea 12X or 30**	*6 hourly*

Symptoms	Remedy	Frequency And Doses
❑ Sparks before eyes; strabismus; eyes hot, tired	**Magnesia phos. 12X or 30**	*4 hourly*
❑ Half sight - upper objects remain invisible	**Aurum met. 200 or 1M**	*weekly (3)*
❑ Visual disturbance with headache	**Natrum phos. 12X or 30**	*4 hourly*
❑ Colours and bright spots before eyes	**Kali bich. 30**	*4 hourly*
❑ Puffiness between eyebrows and lids	**Kali carb. 200 or 1M**	*weekly (3)*
❑ Squinting after convulsions	**Hyoscyamus 200**	*6 hourly*
❑ Eyes drawn backward; twitching in eye-lids; eczema of eye-lids	**Mezereum 30**	*4 hourly*
❑ Styes on eye-lids near internal canthus; day or night blindness; eyes half open during sleep	**Lycopodium 30 or 200**	*6 hourly (3)*
❑ Paralysis of eye-lids	**Causticum 30 or 200**	*6 hourly (3)*
❑ Eye-lids seems too heavy to open; black spots in the field of vision	**Sepia 30 or 200**	*6 hourly*
❑ Soreness of outer canthi; Pustules on cornea and lids	**Antim-crud. 30 or 200**	*4 hourly (3)*
❑ Wild staring look; fear of dark	**Stramonium 200 or 1M**	*6 hourly (3)*

EYES
Burning

☆ Due to acute cold, burning, smarting eyes; with bland discharge	**Allium cepa. 30**	*4 hourly*
☆ With acrid discharge; restlessness and unquenchable thirst for little quantity of water at a time at short intervals	**Arsenic alb. 30**	*4 hourly*
❑ With bodyache, dullness, lethargy, shivering up and down the spine, congestion head, thirstlessness. Desire to lie quietly; better passing urine	**Gelsemium 30**	*4 hourly*

Symptoms	Remedy	Frequency And Doses
❑ Redness and burning; eye-lids swollen, throbbing; worse after lying down	**Belladonna 30**	*4 hourly*
❑ Burning and swelling of lids; discharge acrid	**Euphrasia 30**	*4 hourly*

EYE
Injury

❑ Injuries due to foreign body	**Arnica 200**	*10 min. (3)*
❑ For nerve injuries	**Hypericum 30 or 200**	*10 min. (3)*
Biochemic remedy	**Ferrum phos. 3X or 6X**	*1/2 hourly*

FAINTING
(See Collapse And Unconsciousness Also)

Symptoms	Remedy	Frequency And Doses
❑ Due to severe pain; anger after being scolded; oversensitive patient	Chamomilla 200	1/2 hourly (3)
❑ Collapse; with extreme coldness, blueness and weakness; post-operative shock	Veratrum alb. 30 or 200	1/2 hourly (3)
❑ Due to disturbed emotions; shock or grief (disappointments, etc.)	Ignatia 200 or 1M	1/2 hourly (3)
❑ Due to fear and excitement; nervous tension	Phosphorus 200	1/2 hourly (3)
❑ After being disturbed and touched; sudden realisation of financial losses; due to injury	Arnica 200 or 1M	1/2 hourly (3)
❑ Due to hot stuffy atmosphere; suppression of discharges; jealousy	Lachesis 200	1/2 hourly (3)
❑ Due to sight of pins and needles; ill effects of vaccination	Silicea 200 or 1M	1/2 hourly (3)
❑ Due to loss of sleep; riding in a carriage or on shipboard	Cocculus ind. 200	1/2 hourly (3)
❑ Due to bad news, emotional excitement, fear, apprehension, etc.	Gelsemium 200	1/2 hourly (3)
❑ Due to apprehension, anticipation of coming events	Argent-nit. 200	1/2 hourly (3)
❑ After effects of fear (as after accidents, etc.)	Opium 200 or 1M	1/2 hourly (3)

Symptoms	Remedy	Frequency And Doses
❑ Indignation; wounded honour; rudeness of others	**Staphysagria 200 or 1M**	*1/2 hourly (3)*
❑ Due to excessive joy	**Coffea 200 or 1M**	*1/2 hourly (3)*
☆ Mortification with anger (sometimes the patient goes into coma after suppression of anger)	**Colocynth. 200 or 1M**	*1/2 hourly (3)*
● Intercurrent remedy	**Sulphur 200**	*10 min. (3)*
❑ Due to fear; sudden exposure to dry cold wind	**Aconite 200**	*10 min. (3)*
❑ Due to exhaustive discharges (like - vomiting, diarrhoea, blood or semen loss, etc.)	**China off. 30 or 200**	*1/2 hourly*
❑ In epileptic fits; aura begins at knees and ascends to hypogastrium	**Cuprum met. 30 or 200**	*10 min. (3)*
❑ Due to sun stoke; heat on head; due to working under gas light, etc.	**Glonoine 3X or 6**	*1/2 hourly (3)*
❑ After diarrhoea; taking juicy fruits, etc.	**Arsenic alb. 200**	*1/2 hourly (3)*
Biochemic remedies	**Kali phos. 6X and Magnesia phos. 6X**	*1/2 hourly*

Find the true cause and treat accordingly. In obstinate cases hospitalization is a must.

FATNESS
(See Obesity Also)

❑ With excessive appetite; obesity after abdominal operation; craving for eggs; chilly patient	**Calcarea carb. 200 or 1M**	*weekly (6)*
❑ If Calcarea carb. fails; specific for persons suffering from goitre	**Fucus ves. Q,** 20-30 drops	*4 hourly*
❑ Accompanied with unhealthy skin. Obesity during menopause; stools constipated	**Graphites 200**	*6 hourly*

Symptoms	Remedy	Frequency And Doses
❑ In shy and emotional individuals; loss of thirst; feels better in open air	**Pulsatilla 200**	6 hourly
● When due to malfunctioning of thyroid gland	**Thyroidinum 200 or 1M**	*fortnightly (6)*
❑ To reduce fats from the body (also available in tablet form)	**Phytolacca berry Q,** 10-15 drops	*4 hourly*
❑ Obesity; while flesh decreases, muscles become harder and firmer	**Calotropis 30 or 200**	6 hourly
❑ Fatness; more around buttocks and thighs	**Ammonium mur. 200**	6 hourly
❑ Fatness due to gastric complaints; constipation; tongue thickly whitish coated as if white washed	**Antim-crud. 200**	6 hourly
Biochemic remedies	**Calcarea phos. 6X, Natrum mur. 12X** and **Silicea 30X**	*4 hourly*

FEAR
(See Anxiety Also)

❑ Of falling; downward motion	**Borax 200 or 1M**	*weekly (3)*
❑ Of pointed things; knives and forks, etc.	**Spigelia 200 or 1M**	*weekly (3)*
❑ Of dogs; animals	**Belladonna 200 or 1M**	*weekly (3)*
❑ Being alone; thunder storm, ghosts, etc.	**Phosphorus 200**	*weekly (3)*
❑ Appearing before audience; examination, etc.	**Argentum nit. 30 or 200**	*10 min. (3)*
❑ Fear of failure (examination, etc.)	**Gelsemium 30 or 200**	*4 hourly (3)*
❑ Aeroplanes flying over the head	**Aconite 200**	*10 min. (3)*
❑ Child fears to go to bed alone	**Causticum 30 or 200**	*4 hourly*
❑ Fear to be alone; feels better in open air even though patient is chilly	**Pulsatilla 30 or 200**	*4 hourly*
❑ Fear of poverty	**Calcarea fluor. 200 or 1M**	*weekly (3)*

Symptoms	Remedy	Frequency And Doses
❑ Fear of accidents	**Carbo veg. 200**	*weekly (3)*
❑ If carbo veg. fails	**Psorinum 200**	*weekly (3)*
❑ Fear of being touched	**Arnica 200 or 1M**	*weekly (3)*
❑ Fear of cholera	**Lachesis 200 or 1M**	*weekly (3)*
❑ Fear of consumption; contagious disease, going to a dentist	**Calcarea carb. 200 or 1M**	*weekly (3)*
❑ Fear of cutting face while shaving	**Caladiums. 200 or 1M**	*weekly (3)*
❑ Fear of dark	**Stramonium 200 or 1M**	*weekly (3)*
❑ Fear of death; impending illness, disgust for life	**Pneumococcin. 200**	*10 min. (3)*
● Intercurrent remedy	**Sulphur 200 or 1M**	*weekly (3)*

FEVER (*Simple*)
(*See Hyper-Pyrexia And Other Relevant Chapters Also*)

Symptoms	Remedy	Frequency
☆ Early stage; due to exposure to dry cold wind	**Aconite 30 or 200**	*2 hourly*
☆ High fever; with thirstlessness, changing moods; better in open air	**Pulsatilla 30 or 200**	*3 hourly*
☆ Flushed face with high fever; due to acute tonsillitis, etc.	**Belladonna 30**	*3 hourly*
☆ With headache coming from nape of neck; dullness, loss of thirst, desire to lie quietly; better after passing urine	**Gelsemium 30 or 200**	*3 hourly*
☆ With restlessness and thirst for small quantities of water at short intervals; burning sensation	**Arsenic alb. 30 or 200**	*3 hourly*
☆ With pain all over the body; excessive thirst, drink large quantity of water at a time at long intervals; constipation; worse by motion; better by rest	**Bryonia 30 or 200**	*3 hourly*

Symptoms	Remedy	Frequency And Doses
❑ Due to sun stroke or exposure to heat	Glonoine 6 or 30	4 hourly
❑ Due to urinary infection; frequent micturition with burning	Cantharis 30	4 hourly
☆ With nausea and vomiting; thirstlessness, tongue clean. Irregular pattern of fever	Ipecac 30	2 hourly (3)
☆ Fever after getting wet; with extreme restlessness; better by movements, severe body-ache; triangular tip of tongue red	Rhus tox. 30 or 200	3 hourly
❑ Fever after injury; sore, bruised feeling (as if beaten) all over the body	Arnica 30 or 200	1/2 hourly (3)
❑ Desires cold water during chill, and no thirst during stage of heat; wants fanning	Carbo veg. 30	1/2 hourly (3)
❑ Thirst only during chill stage of fever	Capsicum 30	2 hourly
☆ Disproportion between pulse and temperature; high fever; septic fever	Pyrogenium 200 or 1M	10 min. (3)
❑ Fever with headache; body-ache and constipation; bitter taste in mouth; worse in morning; nausea and vomiting soon after breakfast; burning sensation in hands; fever with chill; worse at night	Amoora rohutika 30	4 hourly
❑ Fever with chill worse 8-10 a.m. and 2-4 p.m.; weakness after fever; white coated tongue; headache better by pressure; thirst for cold water	Caesalpenia bon. 30	4 hourly
❑ Fever with heaviness of eye-lids; laziness, dullness and no desire to work; irritability; worse mental or physical exertion	Sulfonamide 30	4 hourly
Biochemic remedies	Ferrum phos. 6X and Kali sulph. 6X	2 hourly alternate (6)
—	Biocombination No.11	2 hourly

FILARIASIS

A diseased state due to the presence of filaria which burrows in the skin, producing irritation and swelling.

In early filariasis, the onset is manifested by painful swellings of the scrotal contents. Acute swelling of the lymph glands of the inguinal and femoral lesion is common.

Symptoms	Remedy	Frequency And Doses
☆ In cases of recent origin; frequent episodes of adenolymphangitis; worse by exertion; cord like swelling	Rhus tox. 30 or 200	4 hourly
☆ Hot patient; excessive thirst - drinks large quantities at long intervals; worse motion; local oedema of all types, especially fibrotic	Bryonia 30 or 200	4 hourly
☆ With glossy oedema; thirstlessness, burning sensation; worse by heat	Apis mel. 30 or 200	4 hourly
❑ Complaints with intolerance to sun; desire for extra salt in all preparations; thirst increased. Mental irritability; aversion to sympathy; worse at sea shore	Natrum mur. 30 or 200	4 hourly
☆ In hot patients; desire for cold; thirstlessness with dryness of mouth; changing moods; weeps while telling symptoms; gentle, mild disposition	Pulsatilla 30 or 200	4 hourly
☆ With complaints of male genitalia; hydrocele; worse by storms	Rhododendron 200 or 1M	weekly (3)
● With local or generalised burning; better by cold; desire for sweets; cold accompanied by gastric complaints or skin ailments	Sulphur 30 or 200	weekly (3)
❑ Profuse sweat which does not relieve; thirst with moist mouth; suppurative tendency; stools in Q effectual, contains mucous; oedema of legs which becomes hard	Mercurius sol. 30 or 200	4 hourly
❑ Chilly patient; desire for warm food, sweets; flatulent dyspepsia; always in a hurry; worse by heat	Lycopodium 200 or 1M	weekly (3)
Biochemic remedy	**Calcarea fluor. 12X**	4 hourly

Symptoms	Remedy	Frequency And Doses

FISSURE
Anal

● To start the treatment (also intercurrent) — **Tuberculinum k. 1M or 10M** — *fortnightly (6)*

☆ With a sensation of splinters piercing into the anus; foul smelly discharge — **Acid-nit. 30 or 200** — *weekly (3)*

☆ Rectum feels as if full of broken glasses; burns for hours after passing stools — **Ratanhia 6 or 30** — *4 hourly*

☆ Fissure due to severe constipation; hard stools with mucous — **Graphites 30 or 200** — *6 hourly*

❏ Constant smartness in the anus all the time; with much oozing — **Paeonia Q or 30** — *4 hourly*

❏ Fissure due to dryness of all the mucous membranes of the body; watering of mouth or watering from nose or eyes — **Natrum mur. 30** — *4 hourly*

❏ Stools come down with difficulty, with spasm of splinters, when partly expelled recedes back — **Silicea 12X or 30** — *4 hourly*

● Marked redness around anus with constant burning and urging to pass stools — **Sulphur 30 or 200** — *6 hourly*

Biochemic remedies — **Calcarea fluor. 12X** and **Silicea 30X** — *4 hourly*

FISTULA
Ano

Fistula means pipe and Fistula-in-ano means a pipe like canal opening usually at or near the anus. Fistula can be blind, internal or open. The out-come is usually the result of a simple or tubercular abscess in the tissue surrounding the rectum. This abscess opens into the bowel and on the surface of the skin.

● To start the treatment (also intercurrent) — **Tuberculinum k. 200 or 1M** — *fortnightly (6)*

Symptoms	Remedy	Frequency And Doses
❏ Initial stage of pus formation with throbbing pain; redness of anus	**Belladonna 30 and Mercurius sol. 30** *alternate 3 hourly*	
☆ When first stage is over and there is intense pain; abscess turns into pus	**Hepar sulph. 30**	*4 hourly*
❏ When ulcerative stage comes and the passage converts into sinus; fetid, watery discharge	**Silicea 12X or 30**	*4 hourly*
● In tubercular patients (intercurrent remedy) who are susceptible to cold	**Bacillinum 200 or 1M**	*fortnightly (3)*
☆ When there is intense hammering pain in the rectum	**Lachesis 30 or 200**	*4 hourly (3)*
❏ Soreness and intense burning pain; greenish discharge	**Acid-nit. 200 or 1M**	*weekly (3)*
● In blind fistula; yellowish, greenish, painless discharge	**Sulphur 200 or 1M**	*weekly (3)*
❏ With tearing pain around the anus; to improve the drainage of the passage	**Berberis vulg. Q,** 5-10 drops	*4 hourly*
❏ Burning and soreness in the rectum; chronic large piles; better in humid climate	**Causticum 30 or 200**	*4 hourly (3)*
Biochemic remedy	**Calcarea phos. 6X or 12X or Calcarea sulph. 6X** (When there is no pain)	*4 hourly*

For External Use: lotion of Hydrastis or Calendula.

FITS
(See Convulsions)

FLATULENCE (Wind Formation)
(See Dyspepsia Also)

☆ Flatulence with puffiness and loud noise in the abdomen	**Thuja oc. 30 or 200**	*4 hourly (3)*

Symptoms	Remedy	Frequency And Doses
☆ Pain in stomach and flatulence; smell of food aggravates	Colchicum 30 or 200	4 hourly (3)
☆ With distended abdomen effecting lower abdomen; better belching and passing of flatus. Worse 4-8 p.m.	Lycopodium 30	4 hourly
☆ Flatulence in the upper part of the abdomen pressing upwards; (everything eaten converts into wind, better by belching and passing wind) worse night and after lying down	Carbo veg. 30	4 hourly
☆ Flatulence and distention in abdomen; not relieved by passing wind; digestion slow	China 30	4 hourly
❏ When wind formation is around the naval. No emission of flatus by mouth or anus for a long time	Raphanus 30	4 hourly
☆ With loud eructations and belchings	Asafoetida 30	4 hourly
⌐ Flatulence with burning like that of red pepper taste in upper part of abdomen and going upto the throat	Capsicum 30	4 hourly
❏ Every food or drink taken turns into gas; flatulent dyspepsia	Nux mosch. 30	4 hourly
☆ Flatulence due to sedentary life; bad effects of alcohol. Ineffectual urging to pass stools with constipation	Nux vomica 30	4 hourly
❏ Offensive flatus; even small quantity of stools passes with wind; with much rumbling in abdomen	Aloe soc. 30	4 hourly
❏ Accumulation of flatulence in hypochondriac region; worse after anger	Chamomilla 30 or 200	4 hourly
● Flatulence; smells like rotten eggs; *intercurrent and most useful remedy*	Psorinum 30	3 hourly (3)
☆ Abdomen distended, no relief from passing flatus; craving for sweets; loud eructations	Argentum nit. 30	4 hourly
Biochemic remedy	**Biocombination No.25**	4 hourly

Symptoms	Remedy	Frequency And Doses

FOOD AND DRINKS
Aggravation From or Allergic To
(See Allergies Also)

Symptoms	Remedy	Frequency And Doses
❏ Celery (itching)	**Apium gr. 30 or 200**	*4 hourly*
❏ Strawberry (urticaria)	**Fragaria v. 30 or 200**	*4 hourly*
❏ Sugar	**Saccharum 30 or 200**	*4 hourly*
❏ Quinine	**Chin-sulph. 30 or 200**	*4 hourly*
❏ Parsley	**Petroleum 30 or 200**	*4 hourly*
❏ Eggs	**Sulphur 30 or 200**	*4 hourly*
❏ Beer; pickles, sour foods and vinegar	**Ferrum met. 30 or 200**	*4 hourly*
❏ Preserved or cold foods/drinks; over ripen fruits	**Arsenic alb. 30 or 200**	*4 hourly*
❏ Rich, fatty, variety food; non-veg, eggs, etc.	**Pulsatilla 30 or 200**	*4 hourly*
❏ Onions	**Thuja oc. 30 or 200**	*4 hourly*
❏ Oysters	**Lycopodium 30 or 200**	*4 hourly*
● Wheat; milk	**Psorinum 30 or 200**	*weekly (3)*
❏ Cabbage; vegetable and chicken salad	**Bryonia 30 or 200**	*4 hourly*
❏ Scallops	**Pectin 30 or 200**	*4 hourly*

FOOD POISONING

Symptoms	Remedy	Frequency And Doses
☆ Due to eating melons or drinking impure water	**Zingiber 30**	*1/2 hourly*
☆ Eating icy preparations; preserved food or over ripen fruits	**Arsenic alb. 30**	*1/2 hourly*
☆ After eating spoiled or tinted food; patient wants fresh air, fanning	**Carbo veg. 30**	*1/2 hourly*
☆ After eating rich, fatty food; non veg, variety foods, chocolates, etc.	**Pulsatilla 30**	*1/2 hourly*

Symptoms	*Remedy*	*Frequency And Doses*

FOREIGN BODY
Skin

❑ To expell foreign body from the skin in fresh cases — **Hepar sulph. 200 or 1M** *10 min. (3)*

❑ In chronic cases to expell foreign body from the skin — **Silicea 200 or 1M** *4 hourly (6)*

❑ To expell iron nails, etc., pricked into the body — **Ledum pal. 200 or 1M** *4 hourly (6)*

FROZEN
From Cold

When the result is a consequence of exposure to cold (snow, etc.) the patient should be kept in a cool room and he should not be exposed to a current of air. If there are no signs of life the patient should be covered with snow. The mouth and nostrils being left out, the patient should be placed in such a position that the melted snow should be readily run off and the process should be renewed. In case of non-availability of snow a cold bath with a very cold water may be substituted, the body can be immersed in cold water for a short time. After that the body should be covered with clothes wet in cold water covered tightly and then a blanket should be wrapped, due care should be taken and body should be rubbed properly. This process should last for hours together until it becomes apparent that restoration is not possible.

After restoration **Carbo veg. 30, Arsenic alb. 30,** or **Veratrum alb. 30** can be given according to the symptoms.

❑ Though the body is very cold; patient wants fanning, fresh air — **Carbo veg. 30 or 200** *1/2 hourly (3)*

❑ When the body becomes cold; cold sweating and blueness of the body — **Verat. alb. 30 or 200** *1/2 hourly (3)*

❑ Restlessness but can't move because of excessive weakness — **Arsenic alb. 30 or 200** *1/2 hourly (3)*

GAIT
Walking

Symptoms	Remedy	Frequency Doses
Agility; to stimulate the functional activity of all organs	**Coffea 30 or 200**	*weekly (3)*
Spastic; knees knock against each other while walking	**Lachesis 30 or 200**	*fortnightly (6)*
Staggering; unsteady when unobserved	**Argentum nit. 30 or 200**	*fortnightly (6)*
Drags feet while walking	**Nux vomica. 30**	*6 hourly*
Heels do not touch ground while walking	**Lathyrus s. 200**	*fortnightly (6)*
Legs feels heavy as of lead, while walking	**Medorrhinum 200 or 1M**	*fortnightly (3)*
Legs feel heavy as if made of wood or glass	**Thuja oc. 200 or 1M**	fortnightly (6)
☆ Involuntarily thrown back while walking	**Mercurius sol. 30 or 200**	*6 hourly*
Lifts feet higher than usual and brings them down hard	**Heloderma 200**	*weekly (6)*
Limps involuntarily, while walking	**Belladonna 200**	*6 hourly*
Stoops while walking	**Arnica 200**	*weekly (6)*
Walking is very difficult on uneven ground	**Lilium tig. 30 or 200**	*weekly (6)*
Suddenly falls to ground while walking	**Magnesia carb. 30**	*weekly (6)*

When the above mentioned potencies cease to work the next nigher potency should be used accordingly.

Symptoms	Remedy	Frequency And Doses

GALL STONE COLIC

	Symptoms	Remedy	Frequency And Doses
☆	Heady remedy; pain through the lower edge of the right shoulder blade. Liver tender to touch and pressure; dirty yellow face and vomiting	Chelidonium 30	4 hourly
☆	Head remedy for gallstone colic	Cholesterinum 3X	4 hourly
☆	Gall stones; jaundice, uncomfortable fullness in liver region	Carduus m. Q or 6	3 hourly
❏	Violent pain liver region; sensitive to touch, feet constantly cold	Lycopodium 200 or 1M	weekly (3)
❏	Gall stones and jaundice; aversion to food; chilly feeling	Nux vomica 30	4 hourly
❏	Gall stones colic; patient craves for icy cold water/drinks	Phosphorus 200	weekly (3)
❏	Gall stone colic; itching, pain in the region of liver with renal disease. Twitching and shooting pains; spasmodic pain confined to a small spot	Berberis vul. Q or 30	4 hourly
❏	Violent pain; worse by movement or jar, flushed face	Belladonna 30	4 hourly
❏	Great chilliness; darting pain from right to left with profuse sweating	Calcarea carb. 30 or 200	weekly (3)
☆	Periodic recurrence of colic. Stools undigested; liver sensitive to touch and pressure; loss of appetite though feels hungry	China 6, 6 hourly for Ist month in 2nd month 30 potency on alternate days	
❏	Gall stone colic; shifting, cutting pains; better bending backwards	Dioscorea v. 30	4 hourly
❏	Gall stones; discomfort in stomach after eating, constant gagging or empty retching; stools white, loose	Podophyllum 30	4 hourly
❏	Bilious colic; gall-stones; constipation; to prevent formation of gall stones	Chionanthus v. Q or 6	6 hourly

Symptoms	Remedy	Frequency And Doses
● Intercurrent remedy	**Medorrhinum 200 or 1M**	
Biochemic remedy		*fortnightly (3)*
	Magnesia phos 6X and **Natrum sulph. 12X**	*4 hourly*

GANGRENE

Gangrene means the pathologic death of one or more body cells, or of a portion of tissue or organ due to obstruction of blood supply, it may be dry or wet.

❑ Dry; specially of toes and feet, the part becomes cold and numb; better by cold applications	**Secale cor. 30 or 200**	*4 hourly*
❑ Gangrene of the cheek; typhoid fever like symptoms	**Baptisia 30 or 200**	*4 hourly*
❑ Dry; specially of lungs and uterus with soreness and burning sensation; better by warm applications; restlessness and prostration	**Arsenic alb. 30 or 200**	*4 hourly*
❑ When the effected part becomes purple or blue, due to blood poisoning; blood decomposes	**Lachesis 30**	*4 hourly*
❑ Wet; effected part emits foul discharge, oozes freely	**Crotalus h. 30**	*4 hourly*
❑ Wet; purple and icy cold; effected part emits foul discharge; patient desires fresh air, fanning	**Carbo veg. 30**	*4 hourly*
❑ Specially of lungs and uterus in old age; better by warmth	**Kreosote 30**	*4 hourly*
❑ Gangrene of the cheek; aversion to food; hic-cough, frequent putrid eructations; brown tongue, vomiting; discharges foul and dirty	**Acid-mur. 30**	*4 hourly*
❑ Gangrene after mechanical injuries	**Acid-sulph. 30**	*4 hourly*
Biochemic remedy	**Silicea 30X**	*4 hourly*

For External Use: Lotion of Echinacea a.

Symptoms	*Remedy*	*Frequency And Doses*

GASTROENTERITIS
(See Diarrhoea)

GIDDINESS
(See Vertigo Also)

❑ Giddiness seeing flowing water	**Ferrum phos. 6X or 30**	*4 hourly*
❑ From exhaustion and nervous weakness	**Kali phos. 6X or 30**	*4 hourly*

GLANDS
AILMENTS OF
(See Goitre and Tonsillitis Also)

☆ Stony hardness; hard knots in female breast, goitre etc.	**Calcarea fluor. 12X or 30**	*4 hourly*
❑ Ulceration of Cervical glands	**Rhus ven. 30**	*4 hourly*
❑ Induration of parotid glands; enlargement of goitre and other glands	**Bromium 30**	*4 hourly*
❑ Swelling of inguinal glands	**Terebinth. Q or 6**	*4 hourly*
❑ Swelling of sub-maxillary glands	**Pinus syl. 6 or 30**	*4 hourly*
❑ Glands stony hard; progressive debility; especially in old bachelors and maids.	**Conium mac. 200 or 1M**	*weekly (3)*
❑ Left sided glands swollen; hard and red	**Merc-bin-iod. 3X or 6**	*4 hourly*
☆ Enlargement of glands; tonsils, thyroid, etc.	**Calc iod. 3X or 6**	*4 hourly*
❑ Right sided glands swollen; hard and red	**Merc-p-i. 3X or 6**	*4 hourly*
● Intercurrent remedy	**Tuberculinum 200 or 1M**	*weekly (3)*
Biochemic remedies	**Calcarea phos. 6X, Kali mur. 6X** and **Silicea 30X**	*4 hourly*
Scrofulans smelling of glands	**Natrum phos. 6X**	

Symptoms	Remedy	Frequency And Doses

GOITRE

Symptoms	Remedy	Frequency And Doses
❏ At the age of puberty; especially when patient is susceptible to cold	**Calcarea iod. 3X**	*4 hourly*
☆ For obese, constipated patients; exophthalmic, non-toxic goitre	**Fucus ves. Q, 10-30 drops**	*4 hourly*
❏ Exophthalmic goitre; from suppressed menses	**Ferrum iod. 3X**	*4 hourly*
☆ Hard; with a feeling as if the air inhaled is passing through the goitre; pain heart region, chocking feeling in the throat.	**Spongia 30 or 200**	*6 hourly*
● Intercurrent remedy - especially in fatty patients	**Thyroidin. 200 or 1M** *fortnightly (6)*	
❏ Swollen; painful, with emaciation even though eating well; worse during menstrual period, gradual increase in size	**Iodium 30 or 200**	*4 hourly*
☆ With cardiac symptoms; constriction of goitre	**Cactus g. Q or 6**	*4 hourly*
❏ Left sided; with liver disorders, jaundice	**Chelidonium Q or 6**	*6 hourly*
❏ Right sided; patient oversensitive to all impressions; marked chilliness	**Hepar sulph 30 or 200**	*4 hourly*
☆ Goitre quite big; of the size of hen's egg	**Bromium 6 or 30**	*4 hourly*
❏ Hard, swollen; worse during new moon, chilly patient	**Calcarea carb. 200 or 1M** *weekly (6)*	
❏ Nodular; goitre swollen with heat and inflammation	**Phytolacca d. 30 or 200**	*4 hourly*
❏ Pressing pain; round hard swelling on upper right lobe of the goitre	**Natrum carb. 30**	*4 hourly*

Biochemic remedies

For hard and swollen goitre	**Calcarea fluor. 12X and Calcarea phos. 6X**	*4 hourly*

Symptoms	Remedy	Frequency And Doses

GONORRHOEA

Symptoms	Remedy	Frequency And Doses
❑ Suppressed; to restore discharge or to take care of bad effects of suppression or sycotic miasm	Medorrhinum 200 or 1M	weekly (3)
❑ Secondary; history of repeated gonorrhoea and impotency	Agnus cast. 200	weekly (3)
❑ Burning while urinating; frequent urging; spasmodic closure of the sphinctre of the bladder	Cannabis sat. 200 or 1M	weekly (3)
❑ Intense burning; sexual excitement, constant urge to pass urine; urine bloody	Cantharis 30 or 200	4 hourly
❑ Very difficult to begin to urinate; burning and scalding during micturition and straining afterwards	Chimaphilla umb. Q or 200	4 hourly
❑ Frequent urination; burning after urination; urine scanty and reddish, inflammation of urethra	Kali bich. 30 or 200	4 hourly
❑ Cystitics with violent pain in urinary passage and bladder; passing almost blood instead of urine	Acid-nit. 30 or 200	4 hourly
❑ Profuse, slimy discharge due to suppressed gonorrhoea; haematuria; urine acrid, cutting pain while passing urine	Pulsatilla 30 or 200	4 hourly
❑ Retention of urine; urine excoriates; urine white, reddish	Sulphur 30 or 200	4 hourly (3)
❑ Thin, greenish discharge; scalding during micturition; rheumatic complaints	Thuja oc. 200 or 1M	weekly (3)
Biochemic remedies	Ferrum phos. 6X, Kali mur. 6X, Natrum phos. 6X and Silicea 30X	4 hourly

Symptoms	Remedy	Frequency And Doses

GUMS
Ailments Of

Symptoms	Remedy	Frequency And Doses
❑ Gums spongy, bleeds easily; caries of teeth	**Kreosote 30**	*4 hourly*
☆ Ulceration and bleeding of gums; offensive breath, gums unhealthy, sensitive to hot and cold	**Mercurius sol. 30**	*4 hourly*
☆ Gum abscess; due to decayed teeth or otherwise	**Heckla lava 3X or 6X**	*4 hourly*
☆ Inflammation and throbbing pain in the gums with hot feeling	**Belladonna 30**	*4 hourly*
❑ Bleeding of gums; worse morning and pressure; gums purple in colour	**Lachesis 30**	*4 hourly*
❑ Itching of gums; complaints are worse before a storm	**Rhododendron 30**	*4 hourly*
❑ Ulceration and bleeding of gums; blood do not cogulate easily	**Phosphorus 30**	*4 hourly*
❑ Gums retracted and bleed easily; pyorrhoea	**Carbo veg. 3X or 6**	*4 hourly*

Biochemic remedies

Symptoms	Remedy	Frequency And Doses
— Swelling and bleeding of gums	**Ferrum phos. 6X** and **Kali mur. 6X**	*alternate 4 hourly*

For External Use:

Gum paint   Glycerine 70% + Arnica Q, Calendula Q and Echinacea Q 30%

GUMS
BLEEDING
(See Bleeding Gums)

GOUT
(See Arthritis, Etc.)

HAEMATURIA

Symptoms	Remedy	Frequency And Doses

Any condition in which the urine contains blood or red blood cells; (haemorrhage in urinary system can be due to infections, etc.,) is called haematuria. The haemorrhage can be from kidney, ureter, bladder or urethra. So the cause or the source should always be looked first and the treatment should be given accordingly.

Symptoms	Remedy	Frequency And Doses
❏ In the beginning; flow of bright red blood, with fever and anxiety	**Aconite 30 or 200**	*2 hourly*
❏ Due to mechanical injury or infection; bruised pain in the urinary passage	**Arnica 30 or 200**	*4 hourly (3)*
☆ When due to haemorrhage from the kidney; coffee-ground like sediments in urine; pressure in the bladder extending to the kidneys	**Terebinth. Q**, 5-7 drops	*3 hourly*
☆ With red sediments in the urine; due to haemorrhage from kidney, bladder or urethra	**Ocimum can. 30 or 200**	*4 hourly*
❏ With dark, thick, brick dust sediments in urine; retention of urine; at times this medicine replace the use of cathetor	**Thlaspi b-p. Q**, 5-7 drops	*4 hourly*
❏ When urine contains bright red blood; constant nausea, tongue clean	**Ipecac Q or 30**	*3 hourly*
❏ Without pain or any other discomfort; accompanied by subnormal temperature	**China-sulph 30**	*4 hourly*
❏ Patient faints due to excessive haemorrhage; but desires to be fanned; blood dark, clotted	**China off. Q or 6**	*1/2 hourly*
❏ Blood bright red, clotted; comes out suddenly in gushes	**Erigeron Q**, 5-7 drops	*3 hourly*

Symptoms	Remedy	Frequency And Doses
☆ With burning pain before, during, and after urination; more after drinking water; urine comes drop by drop	Cantharis 30	4 hourly
❏ When due to over indulgence of wine and spirituous drinks; or sudden check of the piles; backache and smarting pain in urethra; chilly patient	Nux vomica 30	4 hourly
❏ Bloody urine with burning sensation; pain in kidney and liver region. Patient craves for icy cold drinks	Phosphorus 30 or 200	4 hourly
Biochemic remedies	Ferrum phos. 3X. and Kali phos. 6X	3 hourly

HAEMORRHOIDS
(See Bleeding Piles And Piles-Dry)

HAIR
Affections of
(See Hair Falling Of And Hair Premature Greying Of Also)

Symptoms	Remedy	Frequency And Doses
❏ Unwanted hair (face) in females	Oleum jac-a. 3X	4 hourly
❏ Dry, tangling, matted hair; offensive smell from scalp	Psorinum 200 or 1M	weekly (3)
❏ Soreness of scalp; patient avoids shaving, hair cut and combing of hair	China 6 or 30	4 hourly
❏ Curly; soft, reddish hair; eczema of scalp	Mezereum 30	4 hourly
Biochemic remedies To promote proper growth	Calcarea phos. 6X	4 hourly
Sneezing while combing hair; chilly patient	Silicea 12X or 30	4 hourly

Symptoms	Remedy	Frequency And Doses

HAIR
Falling Of

Symptoms	Remedy	Frequency And Doses
☆ Hair breaks; splits, mats up and ragged, end of the hair dry with loss of natural lustre	Acid-fluor. 200 or 1M	weekly (3)
☆ Falling of hair; due to excessive dandruff; hair fall in bunches leaving big bald patches	Phosphorus 200 or 1M	weekly (3)
❑ Falling of hair from head and other parts of the body; leaving bald, shiny patches	Selenium 6 or 30	4 hourly
❑ Falling of hair; from head and other parts of the body due to weakness	Acid-phos. 6 or 30	4 hourly
❑ Falling of hair eruptions, pimples near-hair; margins	Sepia 30 or 200	weekly (3)
❑ Falling of hair from the head due to eruptions and itching	Zincum phos. 30	6 hourly
❑ Falling of hair with heat in the head, hair stands on its end	Sulphur iod. 6	4 hourly
❑ Hair mats up together and falls; eczema of scalp	Mezereum 30	4 hourly
❑ Falling of hair; unhealthy hair; pulling sensation; itching of scalp	Magnesia carb. 30	4 hourly
❑ Beard, falling off	Sphingurus 6 or 30	4 hourly
❑ Falling of hair, with copious, whitish dandruff	Kali-mur. 6X or 30	4 hourly

Biochemic remedies

Symptoms	Remedy	Frequency And Doses
— When hair becomes very thin and falls	Natrum mur. 6X or 12X	4 hourly
— Falling of hair into bunches	Silicea 12X	4 hourly
— Falling of hair due to weakness or after prolonged ailments	Calcarea phos. 6X	4 hourly
— Falling of hair into bunches; making bald spots with much dandruff	Kali sulph. 6X	4 hourly

In our practice we have found very good results with above biochemic remedies giving separately or mixing together - 2 tablets each of 6X potency, thrice daily for 6 weeks.

Symptoms	Remedy	Frequency And Doses

HAIR
Premature Greying Of

● To prevent pre-mature greying of hair — **Thyroidinum 200 or 1M** — *4 hourly*

☆ Due to weakness; seminal loss; in children — **Acid-phos. 3X or 30** — *4 hourly*

❑ Pre-mature greying of hair; in persons who are under constant mental stress — **Lycopodium 30 or 200** — *weekly (6)*

☆ After exhaustive diseases like typhoid, etc.; fear of dark, noise, etc.; craving for icy cold drinks — **Phosphorus 200 or 1M** — *weekly (3)*

● In psoric patients; when hair turns grey in patches — **Psorinum 200 or 1M** — *weekly (3)*

❑ To darken the hair with speedy growth — **Wiesbaden 30** — *4 hourly*

❑ When there is excessive sweating all over the body; premature greying of hair — **Pilocarpine 1M (Jaborandi 1M)** — *weekly (6)*

❑ Premature grey hair; hyperacidity — **Acid-Sulph. 30** — *4 hourly*

☆ Another well proved remedy — **Ceanothus Q 5-7 drops** — *4 hourly*

Biochemic remedies — **Calcarea phos. 6X** and **Natrum mur. 6X** — *4 hourly*

For External Use:

Arnica Q, Cantharis Q and Jaborandi Q in 10% ratio is Coconut oil or Olive oil.

HANG OVER
(See Alcoholism Also)

❑ Head Remedy for hang over — **Nux vomica 30 or 200** — *1/2 hourly*

❑ Congestion of head after taking wine — **Silicea 200** — *10 min. (3)*

❑ Insatiable craving for liquor which the patient hated earlier — **Medorrhinum 200 or 1M** — *weekly (6)*

Biochemic remedy — **Kali phos. 6X** — *4 hourly*

Symptoms	Remedy	Frequency And Doses

HAY FEVER
(See Allergic Rhinitis, Cold and Catarrh Also)

Symptoms	Remedy	Frequency And Doses
❑ Sudden; after exposure to dry, cold wind	**Aconite nap. 30**	*1/2 hourly (3)*
❑ Coryza with violent sneezing; localised tingling in the throat	**Sabadilla 30**	*2 hourly*
❑ Thin, watery discharge from nose with irritation and violent, painful sneezing; restlessness and unquenchable thirst	**Arsenic alb. 30**	*3 hourly*
☆ Watering of nose and eyes, intense sneezing; soreness of lips and nostrils; worse indoors, morning; better in open air	**Allium cepa 30**	*2 hourly*
☆ Violent sneezing, bland discharge from nose but discharge from eyes burn; worse in open air	**Euphrasia 30**	*4 hourly*
☆ Violent sneezing; running of nose in the morning; excoriating discharge; eyes feel hot and heavy; aching all over the body; loss of thirst; limbs heavy; better after passing urine	**Gelsemium 30**	*4 hourly*
☆ Patient chilly and irritable; irritation in nose, eyes and face; violent spells of sneezing; nose stuffed at night	**Nux vomica 30**	*4 hourly*
● Patient sensitive to cold; chronic catarrh	**Psorinum 200 or 1M**	*3 weekly (3)*
❑ Constant sneezing; nose stuffed up or running of nose and eyes; worse in open air, damp, being chilled when hot	**Dulcamara 30 or 200**	*4 hourly*
☆ Nose stuffed; sneezing; worse at night; pricking in nose with desire to bore into nostrils or watering of nose profusely making nostrils raw and sore	**Arum triph. 30**	*4 hourly*
Biochemic remedy	**Natrum mur. 6X or 12X**	*3 hourly*

Symptoms	Remedy	Frequency And Doses

HEADACHE
(See Migraine And Sinusitis, Etc., Also)

Symptoms	Remedy	Frequency And Doses
☆ With constant nausea; clean tongue	Ipecac 30	3 hourly
☆ With severe throbbing and rush of blood towards head	Belladonna 30	3 hourly
❑ Due to over eating; stomach disorders; tongue thickly whitish coated; worse bathing specially river bathing	Antim-crud. 30 or 200	4 hourly (3)
❑ Due to exposure to dry cold wind; sudden with anxiety	Aconite nap. 30 or 200	1/2 hourly (3)
❑ With watering of eyes with pain and sensitiveness to bright light	Euphrasia 30	3 hourly
❑ Headache; better by bending head backwards; due to nerve injury	Hypericum 30	3 hourly
❑ Headache with humming in the ears; due to nervous weakness	Kali phos. 6X or 30	3 hourly
❑ Hammering headache; worse during menstrual cycle going in sun; school girls	Natrum mur. 30 or 200	4 hourly
☆ Headache starts from the nape of neck and shift over to head; patient desires to lie down quietly; better passing urine	Gelsemium 30 or 200	3 hourly
❑ Violent headache due to working under gas light; sun-stroke	Glonoine 6 or 30	2 hourly
☆ Bursting headache; worse by stooping and movements; excessive thirst, constipation	Bryonia 30 or 200	3 hourly (6)
☆ Nervous headache; after grief, disappointment; worse inhaling smoke	Ignatia 200 or 1M	3 hourly (3)
☆ Headache; due to sinusitis; pressure and pain at root of nose	Kali bich. 30	4 hourly
❑ Due to eating rich fatty food, loss of thirst, better in open cold air	Pulsatilla 30	4 hourly

Symptoms	Remedy	Frequency And Doses
❑ Due to eye strain; disturbances of accomodation of eye sight	**Ruta g. 30**	*4 hourly*
☆ After taking alcoholic drinks; sedentary habits; chilly patient	**Nux vomica 30**	*4 hourly*
❑ Sun headache; aggravation from sun rise to sunset; from cardiac origin	**Kalmia lat. 30 or 200**	*6 hourly*
❑ Of school children; crushing headache, pressure on top of head	**Acid-phos. 30**	*4 hourly*
❑ Headache localised; at the nape of neck; worse by walking and noise	**Pneumococcin. 200**	*10 min. (3)*
❑ Frontal headache; neuralgic pain above and behind the right eye; heaviness of head. Better by rest, lying down and eating	**Penicillinum 30 or 200**	*10 min. (3)*
● Headache worse early morning; empty gone sensation at 10-11 a.m.	**Sulphur 200 or 1M**	*weekly (3)*
Biochemic remedy	**Biocombination No.12**	*4 hourly*

Other Important Remedies:

Spigelia, Sangninaric c., Lachesis, Lycopodium, Magphos., Damiana, etc..

HEART – *Affections of*
(See Other Heart Ailments Also)

❑ Palpitation; lying on the right side	**Alumen 30**	*4 hourly*
❑ Palpitation; better by walking	**Carduus mar. Q or 6**	*4 hourly*
❑ Patient feels as if heart is on the right side	**Borax 30**	*4 hourly*
❑ Pain in the heart before, during or after urination; or at the time of menses	**Lithium carb. 30**	*4 hourly*
❑ Palpitation and dyspnoea in organic heart diseases; worse when thinking of it	**Oxalic acid. 30**	*4 hourly*
❑ Palpitation; after being emotional	**Calcarea ars. 30**	*4 hourly*
❑ Palpitation due to anaemia; restlessness and burning sensations	**Arsenic alb. 30**	*4 hourly*

Symptoms	Remedy	Frequency And Doses
❑ Heart ailments due to suppression of haemorrhoids or menstruation	**Collinsonia 30 or 200**	*4 hourly (3)*
☆ Degeneration of heart; patient craves for icy cold preparations	**Phosphorus 30 or 200**	*6 hourly (SOS)*
❑ Fatty heart; feels as if heart leaped into throat	**Phytolacca 30**	*4 hourly*
❑ Inflammation of heart; pain and aches are worse with slightest movements	**Bryonia 30 or 200**	*4 hourly*
❑ Rapid action of heart; conscious about heart	**Pyrogenium 200**	*1 dose*
❑ Slow action of heart; pulse feeble and rapid	**Latrodectus m. 30**	*1/2 hourly (3)*
❑ Weakness and irritation of heart	**Prunus v. 30**	*6 hourly*
Biochemic remedy	**Kali phos. 6X**	*4 hourly*

HERNIA

The protrusion of an organ or part of an organ or other structure through the wall of the cavity normally containing it is called hernia.

❑ Hiatus; with pain abdomen; worse lying down; patient feels better in open air	**Pulsatilla 30 or 200**	*4 hourly*
❑ Inguinal; painful; stools usually consti-pated, chilly patient	**Silicea 12X or 30**	*4 hourly*
☆ Inguinal; left sided; umbilical; worse in the morning and when constipated; chilly and irritable patient	**Nux vomica 30 or 200**	*4 hourly*
☆ Inguinal or strangulated; right sided; patient prone to gastric complaints	**Lycopodium 30 or 200**	*4 hourly*
● When well selected remedies fail to act	**Cocculus ind. 200**	*4 hourly (3)*
❑ Inguinal; sadness of mind; suicidal thoughts	**Aurum met. 200 or 1M**	*weekly (3)*
❑ Incarcerated; with anxiety and burning pain	**Aconite nap. 200**	*4 hourly*

Symptoms	Remedy	Frequency And Doses
❏ Incarcerated or strangulated; patient can not tolerate touch of clothes on the abdomen	**Lachesis 30 or 200**	*4 hourly*
❏ Incarcerated; with uneasiness and fetid flatus; better by passing flatus or belching	**Carbo veg. 30**	*4 hourly*
❏ Incarcerated; with restlessness and burning sensation; unquenchable thirst, sips little water at a time but frequently	**Arsenic alb. 30**	*4 hourly*
❏ Strangulated; with deathly nausea	**Tabacum 30**	*4 hourly*
❏ Strangulated; other types of hernia; with pain around navel region	**Plumbum met. 30**	*4 hourly*
☆ Incarcerated or strangulated; with vomiting of faecal matter	**Opium 200 or 1M**	*4 hourly (3)*
☆ For all types of hernia; when the walls of abdomen are thin	**Calcarea carb. 200 or 1M**	*weekly (3)*
❏ Hernia of the bladder	**Staphysagria 30**	*4 hourly*
❏ Femoral hernia	**Wiesbaden 30**	*4 hourly*
❏ Umbilical hernia	**Granatum 30**	*4 hourly*

HERPES ZOSTER

An infection caused by Herpes virus varicellae, characterized by an eruption of groups of vesicles on one side of the body following the course of a nerve. The condition is self-limited but may be accompanied by or followed by severe post-herpetic pain.

☆ Head remedy (with fever, restlessness, itching, burning and tingling)	**Rhus tox. 30 or 200**	*3 hourly*
☆ With burning and shooting pain, restlessness and anxiety	**Arsenic alb. 30 or 200**	*4 hourly*
☆ Of right side; with intense burning	**Cantharis 30**	*4 hourly*
❏ On back; sensitive to cold	**Cistus can. 30**	*4 hourly*
❏ On legs; throbbing pain worse by heat	**Comocladia 30**	*4 hourly*
❏ Itching and painful burning with redness of the skin; formation of vesicles and	**Croton tig. 30**	*4 hourly*

Symptoms	Remedy	Frequency And Doses
pustules; desiccation, desquamation and falling off of the pustules		
❑ Burning in the face; inflammed cheeks, with boring, gnawing and digging sensation from gums to ears; itching and tingling in the cheeks	Euphorbia 30	4 hourly
❑ Especially on the left side; oozing of sticky discharge; stools constipated	Graphites 30 or 200	4 hourly
❑ On right side, following with gastric derangement	Iris ver. 30	4 hourly
☆ Facial; in spring and fall; of purple colour	Lachesis 30 or 200	4 hourly
❑ To relieve the burning and to prevent the appearance of new crops. Right sided, extending across the abdomen	Merc-sol. 30 or 200	4 hourly (3)
❑ With pain and itching; burning after scratching; brown scabs on eruptions	Mezereum 30	4 hourly
❑ Worse after taking cold drinks or by tobacco smoke; gastric derangement; evening aggravation and a mild, yielding, tearful disposition	Pulsatilla 30 or 200	4 hourly (3)
❑ With severe burning pain and itching; worse by touch or motion; preceding interco-stal neuralgia due to alcoholism	Ranun-bulb. 30	4 hourly
● Due to suppressed gonorrhoea; burning after scratching	Thuja oc. 200	3 hourly (3)
❑ With lancinating pain; suppurating herpes	Zincum met. 30	4 hourly
❑ Eruptions; large, swollen; burns and stings; better by cold applications	Apis mel. 30	4 hourly
❑ Due to digestive disturbances; sedentary habits; indulgence of women and wine	Nux vomica 30	4 hourly
❑ Violent; worse by taking hot drinks; fear of dark	Stramonium 30	4 hourly
❑ Herpes of labialis pudendi	Terebinth. 30	4 hourly
❑ Facial neuralgia after herpes zoster	Kalmia lat. 30	4 hourly
Biochemic remedy	Kali mur. 6X and Natrum mur. 12X	4 hourly

Symptoms	Remedy	Frequency And Doses

HICCOUGH

✩ After smoking; eating or emotional disturbances	**Ignatia 200 or 1M**	*10 min. (3)*
✩ After smoking; worse after hot drinks	**Veratrum alb. 30 or 200**	*10 min. (3)*
❏ After smoking; worse after cold drinks or during fever; restlessness	**Arsenic alb. or 200**	*1/2 hourly*
✩ Due to gastric origin; chilly patient	**Nux vomica 30 or 200**	*1/2 hourly (3)*
❏ After slightest provocation; such as laughing, talking or taking food	**Cajuput. 30**	*3 hourly*
❏ Violent and noisy; associated with convulsions	**Cicuta v. 30 or 200**	*2 hourly*
❏ After eating; associated with convulsions; worse at night, post - operative; hysterical	**Hyoscyamus 30 or 200**	*3 hourly*

Biochemic remedy

Spasmodic with soreness	**Magnesia phos. 6X** in warm water	*1/2 hourly*

HOARSENESS
(See Laryngitis Also)

An unnaturally deep and harsh quality of the voice.

❏ Hoarseness; due to sudden exposure to dry cold wind	**Aconite 30 or 200**	*2 hourly*
✩ Due to over use of voice; of politicians, singers, etc.	**Arnica 30 or 200**	*3 hourly*
✩ In professional singers; chronic laryngitis	**Argentum nit. 30 or 200**	*4 hourly*
❏ When Arg-nit. fails	**Manganum acet. 30**	*4 hourly*
✩ Sudden; violent hoarseness with scrapping feeling in the throat	**Belladonna 30**	*4 hourly*

Symptoms	Remedy	Frequency And Doses
❏ Due to paralytic effects; can't tolerate touch of clothes around throat	**Lachesis 30**	*4 hourly (3)*
☆ Due to catarrh; involunatry urination while coughing; constant hawking	**Causticum 30**	*4 hourly (3)*
☆ Due to hysteria; emotional disturbances; inhaling smoke	**Ignatia 30 or 200**	*4 hourly (3)*
❏ Due to paralysis of vocal cord	**Oxalic acid. 6 or 30**	*4 hourly*
☆ Hoarseness with sore throat; worse by eating sweets; clears throat constantly	**Spongia 30**	*4 hourly (3)*
☆ Complete loss of voice; accompanied with loose cough; loss of thirst with dry throat; better in open and cold air	**Pulsatilla 30**	*4 hourly*
❏ Hoarseness of singers; as soon as they begin to sing	**Selenium 30 or 200**	*10 min. (3)*
❏ Tendency to get hoarseness off and on	**Wyethia 6 or 30**	*4 hourly*
☆ Hoarseness with constant hawking in public speakers. Worse by singing, talking, due to sudden exposure	**Arum triph. 30**	*4 hourly*
☆ Hoarseness due to exposure, with profuse clammy perspiration; worse in the evening; desire for icy cold drinks	**Phosphorus 30 or 200**	*4 hourly (3)*
☆ Hoarseness during Menstrual cycle; feverish and lethargic feeling	**Gelsemium 30**	*4 hourly*
● Intercurrent remedy for psoric patients (over-sensitive and prone to colds)	**Psorinum 200 or 1M**	*weekly (3)*
❏ Hoarseness due to sudden exposure	**Borax 1X or 30**	*10 min. (3)*
❏ Hoarseness due to exposure to heat	**Antimonium crud. 30**	*4 hourly*
❏ Hoarseness; better by talking	**Rhus tox. 30**	*4 hourly*
❏ Hoarseness, from cold or congestion of vocal cords; tongue clean; persistent nausea	**Ipecac 30**	*4 hourly*
❏ Hoarseness due to exposure; accompanied by vomiting and excessive hunger	**Cina 30 or 200**	*4 hourly*

Symptoms	Remedy	Frequency And Doses
❏ Complete loss of voice; burning in throat, as from hot vapors, excessive salivation	Mercurius sol. 30	4 hourly
❏ With irritation of throat; localised irritation at one point	Sabadilla 30	4 hourly
● When well selected remedies fail; patient feels discomfort at night	Syphilinum 1M	weekly (3)
Biochemic remedy	Calcarea phos. 6X Ferrum phos. 6X and Kali mur. 6X	4 hourly

HYDROCELE
(See Orchitis Also)

A collection of serous fluid in a sacculated cavity; specifically, such a collection in the tunica vaginalis testis is called hydrocele.

Symptoms	Remedy	Frequency And Doses
☆ Due to injury, stitches in scrotum; testes hard, swollen and tender	Arnica mont. 200 or 1M	weekly (6)
☆ Congenital; testes swollen; soreness, tearing pain; testicles hang down; left hang low	Pulsatilla 200 or 1M	weekly (6)
❏ With induration of testes; specially in boyhood	Sulphur iod. 3X or 6	4 hourly
☆ Testes heavy and sore; enlarged, hard, specially after injuries	Conium mac. 200 or 1M	weekly (6)
☆ Testes drawn up; swollen, painful, hard; worse right side; when air become cold and before storms	Rhododendron 200 or 1M	weekly (6)
☆ Swelling and tensive pain in right testicle as if bruised; atrophy of testicles; sadness in mind	Aurum met. 200 or 1M	weekly (6)
❏ Stitches in testicles while sitting; painful tension from right testicle along spermatic cord in groin	Bryonia alb. 200	6 hourly
❏ Lassitude; it seems as if he should walk for ever; pain better by walking	Acid-fluor. 200 or 1M	weekly (6)

Symptoms	Remedy	Frequency And Doses
❑ Hydrocele with skin ailments; constipation	**Graphites 200 or 1M**	*weekly (6)*
❑ Sticking through testicles; pain worse after lying down and at night, pressure in sperm-atic testes cords; hang down	**Silicea 200 or 1M**	*weekly (6)*
● Intercurrent remedy	**Sulphur 200 or 1M**	*fortnightly (3)*
Biochemic remedy	**Calcarea fluor. 12X**	*4 hourly*

HYDROCEPHALUS

Abnormal accumulation of cerebro-spinal fluid within the skull, which may involve ventricular cavities and the general spaces. Due to this distension the cranial bones may expand and the skull becomes enlarged. This complication may be congenital or acquired.

❑ Rush of blood to face and head; face red; fever, violent headache	**Belladonna 30**	*4 hourly*
☆ Accumulation of fluid rapid; patient cries with intense pain; loss of thirst	**Apis mel. 30 or 200**	*4 hourly*
☆ Bulging of the fontanelles; suppression of urine; constant involuntary motion of one leg	**Apocynum can. Q or 30**	*4 hourly*
● When there is tubercular history in the family or the patient	**Tuberculinum k. 1M**	*fortnightly (3)*
❑ Rolling of head; jerking of muscles during sleep; fidgety feet; patient bores his head in the pillow and screams	**Zincum met. 30 or 200**	*6 hourly*
❑ Suspension of senses; unconsciousness with screaming; urine suppressed; eyes do not react to light; involuntary motion of one half of the body; beginning of paralytic stage	**Helleborus 30 or 200**	*6 hourly*
❑ After measles or scarlatina; head-sweats which do not relieve; moaning; patient rattles head	**Mercurius sol. 30 or 200**	*6 hourly*

Symptoms	Remedy	Frequency And Doses
● Tubercular or syphilitic history in the family; violent headache; better in open air	Kali iod. 30 or 200	6 hourly
● Stupor; cold sweat; patient cries in sleep; history of suppression of eruptions	Sulphur 200 or 1M	10 min. (3)
❑ Sweating of entire head; face and hands cold; offensive foot sweat; startlings in sleep; chilly patient	Silicea 30 or 200	4 hourly
❑ In chronic cases; patient feels worse during and after sleep	Lachesis 200 or 1M	weekly (3)
❑ Sweating on scalp during sleep; head large; desire for eggs. Child weak though fatty	Calcarea carb. 200 or 1M	fortnightly (3)
Biochemic remedy	Calcarea phos. 6X	4 hourly

HYDROPHOBIA
Rabies

There is no set treatment for hydrophobia in homoeopathy. The patient should be rushed to the hospital.

The developed disease requires first of all "the removal of every cause of excitement; the separation of the patient from everything calculated to disturb or render him anxious; the maintenance of the utmost quiet; the employment of a friendly tone of address (in place of coercive measures); and the endeavour to calm the sufferer by kind treatment" (Bollinger.).

The following medicines can be tried till patient is hospitalized.

❑ Congested face; wild staring look, pupils dilated, sensitive to sunlight or shining objects; throat sore, spasms of throat, hoarse, barking voice; inability to swallow; oppression; anxiety, hallucinations; biting and snapping; convulsions	Belladonna 30 or 200	1/2 hourly
❑ When swallowing is prevented by inflammation; and not only from spasms of the throat; spasms follow the pain caused by swallowing; also when there is priapismus	Cantharis 200 or 1M	10 min. (3)
❑ When the skin becomes bluish-red, with edges hard and swollen. Fear of water	Hydrophobinum 200 or 1M	10 min. (3)

Symptoms	Remedy	Frequency And Doses
❏ General convulsions more prominent than spasms of the throat; abuses those around. Sleep is interrupted as if by a sudden fright followed by convulsions.	**Hyoscyamus 200 or 1M**	*10 min. (3)*
❏ Fear of imaginary objects; and the great mobility and restlessness, with screaming; Fear of dark	**Stramonium 200 or 1M**	*10 min. (3)*
❏ In the worse state of the developed disease	**Lachesis 200 or 1M**	*10 min. (3)*

HYPER ACIDITY
(See Acidity)

HYPER-PYREXIA
(See Fever)

HYPERTENSION
High Blood Pressure

Symptoms	Remedy	Frequency And Doses
☆ Head remedy; With nervousness (during pregnancy use with care)	**Rauwolfia s. Q**, 5-10 drops	*4 hourly*
☆ With depression; suicidal tendency and cardiac symptoms	**Aurum met. 200 or 1M**	*10 min. (3)*
☆ With arteriosclerosis and senile paresis	**Aurum iod. 30**	*6 hourly*
☆ With senility and senile behavioural changes	**Baryta carb. 200 or 1M**	*weekly (3)*
☆ Systolic pressure high and diastolic very low	**Baryta mur. 3X or 6X**	*4 hourly*
☆ With constriction is heart region and anginal pain	**Cactus g. Q or 30**	*3 hourly*
☆ For fat and flabby patient; sweat on head, palms and soles, craving for eggs; chilly patient	**Calcarea carb. 200 or 1M**	*weekly (3)*
❏ In old age; old bachelors and old maids	**Conium mac. 200 or 1M**	*weekly (3)*

Symptoms	Remedy	Frequency And Doses
☆ Palpitation on slight exertion; dyspnoea, insomnia and gastric complaints	Crataegus ox. Q or 30	4 hourly
❑ Due to shock (broken love affair, etc.); emotional disturbances	Ignatia 200 or 1M	4 hourly (3)
❑ Due to congestion in brain; severe headache, lassitude and dizziness	Glonoine 3X or 6	1/2 hourly
❑ Due to syphilitic origin; lancinating pain in head and bones	Kali iod. 30 or 200	4 hourly (3)
❑ Due to gastric origin; flatulence; craving for sweets and warm food; worse 4-8 p.m.	Lycopodium 30 or 200	4 hourly
❑ Due to shock or grief; hyperthyroidism, goitre, addison's disease, diabetes, etc. Desire for salt preparations	Natrum mur. 200 or 1M	10 min. (3)
❑ In syphilitic cases; angina pectoris; vertigo, dyspnoea and endocarditis	Natrum iod. 30 or 200	10 min. (3)
❑ In tall, intelligent, hypertensive people; craves for icy cold things, fear of dark and storms, etc.	Phosphorus 30 or 200	10 min. (3)
❑ With sclerotic degeneration specially of spinal cord	Plumbum iod. 30 or 200	6 hourly
❑ Due to grief; apprehension, dullness, loss of thirst, etc.	Gelsemium 30 or 200	3 hourly
☆ During menopausal stage; worse after sleep; great loquacity	Lachesis 30 or 200	4 hourly
❑ Bursting pain in head; better by cold application, pressure; vertigo; palpitation of heart; worse when alone; sleeplessness with heaviness in head; oedematous swelling on face and legs	Boerhaavia diffusa Q or 6	4 hourly
Biochemic remedy	Calcarea fluor. 12X, Silicea 12X and Kali phos. 6X	4 hourly

Symptoms	Remedy	Frequency And Doses

ESSENTIAL HYPERTENSION

☆ Essential hypertension (hypertension without any marked symptoms)	*Crataegus Q, Glonoine Q*, and *Passiflora Q*, 5 drops each	*4 hourly*
❑ For high systolic and low diastolic pressure	*Viscum alb. Q*, 5-7 drops	*4 hourly*

For essential hypertension constitutional treatment should be given.

HYPOCHONDRIASIS
(See Different Ailments)

Exaggerated attention to any unusual bodily or mental sensation, a false belief that one is suffering from some disease. As in homoeopathy the treatment is always sick oriented so any medicine which is constitutional for the concerned person will help.

HYPOTENSION
Low Blood Pressure

☆ Due to fluid loss; exhaustive discharges (excessive vomiting, diarrhoea, blood loss or semen loss, etc.)	China off. 30	*4 hourly*
☆ Due to low vitality; flatulence in upper part of abdomen, desire for fresh air	Carbo veg. 6 or 30	*4 hourly*
❑ Faints in hot sun, craves for salt; excessive thirst and constipation	Natrum mur. 12X or 30	*4 hourly*
❑ Craves for sweets; flatulence in lower part of abdomen; uric acid diathesis	Lycopodium 30 or 200	*4 hourly (3)*
❑ When pulse is slow and weak; vertigo, weight and oppression of heart as if being squeezed	Viscum alb. Q or 30	*4 hourly*
☆ With irregular heart beating and palpitation; feels as if heart would stop beating if do not move about	Gelsemium 30	*4 hourly*

Symptoms	Remedy	Frequency And Doses
❑ Due to excessive sexual indulgence	Acid-phos. 30	4 hourly
Biochemic remedy Far fast growing young people	Calcarea phos. 6X	3 hourly

HYPOTHYROIDISM

Thyroid gland synthesize, store and secrete two hormones – Thyroxine and tri-iodo thyroxine; iodine is an essential constituent of these hormones. The decreased function of thyroid gland is called hypothyroidism. The main symptoms are oedema, weight gain and thickening of skin and mental derangements, it is more common in ladies during the age of 30 to 50 years.

☆ Lack of self confidence; absent minded, easily offended; loss of memory; feels better after eating	**Anacardium or. 30 or 200**	6 hourly
☆ Shy; childish behaviour; aversion to strangers; chilly patient	**Baryta carb. 200 or 1M**	weekly (3)
❑ History of abortions; weight gain; oedema of extremities and face	**Pyrogenium 200 or 1M**	weekly (3)
● In chronic cases; as an intercurrent remedy	**Tuberculinum k. 1M**	fortnightly (3)
☆ In unmarried persons; forced to celibacy; old bachelors and maids	**Conium mac. 200 or 1M**	weekly (3)
☆ Melancholy, irritability and restlessness; desires sweets; cannot stand opposition	**Thyroidin. 3X or 30**	4 hourly
❑ With restlessness; eats well yet emaciates	**Iodium 30**	4 hourly
☆ Fear of darkness and thunder storms; delicate, anaemic patients; craves for cold and salt preparations	**Phosphorus 200**	weekly (3)
❑ For hot patients; sweats easily; worse in warm damp weather. Better from any motion, exercise and at sea	**Bromium 30**	4 hourly
Biochemic remedies	**Calcarea phos. 6X, Silicea 6X and Calc-flour. 12X**	4 hourly

Symptoms	Remedy	Frequency And Doses

HYSTERIA

Symptoms	Remedy	Frequency And Doses
☆ Changing moods; laughing and crying alternately	**Ignatia 200 or 1M**	*10 min. (3)*
☆ Due to sudden suppression of discharge	**Asafoetida 200**	*4 hourly (3)*
❏ Jaws clenched; psychic causes of disease; ill effects of grief, fright, anger, etc.	**Natrum mur. 200**	*4 hourly (3)*
❏ Breath suddenly arrested; worse ascending; disfunction of pituitary and thyroid gland.	**Calcarea carb. 200 or 1M**	*10 min. (3)*
❏ With forward jerking of head; fainting fits	**Nux mosch. 30 or 200**	*6 hourly*
❏ Deep stupor; attempt to run away; obscene, lascivious mania; patient uncovers body	**Hyoscyamus 200**	*4 hourly*
Biochemic remedy	**Calcarea phos. 6X, Kali phos. 6X and Natrum mur. 12X**	*4 hourly*

IMPOTENCY
Male

Symptoms	Remedy	Frequency And Doses
☆ Absence of erection and desire; to tone up the sexual system	**Nuphar lut. Q,** 5-10 drops	4 hourly
☆ Due to masturbation; erections only when half - asleep	**Caladium s. 30 or 200**	6 hourly
☆ Due to old age; complete loss of desire (even in young man); premature emission	**Lycopodium 200 or 1M**	fortnightly (3)
☆ Due to sexual excesses; debility and impotency	**Kali brom. 30**	6 hourly
☆ Due to excessive indulging in sex; penis shrivelled; spermatorrhoea; guilty look	**Staphysagria 30 or 200**	6 hourly
❏ Due to injury	**Arnica 200 or 1M**	weekly (3)
❏ In fat and flabby persons; due to frequent coitus; increased desire	**Calcarea carb. 200 or 1M**	fortnightly (3)
❏ Due to syphilis; in humorous (jolly) persons	**Kali iod. 30 or 200**	6 hourly
❏ Impotency due to debility; enlargement of prostate gland	**Sabal ser. Q,** 5-10 drops	4 hourly
❏ Due to spinal injury	**Hypericum 200 or 1M**	fortnightly (3)
☆ In young boys who are afraid of marriage due to their past of free sexual indulgence	**Anacardium or. 200**	weekly (3)
❏ Impotency with diabetes melitus	**Moschus 30 or 200**	fortnightly (3)
☆ Due to excessive loss of seminal fluid (chronic); due to onanism	**Acid-phos. Q or 30**	4 hourly
❏ Due to excessive loss of seminal fluid (acute); excited lascivious fancy	**China 30**	4 hourly

Symptoms	Remedy	Frequency And Doses
❏ Impotency with lascivious thoughts. Stools constipated, can be passed by mechanical aid - by finger, etc., only	Selenium 30	4 hourly
❏ Premature old age, due to abuse of sexual power. Genitalia cold, relaxed, no desire, no erection; after suppressed gonorrhoea	Agnus cast. 30 or 200	4 hourly
❏ Sexual debility due to nervous prostration; to tone up the sexual system	Damiana Q, 5-10 drops	4 hourly
❏ Neurasthenic impotence. Strong and lasting erections	Yohimbinum Q, 5-10 drops	4 hourly
● With nocturnal emissions followed by great weakness	Medorrhinum 200 or 1M	fortnightly (3)
☆ Due to suppression of desire (chronic bachelors) or excessive indulgence	Conium mac. 200 or 1M	fortnightly (3)
Biochemic remedies	Calcarea phos. 30X and Kali phos. 30X	4 hourly

INDIGESTION

Indigestion may be the result of faulty habits of eating or drinking; dietary indiscretion, either episodic or habitual. Mental tension, inadequately countered by a healthy nonchalance and proper periods of leisure and relaxation; fear and anxiety; rage and resentment; impatience and irritation; these and allied harmful emotions are potent disturbers of digestive rhythm and well-being. These tensions cause indigestion in three ways. They interfere with the tone of the muscle in the wall of the stomach and gut which leads to spasm or over-distension.

❏ Indigestion from taking tea in excess	Thuja oc. 30 or 200	4 hourly
❏ With constriction of oesophagus	Abies nig. 30	4 hourly
☆ Accompanied with flatulence; better passing flatus	Carbo veg. 30	4 hourly
☆ From over eating; sedentary habits	Nux vomica 30 or 200	4 hourly
☆ After being angry; better doubling up	Colocynth. 30 or 200	4 hourly (3)
☆ Due to anticipation; taking sweets	Argentum nit. 30 or 200	4 hourly (3)

Symptoms	Remedy	Frequency And Doses
❏ While going somewhere or hearing any sudden news, etc.; due to apprehension	**Gelsemium 30 or 200**	*1/2 hourly (3)*
❏ After taking coffee; excessive thirst and constipation	**Natrum mur. 30 or 200**	*3 hourly (3)*
☆ Eating vegetables, preserved food; unquenchable thirst; burning sensation in the stomach or abdomen with restlessness	**Arsenic alb. 30 or 200**	*4 hourly (3)*
☆ Heartburn; pain and fullness in pit of stomach 2 to 3 hours after eating; foul breath, bad taste in mouth; hollow sinking feeling or "plug" sensation in belly; worse after taking cold drinks, emotional stress; better after eating	**Anacardium or. 30 or 200**	*4 hourly*
☆ Distress in stomach pit soon after food, with heaviness 'like a stone'; water-brash; biliousness; dull pain in liver region; heartburn; hiccough; thirst for large quantities but warm drinks are vomited; better lying quiet still on back; thoughts of business	**Bryonia 30 or 200**	*4 hourly*
❏ Constrictive pain in pit of stomach about 2 hrs. after eating; constant desire to retch or swallow; saliva dribbles during sleep; eructations tasting of food or acid; feels nauseated and weak; trembling in the morning; much burning, griping and bloating	**Graphites 30**	*4 hourly*
❏ Burning, heaviness and pressure in stomach pit, even after eating small meal; severe bloating; frequent belching; faintness in morning; bilious attacks; sticking pain in liver region; desire for vinegar, wine, spicy food; worse when walking; better after eating	**Hepar sulph. 30**	*4 hourly*
❏ Constant pain in pit of stomach; as from a hard-cornered object; feels horribly ill;	**Hydrastis can. 6 or 30**	*4 hourly*

Symptoms	Remedy	Frequency And Doses
nothing tastes right, vomits every thing taken, tongue feels burnt; worse after breakfast and eating vegetables		
❑ Heartburn and weight in stomach immediately after taking food with pain which spreads to back between shoulder-blades; may be small spot of soreness and tenderness below ribs on left side; better after eating food	**Kali bich. 30**	*4 hourly*
☆ Much bloating, sensation as if 'had eaten too much' or 'a stone in stomach', 1 to 2 hours after eating; food regurgitates; eructations tasting of food; raw, burning in stomach; vomiting of food taken some hours before; worse in a warm room, eating warm and rich food; better temporarily from taking cold things	**Pulsatilla 30 or 200**	*4 hourly*
❑ Due to nervousness; grief or dis-appointment	**Ignatia 30 or 200**	*4 hourly*
Biochemic remedies	**Calcarea phos. 6X** and **Silicea 12X**	*4 hourly*

INFLUENZA
(See Cold, Catarrh Also)

Symptoms	Remedy	Frequency And Doses
☆ Head remedy; restlessness with prostra-tion and excessive thirst at short intervals	**Arsenic alb. 30**	*4 hourly*
● Intercurrent remedies	**Influenzinum 200 and Sulphur 200**	
☆ Early stage with chill and sneezing; heaviness and tiredness of body and limbs; loss of thirst; bursting headache; relief from passing large quantities of pale urine	**Gelsemium 30 or 200**	*4 hourly*
☆ Severe pains in limbs and back; bones feel 'broken', bursting headache; shivering, and chills in back; eyeballs sore	**Eupatorium perf. 30 or 200**	*3 hourly*

Symptoms	Remedy	Frequency And Doses
❑ Rapid prostration; high fever, gastric symptoms; dull red face; nervousness	**Kali phos. 6X or 30**	*4 hourly*
❑ With dry, hacking cough; headache is worse after least movement; wants to lie still and alone; better by pressure; tongue is coated white; great thirst	**Bryonia alb. 30 or 200**	*4 hourly*
☆ Patient very chilly; feels cold even in bed; least movement or exposure intensifies the sensation of cold; fresh shivering and chill after drinking; aching in limbs and back; nose stuffed up at night	**Nux vomica 30 or 200**	*4 hourly*
❑ Severe pains in back and thighs; chilliness no fire or heat can warm the patient; rapid pulse with temperature not proportionately high; restlessness; violent pulsations; bruised feeling all over	**Pyrogenium 200**	*3 hourly (3)*
Biochemic remedies	**Ferrum phos. 6X, Kali mur. 6X and Natrum sulph. 12X**	*3 hourly*

INJURY
Trauma, Cuts, Wounds, etc.

Symptoms	Remedy	Frequency And Doses
☆ Head remedy; covers even unconsciousness; bruised pains and tumefication of soft parts	**Arnica 200 or 1M**	*3 hourly (3)*
☆ Injury of deeper tissues; sprains and bruises	**Bellis p. 6 or 30**	*4 hourly*
❑ Bad effects of head injury; Sheershaasan (head-stand) or a fall on head	**Natrum sulph. 200 or 1M**	*10 min. (3)*
❑ Injury to fibrous tissues; tendons and muscles; sprains and over strain	**Rhus tox. 30 or 200**	*4 hourly*
❑ Injury to periosteum and bones; sprains of ankles and wrist; house maid's knee	**Ruta g. 30 or 200**	*6 hourly*

Symptoms	Remedy	Frequency And Doses
❏ Open/ragged wounds due to injuries	**Calendula 30**	*4 hourly*
❏ Wounds turns black; instead of healing	**Carbo veg. 30**	*4 hourly*
☆ To avoid tetanus; punctured wounds due to splinters, insect bites, nail-prick, etc.	**Ledum pal. 200 or 1M**	*10 min. (3)*
❏ For wounds which are very painful and do not heal	**Acid-nit. 30**	*4 hourly*
❏ Injury of cornea	**Opium 30 or 200**	*4 hourly (3)*
❏ To aid speedy union of fractured bones; eye injury without any marked sign	**Symphytum 6 or 30**	*4 hourly*
❏ Corneal ulceration by a blow; sharp cut wounds	**Staphysagria 30 or 200**	*4 hourly*
☆ Spinal injury; injury of nerves, crushed fingers in a door or machine, etc.	**Hypericum 200 or 1M**	*10 min. (3)*
❏ When small wounds bleed much; blood bright red as after extraction of tooth, etc.	**Phosphorus 30 or 200**	*10 min. (3)*
❏ Oozing of blood through bandage	**Strontium carb. 30**	*4 hourly*
❏ Stage of toxaemia and septicaemia with fever and restlessness	**Pyrogenium 200 or 1M**	*10 min. (3)*
☆ Neuralgia in stump; exposed nerves; after amputation,	**Allium cepa 30 or 200**	*4 hourly*
❏ When patient becomes unconscious; due to shock after injury and body becomes cold	**Camphor. Q,** 5 drops	*15 min. (3)*
❏ When Camphor. Q do not respond and body remains cold; patient desires fanning	**Carbo veg. 30 or 200**	*15 min. (3)*
❏ When Carbo veg. also fails and body remains cold	**Veratrum alb. 30 or 200**	*15 min. (3)*
❏ Cataract after injury	**Conium 30 or 200**	*fortnightly (3)*
Biochemic remedies	**Calcarea phos. 6X** and **Kali phos. 6X**	*4 hourly*

For External Use:

Ferrum phos. 1X should be sprayed on the cuts/wounds to check the bleeding (dressing should be done with Calendula lotion or Calendula ointment).

Symptoms	Remedy	Frequency And Doses

INOCULATION
Ill Effects Of

❑ Dick serum	**Ailanthus g. 200**	*10 min. (3)*
❑ Diphtheria	**Merc-cy. 200**	*10 min. (3)*
❑ Typhoid fever	**Bryonia alb. 200**	*10 min. (3)*
❑ Whooping cough	**Pulsatilla 200**	*10 min. (3)*
❑ Yellow fever	**Arsenic alb. 200**	*10 min. (3)*

INSANITY
Madness
(See Mania Also)

❑ Dictatorial patient; envy; easily aroused to anger with violence	**Lycopodium 200 or 1M**	*weekly (3)*
❑ Due to head injury; melancholy from hearing music; thinks and tries to shoot himself	**Natrum sulph. 200 or 1M**	*weekly (3)*
❑ Due to fright or grief; attempts to escape; sadness and crying at slightest provocation	**Arsenic alb. 200 or 1M**	*weekly (3)*
❑ With paralysis and Loquaciousness; quarrelsome; patient becomes violent, scolds and insults others due to jealousy; intolerance of noise	**Nux vomica 200 or 1M**	*weekly (3)*
❑ Due to intolerable pain; with convulsions; suspicious, delirious and quarrelsome	**Veratrum alb. 200 or 1M**	*weekly (3)*
❑ Due to sexual excesses; exaggerated idea of one's own importance, of his grandeur and riches	**Phosphorus 200 or 1M**	*weekly (3)*
❑ With increased strength; threatens death and destruction; quarrelsome and mischievous; sensitive to music	**Tarentula h. 200 or 1M**	*weekly (3)*

Symptoms	Remedy	Frequency And Doses
❏ Abnormal impulses; sleeplessness, lies awake for hours in bed; uncovers the whole body without shame	**Hyoscyamus 200 or 1M**	*10 min. (3)*
❏ Imagines as if under superhuman power; fear of being poisoned; thinks others are talking about him	**Lachesis 200 or 1M**	*10 min. (3)*
● Plays and wears rags and thinks as if he is not less thán a king; monomania	**Sulphur 200 or 1M**	*10 min. (3)*
❏ Patient becomes wild; fear of dark	**Stramonium 1M**	*10 min. (3)*
❏ Imagines that he hears music; shuts his eyes and is lost in delicious thought melody; excitement with dancing, laughing; talks nonsense	**Cannabis ind. 200 or 1M**	*10 min. (3)*
❏ Excessive anger at slight offence; breaking out in personal violence; conscious of double ego	**Anacardium or. 200 or 1M**	*10 min. (3)*
● Intercurrent remedy	**Bacillinum 1M or 10M**	*fortnightly (3)*
Biochemic remedy	**Kali phos. 6X**	*4 hourly*

INSOMNIA
Sleeplessness

Symptoms	Remedy	Frequency And Doses
❏ Sleeplessness during menopausal stage	**Senecio aur. 30**	*4 hourly*
☆ Can not sleep in the early hours of night; utterly wide awake, mind active; sleeplessness due to excitement	**Coffea 30**	*6 hourly*
☆ Cannot sleep after 3 a.m.; sleeplessness due to mental strain or sedentary habits; sleep dreamy and restless	**Nux vomica 30**	*at bed time for 7 days*
❏ Due to fear or panic; insomnia after shock or fright; restlessness and tossing in bed	**Aconite nap. 30**	*4 hourly*

Symptoms	Remedy	Frequency And Doses
❑ Due to tiredness; either physical or mental; bed feels too hard; must keep moving in search of soft portion for relief in bed	**Arnica mont. 30 or 200**	*1/2 hourly (3)*
❑ Sleeplessness after midnight from anxiety and restlessness; has to get up and walk	**Belladonna 30**	*4 hourly*
❑ Sleepy yet unable to sleep; child tosses, kicks clothes off, twitches; restless sleep with frightful dreams	**Arsenic alb. 30 or 200**	*4 hourly (3)*
❑ Sleeplessness and restlessness, especially in first part of night; gets up and walks the floor; as soon as bed time comes patient is wide awake	**Chamomilla 30 or 200**	*4 hourly*
❑ Sleeplessness due to old grief; after dreams of thieves or robbers	**Natrum mur. 200 or 1M**	*10 min. (3)*
❑ Sleeplessness due to sudden shock; disappointment	**Ignatia 200 or 1M**	*10 min. (3)*
❑ Feels sleepy but cannot sleep; clocks striking at a distance keep him awake; bed feels hot; moves about in vain to find a cool spot in bed	**Pulsatilla 30 or 200**	*4 hourly*
❑ Restlessness during early part of sleep; sound sleep when it is time to rise; gets too hot in bed; throws off covers, gets chilly and puts them on again; puts arms above the head during sleep	**Opium 30 or 200**	*4 hourly*
Biochemic remedies	**Kali phos. 6X** and **(Ferrum) phos. 30X**	*daily at bed time*

IRITIS

Inflammation of the Iris.

❑ Due to exposure to dry cold winds	**Aconite nap. 30 or 200**	*2 hourly.*
❑ Due to mechanical injury	**Arnica mont. 200**	*4 hourly (3)*

Symptoms	Remedy	Frequency And Doses
❏ Complaints due to syphilitic origin; wart like growth on the iris	**Thuja oc. 200**	*4 hourly (3)*
❏ After getting wet or after cataract operation; eye-lids swollen; watering from eyes on opening	**Rhus tox. 30 or 200**	*4 hourly*
❏ Severe pains in and around the eyes; worse at night and in damp weather; sensitive to light; iris discoloured; pupil contracted	**Mercurius sol. 30**	*4 hourly*
❏ Marked inflammation; syphilitic origin, specially after mercurial treatment	**Kali iod. 6 or 30**	*6 hourly*
❏ With severe pain; which seems deep in the bones surrounding the eyes	**Aurum met. 200**	*4 hourly (3)*
❏ Pain occurs in inner canthus and extends across the eye brows or even passes around eyes	**Cinnaberis 200**	*4 hourly (3)*
❏ When the inflammation extends to the neighbouring tissues and cornea; and pus forms in the anterior chamber; better by warmth	**Hepar sulph. 200**	*4 hourly (3)*
❏ After exposure to cold; sharp and shooting pain in the eyes extending to the head or face; worse by motion	**Bryonia alb. 30**	*3 hourly*
❏ Burning pains; worse at night; better by warmth	**Arsenic alb. 30**	*3 hourly*

Other Useful Remedies:

Argentum nit., Asafoetida, Belladonna, Cedron, China, Croton tig., Nux vomica, Pulsatilla, Silicea, Staphysagria, Sulphur, Terebinth. and Zinc-met., etc..

ITCHING
(See Scabies and Pruritus Also)

❏ Itching all over the body without eruptions	**Dolichos 30**	*4 hourly*
● Itching worse after undressing; scratching is pleasurable but results in burning	**Sulphur 30**	*4 hourly*

Symptoms	Remedy	Frequency And Doses
☆ Barber's itch; arms covered with itching and rash; itching on ears, nose and in urethra	Sulphur iod. 6 or 30	4 hourly
☆ Scrotal itching; worse by touch or walking	Croton tig. 30 or 200	4 hourly
● Hot bath ameliorates the itching; worse at night	Syphilinum 200 or 1M	weekly (3)
● Intense and incessant itching; worse at night and when thinking of it	Medorrhinum 200 or 1M	10 min. (3)
● Itching with soreness; body has always filthy smell even after a bath; skin dirty, usually moist as if bathed in oil and at times dry also	Psorinum 200 or 0/6 or above (50 millesimal)	6 hourly
❏ Burning and itching; worse by warmth; urticaria like eruptions	Rhus tox. 30	4 hourly
Biochemic remedy	**Biocombination No. 20**	4 hourly

JAUNDICE

Symptoms	Remedy	Frequency And Doses
❏ Jaundice in new born baby; during pregnancy. Acute pain in liver region with fever and anxiety	**Aconite nap. 30**	3 hourly
❏ Jaundice in new born baby. Child cries a lot; better by carrying	**Chamomilla 30 or 200**	4 hourly
☆ In the beginning when there is nausea and indigestion with clean tongue	**Ipecac 30**	3 hourly (6)
☆ With shooting, stitching pains in the abdomen; complaints after eating non-veg; excessive thirst and constipation	**Bryonia 30 or 200**	4 hourly (6)
☆ With bad taste; vomiting and dull headache; dragging pain-right hypochondriasis after lying down on left side. White coated tongue especially in centre	**Carduus m. Q or 30**	4 hourly
☆ With inflammation and shooting pain in liver radiating to every direction of liver; liver sensitive to touch; eyes pale	**Chelidonium Q or 30**	4 hourly
❏ With constant nausea; Jaundice especially during climacteric age. Foaming black urine	**Lachesis 30 or 200**	4 hourly (3)
☆ When jaundice is due to gastric catarrh; liver swollen and sensitive; digestion slow; Jaundice due to sexual excesses; loss of vital fluids	**China off. 6 or 30**	4 hourly
❏ Jaundice due to gastric complaints; too high living. Frequent but ineffectual urging to pass stools; chilly patient	**Nux vomica 30 or 200**	4 hourly

Symptoms	Remedy	Frequency And Doses
● Intercurrent remedy	**Sulphur 30 or 200**	*weekly (3)*
❑ After abuse of Quinine; unquenchable thirst and restlessness	**Arsenic alb. 30**	*4 hourly*
❑ Jaundice in complication with liver affection; Chalk like, dirty, watery, offensive stools	**Podophyllum 30**	*4 hourly*
❑ Flow of dark blood from nose, mouth, uterus, bowels, etc.. Malignant black Jaundice	**Crotalus h. 30 or 200**	*4 hourly (3)*
❑ Yellow dirty skin, dark brown colour of face; canine hunger	**Iodium 30**	*4 hourly*
❑ Jaundice with liver disorders. Black, tar like stools	**Leptandra 30**	*4 hourly*
❑ Jaundice with deep seated brain and lung diseases associated with Anaemia	**Phosphorus 30 or 200**	*4 hourly (3)*
❑ Loss of appetite; with nausea and vomiting; indigestion from milk; pain in right hypochondrium; dry hard stools; conjunctiva yellow	**Carica papaya Q or 30**	*4 hourly (3)*
❑ For 'Haemolytic jaundice'	**T.N.T. 200**	*weekly (3)*
Biochemic remedies	**Ferrum phos. 6X, Kali mur. 6X** and **Natrum sulph. 12X**	*4 hourly*

KELOIDS

A fibrous growth almost like a tumor usually occuring at the site of a scar.

Symptoms	Remedy	Frequency And Doses
☆ Head remedy; to dissolve the scar tissues	**Thiosinamine. 3X**	*4 hourly*
❑ When there are deep cracks in keloids; constipated stools	**Graphites 30 or 200**	*4 hourly*
☆ To dissolve the scar tissues; in chilly patients	**Silicea 200 or 1M**	*weekly (6)*
● In tubercular constitutions; when there is tubercular history in the family	**Tuberculinum k. 1M**	*fortnightly (6)*
❑ Edges of keloids red; itching; worse by warmth; offensive sweat	**Acid-fluor. 30 or 200**	*6 hourly*
● When the love of life is lost due to ugly look of keloids; suicidal thoughts	**Aurum met. 200 or 1M**	*weekly (3)*
❑ Due to old injury or burns	**Causticum 30 or 200**	*6 hourly*
● Intercurrent remedy when there is pain in keloids	**Acid-nit. 200 and** above	*fortnightly (6)*
Biochemic remedy	**Calcarea fluor. 12X**	*4 hourly*

KERATITIS

Inflammation, thickening and haziness of cornea without ulceration is called Keratitis.

Symptoms	Remedy	Frequency And Doses
❑ When discharge from eyes is sticky, profuse and whitish	**Kali bich. 30 or 200**	*4 hourly*
❑ With over sensitivity to light; ciliary neuralgia	**Lac-fel. 30 or 200**	*4 hourly (3)*

Symptoms	Remedy	Frequency And Doses
❏ With acrid tears and intolerable pain in cornea	Merc-sol. 30 or 200	4 hourly
❏ When eyes are very sensitive to touch and to light; discharge yellowish, thick with corneal opacity	Hepar sulph. 30 or 200	4 hourly
❏ Corneal opacity; profuse, acrid tears; severe pains; worse at night. Superficial tendency of ulceration	Acid-nit. 30 or 200	4 hourly
❏ With pain worse at night; better after bathing with cold water	Syphilinum 200 or 1M	weekly (3)
❏ In fat, flabby and chilly patients; worse by cold	Calcarea carb. 200 or 1M	weekly (3)
● Intercurrent remedy	Sulphur 200 or 1M	weekly (3)
Biochemic remedy	Kali mur. 6X or 12X	4 hourly

KIDNEY
Affections Of

Symptoms	Remedy	Frequency And Doses
❏ Acute nephritis. Urine dark, scanty; retention of urine with stitching pains in kidney. Fever with anxiety	Aconite nap. 30 or 200	3 hourly
☆ Urine scanty with albumen; acute nephritis; albuminuria; thirstlessness	Apis mel. 30 or 200	4 hourly (3)
☆ Severe pain in kidneys extending to bladder and urethra	Berb-vul. Q or 30	4 hourly
☆ Nephritis with irritation of bladder; intolerable burning, urine hot, bloody, albuminous. Constant urging to urinate	Cantharis 30 or 200	4 hourly (3)
☆ Pain in upper part of right kidney extending downward and forward	Ocimum can. 30	4 hourly
❏ Scanty urine with albumen. Difficulty in breathing especially after midnight and on	Arsenic alb. 30 or 200	4 hourly (3)

Symptoms	Remedy	Frequency And Doses
lying down. Excessive exhaustion from slight exertion		
❑ In early stage; bloody urine, violent burning and pain in urethra and kidney region while passing urine; coffee ground like sediment in urine	**Terebinth. Q,** 5-7 drops	*4 hourly*
❑ Dropsy with nephritis. Pulse slow and weak; sensation as if heart stood still. Scanty, dark urine.	**Digitalis 30**	*4 hourly*
❑ Nephralgia of right kidney. Pain right side of body with ineffectual urging to urinate	**Nux-vom. 30 or 200**	*4 hourly*
❑ Suppression of urine which passes drop by drop only. Spasmodic, crampy pain which appear and disappear suddenly with sensation of a warm feeling in the bladder.	**Belladonna 30**	*4 hourly*
❑ Kidney affections associated with pneumonia or pulmonary catarrh. Constant pain in region of right kidney with bloody urine.	**Phosphorus 30 or 200**	*4 hourly (3)*
☆ Repulsive odour of urine; dark brown sediments in urine. Severe kidney pain which penetrate into the chest	**Acid-benz. 30**	*4 hourly*

KIDNEY STONE
(See Renal Calculi)

LABOR

The process of expulsion of a fetus from the uterus at the normal termination of pregnancy.

Symptoms	Remedy	Frequency And Doses
☆ Os rigid, large, thick, hard, band like; nervousness; unrythmical, spasmodic, severe pains which often become weak after initial stage	**Caulophyllum 200**	*10 min. (3)*
☆ Restlessness and fear; patient becomes violent being upset by examination, etc.	**Aconite 200 or 1M**	*10 min. (3)*
❑ After prolonged restlessness; when patient becomes weak and exhausted; wants heat and to be covered	**Arsenic alb. 200**	*10 min. (3)*
☆ Patient nervous, cross and easily excited; hard to manage says nasty things and shouts	**Chamomilla 200 or 1M**	*10 min. (3)*
❑ Feels pain severely; cries, begs to be helped and generally makes a lot of noise and fuss, but not so cross and irritable as Chamomilla	**Coffea 200**	*10 min. (3)*
❑ Patient sad; weeps and sighs, always takes very deep breath. Patient does not seem to be able to get the air deep enough into her lungs	**Ignatia 200 or 1M**	*10 min. (3)*
❑ Nausea very prominent; especially accompanied by sharp cutting pains about navel region	**Ipecac 30 or 200**	*10 min. (3)*
☆ Patient keeps one foot jiggling against the floor, bed or chair and moves during the pains. Weeps and complains a great deal	**Actaea racemosa 30 or 200**	*4 hourly*
❑ Patient sad; weeps, feels faint and wants lots of open, fresh air	**Pulsatilla 200**	*10 min. (3)*

Symptoms	Remedy	Frequency And Doses
❑ Patient wants to be covered; pains accompanied by shuddering; old history perhaps of car sickness and bearing down or prolapsus	**Sepia 200 or 1M**	*10 min. (3)*
❑ After pains, excited by least motion, even by taking a deep breath; parched lips, mouth dry; headache as if head would split	**Bryonia 200 or 1M**	*10 min. (3)*
❑ To be given during last stage (and another dose after placenta is removed on account of bruised condition of genital organs)	**Arnica 200 or 1M**	*10 min. (3)*
❑ After pains; excited by putting baby to breast; pains extending from left to right	**Conium mac. 200**	*10 min. (3)*
❑ After pains; at night; hardly any during day; better from changing position and from being properly covered	**Rhus tox. 200 or 1M**	*10 min. (3)*
❑ After pains, spasmodic with severe cramping, contractions of os uteri; pains radiating down the legs	**Viburnum op. 30 or 200**	*10 min. (3)*

LACHRYMATION
Tears

❑ Tears bland; worse indoors; better open air	**Allium cepa 30**	*4 hourly*
❑ Tears acrid; irritates the eyes	**Euphrasia 30**	*4 hourly*
❑ Tears burning; due to blockage of naso - lachrymal duct; worse by cold	**Rhus tox. 30 or 200**	*4 hourly*
❑ When *Rhus tox.* fails; chilly patient	**Silicea 30 or 200**	*4 hourly*
Biochemic remedy	**Natrum mur. 6X or 12X**	*4 hourly*

Other Important Remedies:

Merc-cor., Petroleum, Acid-fluor., Sulphur, Nat-mur., Arsenic alb. and Hydrastic can., etc..

Symptoms	Remedy	Frequency And Doses

LACTATION

Symptoms	Remedy	Frequency And Doses
❑ Profuse flow of milk; breasts inflammed, red, hot, swollen, tender, at times stony hard; face flushed; skin hot and dry	**Belladonna 30 or 200**	*4 hourly*
☆ Copious flow of watery milk; refused by infant; or milk scanty with distended breasts; patient chilly, aversion to cold air; pale, flabby, weak, apt to perspire, especially on head at night	**Calcarea carb. 200**	*4 hourly (3)*
☆ Diminished secretion of milk; decrease in size of breasts; feels very depressed and despondent; very thirsty	**Lac def. 30 or 200**	*6 hourly*
☆ Flow of milk excessive; nipples extremely sore, nursing painful, pain radiates all over the body; breasts hard, lumpy, possibly due to formation of pus	**Phytolacca d. 30**	*4 hourly*
☆ Milk scanty; nursing painful, pains extend to chest, neck and back; or continued secretion of milk after weaning and breasts feel stretched, tense and sore; mild, and tearful patient; aversion to stuffy heat and desire for cool, open air	**Pulsatilla 30 or 200**	*4 hourly*
❑ Milk suppressed; discharge of blood from nipples when attempts to nurse the infant; child refuses milk or vomits after feed; breasts inflammed, deep red in centre and rose coloured elsewhere breasts hard and sensitive to touch	**Silicea 30 or 200**	*4 hourly*

LARYNGITIS
(See Hoarseness Also)

Symptoms	Remedy	Frequency And Doses
❑ With inflammatory fever; larynx sensitive to touch and to inspired air; voice husky	**Aconite nap. 30**	*4 hourly*

Symptoms	Remedy	Frequency And Doses
☆ Laryngitis of singers; loss of voice; better from getting overheated, in a warm room; worse after rest	**Antim-crud. 30 or 200**	*4 hourly*
☆ Acute laryngitis; vocal cords bright-red; pain in larynx when talking	**Belladonna 30**	*4 hourly*
☆ Chronic laryngitis of singers; raising the voice causes cough; inflammation and swelling of the posterior wall and lining of the larynx; hoarseness and loss of voice	**Argentum nit. 30 or 200**	*4 hourly*
❑ Burning pain in larynx; short, dry, hoarse cough in rapid paroxysms, mostly in daytime, less at night and in warm bed	**Arsenic alb. 30**	*4 hourly*
☆ Inflammation of larynx and pharynx; constant pain and internal swelling; voice hoarse, deep and weak or aphonia	**Arum triph. 30**	*4 hourly*
☆ Laryngeal catarrh of singers; the laryngeal muscles refuse to act, cannot speak a loud word; worse morning and evening	**Causticum 30 or 200**	*4 hourly*
❑ Violent catarrhal laryngitis; hoarse cough, seems to split and tear the larynx	**Allium cepa 30**	*4 hourly*
❑ Constriction in larynx when talking; sensation of a feather in larynx	**Drosera 30 or 200**	*10 min. (3)*
☆ Stitches and pains extending from ear to ear while swallowing; great hoarseness with rough barking cough; scanty, tenacious, muco-purulent secretion, difficult to expectorate; aphonia with slight suffocative spasms; worse morning	**Hepar sulph. 30 or 200**	*4 hourly*
❑ Laryngeal and tracheal ulceration; voice altered, husky; dry, irritating cough with dyspnoea; tightness and constriction about larynx and trachea with soreness and hoarseness	**Iodium 30**	*4 hourly*
❑ Chronic laryngitis; great irritation of the air-tubes; dry, tormenting cough chiefly at night; fat, flabby and chilly patient	**Calcarea carb. 30 or 200**	*4 hourly (3)*

Symptoms	Remedy	Frequency And Doses
❑ Oedematous laryngitis; hoarseness, rawness and dryness of larynx; sensitive to touch; feeling of a lump in throat with sensation of suffocation	Lachesis 30 or 200	4 hourly
☆ Syphilitic laryngitis; parts much swollen, dark-coloured with much hawking and cough	Merc-sol. 30 or 200	4 hourly
❑ Chronic laryngeal cough; without expectoration; stinging, smarting sensation as if a small ulcer were there, generally felt on one side; long standing, short, dry cough, continuing all day	Nitric acid. 30 or 200	4 hourly
❑ Violent tickling in larynx when speaking; dry, spasmodic cough with constriction of throat; stitches in larynx; chilliness with cough	Phosphorus 30 or 200	4 hourly (6)
☆ Dry, irritating cough with burning and tickling in larynx; swelling of submaxillary glands; larynx swollen; difficult respiration as due to a plug in throat; great dryness of larynx with short or barking cough	Spongia 30	4 hourly
❑ Laryngeal phthisis with constant short, irritating and hacking cough	Stannum met. 30	4 hourly
☆ Hawking of mucous from larynx; voice hoarse, tickling in throat; cough increased by pressure on larynx; worse evening	Rumex 30	4 hourly
❑ Acute oedematous laryngitis; dryness in throat with soreness, swelling and redness; expectoration of thick mucous	Sanguinaria c. 30 or 200	4 hourly
❑ Chronic laryngitis with congestion; swelling of the tissues and increased secretion of a glutinous fluid; worse morning; follicular laryngitis with ropy and stringy discharge	Kali bich. 30 or 200	4 hourly

Symptoms	Remedy	Frequency And Doses
❑ Follicular inflammation; laryngeal irritation and dry cough; burning and tickling in throat; oedema of larynx	**Kali iod. 30 or 200**	*4 hourly*
❑ Fetid breath; loss of voice; hoarseness with white and viscid expectoration	**Kali mur. 12X or 30**	*4 hourly*
● Intercurrent remedy	**Sulphur 200**	*weekly (3)*
Biochemic remedies	**Ferrum phos. 6X** and **Kali mur. 6X**	*4 hourly*

LEFT SIDED REMEDIES

Medicines which have special affinity to the left sided organs of the body have been given here. For repetition, etc., see ailments accordingly.

❑ Affects left arm, left leg, left sided abdomen, etc.	**Asafoetida 30 or 200**
❑ Pain from left side of stomach through to back	**Alstonia 30 or 200**
❑ Symptoms appear to the left side and then right	**Benzoic acid. 30 or 200**
❑ Left sided complaints - stitches in spleen	**Bellis perennis 30 or 200**
❑ Oedema of left hand and foot	**Cactus g. 30 or 200**
❑ Left sided sciatica, following influenza	**Iris versicolor 30 or 200**
❑ Sweating mostly on left side	**Jaborandi 30 or 200**
❑ Left sided intercostal neuralgia with numbness of the whole left arm	**Kalmia lat. 30 or 200**
❑ Left sided rheumatism; sharp pains through the lower lobe of left lung	**Oxalic acid. 30 or 200**
❑ Left half of face red and hot and the right half pale and cold	**Paris quadrifolia 30 or 200**
❑ Left sided symptoms; worse 3 p.m.	**Thuja oc. 30 or 200**

Symptoms	Remedy	Frequency And Doses
❏ Paroxysmal neuralgias mostly on the left side though the sciatica is right sided	Colocynth. 30 or 200	
❏ Neuralgias about the abdomen; worse left side	Nux vomica 30 or 200	
❏ Left sided pains	Colchicum 30 or 200	
❏ Left infra-mammary pains suggesting ovarian troubles	Cimicifuga 30 or 200	
❏ Left sided throat complaints; diphtheria, sore throat, ulceration, etc.	Merc-bin iod. 30	
❏ Left sided headache; neuralgia of the fifth nerve	Spigelia 30 or 200	
❏ Left sided throat complaints	Lachesis 30 or 200	

LEPROSY

Chronic granulomatous infection caused by the **Mycobacterium leprae** is called leprosy. Leprosy occurs in two relatively stable types; lepromatous and tuberculoid. The first sign of infection is the appearance of eruption on the skin and slowly the disease progress and later on the sensation in the effected area is diminished or lost.

Symptoms	Remedy	Frequency And Doses
✫ Head remedy (to start the treatment)	Sulphur CM	monthly (3)
● Intercurrent remedy	Bacillinum 1M	fortnightly (6)
❏ Thickening of skin; scale formation	Hydrocotyle 30 or 200	4 hourly
❏ With depression; love of life lost and suicidal tendency	Aurum met. 200 or 1M	monthly (3)
❏ Dropping off of fingers and toes; night sweats	Arsenic iod. 30 and above	6 hourly
✫ Cracks and oozing of sticky fluid; music makes the patient to weep	Graphites 200 or 1M	fortnightly (6)
❏ Complaints with numbness in hands and feet	Hoang nan Q, 5-7 drops	4 hourly
● Thickening of skin; syphilitic origin	Thyroidinum 200 or 1M	weekly (6)

Symptoms	Remedy	Frequency And Doses
❑ Effected parts cold; loss of sensation	**Secale cor. 200 or 1M**	*fortnightly (6)*
❑ Pimples on all projecting portions of bones	**Hura br. CM**	*monthly (3)*
☆ Gangrenous tubercles; thickening of skin; heat in stomach	**Calotropis 200 or 1M**	*weekly (6)*
● Intercurrent remedy; when there is tubercular history in the family	**Tuberculinum k. 1M**	*weekly (6)*
Biochemic remedies	**Calcarea fluor. 12X** and **Silicea 30X**	*4 hourly*

Other Important Remedies:

Anacardium or., Arsenic alb., Elaeis, Crotalus hor., Syphilinum, etc..

LEUCODERMA
Vitiligo
Whitish Discoloration Of The Skin

❑ Head remedy	**Arsenic sul-fl. 3X**	*4 hourly*
❑ Intercurrent remedy	**Tuberculinum bov. 1M**	*fortnightly (6)*

Aurum met., Bacillinum, Hydrocotyle, Lycopodium, Natrum mur., Nitric acid., Sepia, Thuja oc. and other constitutional medicines are useful. Leucoderma is a disease which requires deep study and only constitutional treatment can help.

LEUCORRHOEA
White Discharge From The Vagina

❑ Leucorrhoea associated with diabetes mellitus; thick whitish discharge; stains the linen; irregular, painful, scanty, dark and clotted menstruation with backache; worse by movement; better by rest	**Abroma augusta 30**	*4 hourly*

Symptoms	Remedy	Frequency And Doses
❑ Discharge leaves yellow spot on clothes	**Chelidonium 6 or 30**	*4 hourly*
☆ Acrid, yellow discharge due to trichomonas infection; causing low backache; worse between periods	**Kreosote 30 or 200**	*4 hourly*
☆ Acrid, curd like or like white of egg; with sensation as if warm water was flowing	**Borax 3X or 30**	*4 hourly*
☆ Head remedy; leucorrhoea with backache	**Ova tosta 3X**	*4 hourly*
❑ Acrid, excoriating, yellowish or greenish discharge with constipation. Bearing down sensation as if everything will come out from vagina	**Sepia 200 or 1M**	*weekly (3)*
❑ Milky, creamy, bland or acrid discharge; sometimes with burning. In mild, tearful women; loss of thirst with dry mouth	**Pulsatilla 30 or 200**	*6 hourly*
❑ Leucorrhoea with burning, itching and rawness; worse at night	**Mercurius sol. 30 or 200**	*4 hourly*
☆ Leucorrhoea like milk with burning and itching of parts before and after menstruation; in little girls; feet cold and damp; chilly patient	**Calcarea carb. 200 or 1M**	*weekly (3)*
☆ Acrid, ropy, profuse, transparent discharge, running down to heel with burning; worse during day time and after menstruation; better by washing	**Alumina 0/7 or above**	*6 hourly*
❑ In obese females profuse discharge of white colour; with itching around genitals and constipation	**Graphites 200 or 1M**	*weekly (3)*
❑ Whitish, non-irritating discharge; menses late and scanty	**Penicillinum 200**	*4 hourly (3)*
● Intercurrent remedy; patient feels worse at night; when there is history of miscarriage	**Syphilinum 200 or 1M**	*fortnightly (3)*

Symptoms	Remedy	Frequency And Doses
Biochemic remedies	Calcarea phos. 6X, Kali mur. 6X, and Natrum mur. 12X	4 hourly

LEUKEMIA

Progressive proliferation of abnormal leukocytes found in hemo tissues, other organs, and usually in the blood in increased numbers; occurring due to acute infection, with severe anaemia, haemorrhages, and slight enlargement of lymph nodes or the spleen is known as leukemia.

For homoeopathic treatment find the suitable remedy based on the totality of symptoms of the sick. **Arsenic alb., Arsenic iod., Calcarea iod., Calcarea phos., China off., Ferrum phos., Ceanothus, Natrum mur., Natrum sulph., Ocimum sanc., Phosphorus, Bacillinum, Malaria off., Ocimum can., Tuberculinum, Sulphur, Syphilimum, Radium brom., Medorrhinum and Carcinocin, etc.,** are the main remedies.

The treatment should be under an expert Homoeopath.

LICE

	Symptoms	Remedy	Frequency
☆	For head lice and also for lice of private parts	**Staphysagria Q or 30**	4 hourly
❑	Lice in skin; difficult to cure; breeds very fast	**Lycopodium 30 or 200**	4 hourly
●	Hair lustreless and dirty; head lice. Intercurrent remedy	**Psorinum 200 or 1M**	weekly (3)
☆	Head-lice. Acuteness of smell is a prominent symptom	**Carbolic acid. 30**	4 hourly
❑	Head-lice; scalp offensive; moist and eruptions on head	**Vinca min. 30**	4 hourly
●	Intercurrent remedy	**Bacillinum 200 or 1M**	weekly (3)

For External Use:

Staphysagria Q in oil: ratio-1: 9 (Coconut, Mustard or Olive oil, etc., can be used).

Symptoms	Remedy	Frequency And Doses

LUMBAGO
(See Backache)

LUPUS

Erosion of the skin.

	Symptoms	Remedy	Frequency And Doses
●	Head remedy; Intercurrent also	**Radium brom. 30 or 200**	*4 hourly*
❑	Brown saddle across the nose; aversion to loved ones and family members	**Sepia 30 or 200**	*6 hourly*
❑	Worse going in the sun. Disseminated erythematous lupus	**Natrum carb. 30 or 200**	*4 hourly*
❑	Lupus with burning sensation, restlessness and exhaustion; better by hot; worse by cold. Unquenchable thirst	**Arsenic alb. 30 or 200**	*4 hourly*

Other Important Remedies:

Calcarea carb., Graphites, Lycopodium, Merc-sol., Natrum mur., Rhus tox., Silicea, Staphysagria, Sulphur and Syphilinum, etc..

Symptoms	Remedy	Frequency And Doses
❏ Fever comes every other day or every week. Great thirst before chill which ceases as soon as chill begins; no thirst during stage of heat which returns again during stage of sweat; worse by motion; better by warmth	**China off. 30 or 200**	*3 hourly*
☆ Paroxysms regular; thirst in all stages; severe shaking chill continues for long. Tongue clean; profuse, exhausting sweat. Pain in back (spine); worse during stage of chill (almost a specific)	**China sulph. 1X** and **above**	*4 hourly (6)*
☆ Severe aching bone pains, as if bones are broken. Nausea and vomiting as the chill passes on. Great thirst; drinking excites nausea and vomiting in every stage (chill, heat and sweat); better after sweating, except headache. Tongue thickly (yellowish) coated; taste bitter	**Eup-perf. 30 or 200**	*4 hourly*
☆ Chill without thirst (thirst almost absent in all the stages); violent shaking; chill runs up and down the spine (back), patient wants to be hold. Heat and sweat stage long and exhausting; pain in the nape of neck. Soreness of muscles, muscular power weakened; desire to lie down quietly and to sleep; drowsy; sweat absent; better after passing urine	**Gelsemium 30 or 200**	*3 hourly*
☆ When there are no clear cut indications for a medicine (paroxysms not clear) - a	**Ipecac 30 or 200**	*3 hourly*

Symptoms	Remedy	Frequency And Doses
few doses of Ipecac 30 opens up the case, especially after (suppression)/abuse of quinine or relapse. Nausea, vomiting and dyspnoea in all the stages and clean tongue		
☆ Great thirst with throbbing headache, before chill and during stage of heat. Severe long lasting chill between 10-11 a.m., even lips and nails become blue because of shivering. Profuse sweat, which relieves all the symptoms except headache.	Nat-mur. 30 or 200	4 hourly (6)
☆ Chill with thirst; worse by warmth and motion. Fever (heat stage) without thirst or very little thirst. Sweating alternate with dry heat or little sweat	Apis mel. 30 or 200	4 hourly
❑ Paroxysms irregular; chill absent or very little; sweat usually absent; great restlessness; unquenchable thirst, drinks frequently but little at a time; better after sweating and by warmth	Arsenic alb. 30 or 200	4 hourly
❑ Chill with great thirst and external coldness, drinks at long intervals but large quantities at a time; stools constipated. Stitching pains in chest and in the region of spleen; sour sweat after slightest exertion. Irritable; desires to lie quietly	Bryonia 30 or 200	3 hourly
❑ Chill followed by sweat. Icy coldness, one feet cold and the other hot. Thirst during stage of heat for warm drinks (vomits after taking cold drinks); worse 4 to 8 p.m.	Lycopodium 30 or 200	4 hourly
❑ Chill without thirst. Great heat (with thirst) yet patient cannot move or uncover, feels very chilly; better by warmth and after sweating	Nux vomica 30 or 200	4 hourly
☆ Paroxysms ever changing; chill at 4 p.m. without thirst; sweating worse left side;	Pulsatilla 30 or 200	4 hourly

Symptoms	Remedy	Frequency And Doses
feels very hot in bed, desires to uncover; thirst during stage of heat, licks the lips (with water) only; thirst during stage of sweat only		
❑ Dry exhausting cough an hour before chill and continues till chill lasts. Extreme chill and heat. Chill starts in thigh and between shoulders or over one scapula, small of back, running up spine. Restlessness, changing position constantly; urticarial rashes; better during sweat stage and by warmth	**Rhus tox. 30 or 200**	*4 hourly*
❑ Chill with clock like periodicity with pain in long bones; chill lasts for long - throughout day and night	**Aranea dia. 30 or 200**	*4 hourly*
❑ Paroxysms regular; at clock like periodicity (at same hour). Thirst during stage of heat for warm drinks; tearing pain and/or numbness in legs or whole body during stage of heat; eyes red	**Cedron 30 or 200**	*4 hourly*
❑ Thirst before chill; shivering and chilliness after every drink, chill starts in back and spreads over the whole body; after chill, heat without thirst and cold sweat	**Capsicum 30 or 200**	*4 hourly*
❑ Paroxysms irregular; chill with thirst, heat without thirst. Patient wants fanning instead of drinking water during heat stage; coldness of legs even after covering with blanket. Sweat profuse, sour and offensive	**Carbo veg. 30 or 200**	*4 hourly*
❑ Chronic, spoiled cases; paroxysm irregular; chill, heat, sweat all erratic. Fever followed by severe heat - making one almost senseless followed by profuse sweating. Feet cold and wet, shivering with thirst; worse in the evening	**Sepia 30 or 200**	*4 hourly*

Symptoms	Remedy	Frequency And Doses
● Intercurrent remedy. Chronic cases, when symptoms are not clear. Chill with shivering, without heat or thirst; palms and soles hot and burns	Sulphur 200	4 hourly (3)
❑ Fever worse at night; tongue thickly whitish coated. Desire for acids and pickles, etc., Patient desires to sleep; chill quite often with gastric complaints	Antim-crud. 30 or 200	6 hourly (6)
● Paroxysms irregular. During heat stage body is covered with boiling and offensive sweat	Psorinum 200 or 1M	10 min. (3)
❑ Chill begins in back; fever rises quickly, great heat with profuse sweat; fever do not come down with sweat. Restlessness. Fever and pulse improportionate	Pyrogenium 200 or 1M	10 min. (3)
Biochemic remedies	Kali phos. 6X, Natrum mur. 12X and Natrum sulph. 12X	4 hourly

Other Important Remedies:

Acid-fluor., Arnica, Caladium, Calcarea carb., Causticum, Chamomilla, Chelidonium, Cimex, Ferrum ars., Cina, Iodium, Malaria off., Nyctanthes ar., Stramonium, Verat-v., Wyethia, etc..

MAMMARY GLANDS
(Breast) Affections Of

❑ Undeveloped; with infantile uterus and ovaries. For proper growth of female organs	Pituitary g. 200	fortnightly (6)
☆ Breasts undeveloped and shrivelled; with infantile uterus and ovaries; general and sexual debility	Sabal ser. Q, 5-10 drops	4 hourly
☆ Breasts undeveloped with infantile uterus and ovaries; aching in breasts and itching of nipples	Onosmodium CM	monthly (3)

Symptoms	Remedy	Frequency And Doses
☆ Atrophy; mammae lax and shrunken, painful to touch.	Conium 200 or 1M	weekly (6)
☆ Atrophy; painful tumours, with undue secretion of milk. Very large breasts with tumor	Chimaphila Q or 30	4 hourly
❑ Abscess; fistula of mammary glands; stitching pain. Desire for cold drinks	Phosphorus 200	4 hourly (3)
❑ Eruptions on mammary glands; sensation of burning and pressure everywhere	Piper nig. 30	4 hourly
☆ Pain behind mammary glands; worse by heat; loss of thirst; desires cold open air	Pulsatilla 30 or 200	4 hourly
● Mammary glands sensitive; sharp, cutting pains in ovaries; worse at night	Syphilinum 200 or 1M	weekly (3)
❑ Soreness of mammary glands	Symphytum 6 or 30	4 hourly
❑ Ulceration of mammary glands; itching and burning	Paeonia Q or 6	4 hourly
❑ Pain between the space of breasts; below the mammary glands; sexual insomnia and gastric complaints	Raphanus 30 or 200	4 hourly
☆ Tumors of the breasts; hard and sensitive; when child nurses pain goes from nipple all over the body	Phytolacca 30 or 200	4 hourly
❑ Sinuses in mammary gland; chilly patient	Silicea 12X or 30	4 hourly

MANIA
(See Insanity Also)

An emotional disorder characterized by great psychomotor activity and excitement is called Mania.

❑ Patient moves constantly; can not sit at one place; uncontrollable laughter	Cannabis ind. 200 or 1M	10 min. (3)
❑ Abusing everyone; destructive, tears clothes; sings songs and loves music	Tarentula h. 200 or 1M	10 min. (3)

Symptoms	Remedy	Frequency And Doses
❑ After sexual excesses; with an exaggerated idea of one's own importance	**Phosphorus 200**	*10 min. (3)*
❑ After injury; fears to be touched or approached by anyone	**Arnica mont. 200**	*10 min. (3)*
❑ Due to sun stroke; great loquacity; worse after sleep	**Lachesis 200 or 1M**	*10 min. (3)*
● Intercurrent remedy; monomania; worse early morning	**Sulphur 200 or 1M**	*weekly (3)*
Biochemic remedy	**Kali phos. 6X**	*4 hourly*

MARASMUS
(See Emaciation Also)

Symptoms	Remedy	Frequency And Doses
☆ Marked emaciation of legs; ascending muscles; neck weak, can not hold the head; flabby, loose skin; better when diarrhoea occurs	**Abrotanum 30 or 200**	*6 hourly (3)*
☆ Marked emaciation of neck; dehydration; constipation; desire for extra salt	**Natrum mur. 30 or 200**	*4 hourly*
❑ Emaciation with good appetite; weakness after physical or mental exertion	**Acid-picric. 30**	*4 hourly*
☆ Emaciation with glandular swelling and enlargement of abdomen; nature shy	**Baryta carb. 200 or 1M**	*weekly (3)*
❑ Though eats well but emaciates; joints swollen and deformed	**Iodium 30 or 200**	*4 hourly*
● Intercurrent remedy; when there is tubercular family history; susceptible to changes of weather	**Tuberculinum 200 or 1M**	*weekly (3)*
❑ Emaciation of children; mentally deficient; excitable and nervous	**Ambra gr. 30 or 200**	*4 hourly*
☆ Progressive emaciation; craves for sweets which do not suit; much flatulence	**Argentum nit. 30 or 200**	*4 hourly*

Symptoms	Remedy	Frequency And Doses
❏ Rapid emaciation; diarrhoea soon after drinking or eating anything; burning in stomach	**Arsenic alb. 30**	*4 hourly*
☆ Emaciation of neck and face; much flatulence; desires sweets and hot drinks	**Lycopodium 30 or 200**	*4 hourly*
❏ Emaciation; can not digest milk though desires it; craves for meat	**Magnesia carb. 30 or 200**	*4 hourly*
❏ Emaciation due to defective assimilation; offensive foot sweat chilly patient	**Silicea 30 or 200**	*4 hourly*
❏ In bottle fed babies	**Natrum phos. 6X or 30**	*4 hourly*
Biochemic remedies	**Calcarea phos. 6X and Natrum mur. 12X**	*4 hourly*

MASTOID PROCESS

Symptoms	Remedy	Frequency And Doses
☆ Inflammatory stage; affected part red and hot	**Belladonna 30 or 200**	*4 hourly*
☆ Pain and swelling with threatening deep - seated abscess and caries of mastoid	**Capsicum 30** *in acute cases and higher potencies in chronic cases*	*3 hourly (6)*
❏ In diabetic patients; to check destructive processes	**Acid-fluor. 30 or 200**	*6 hourly*
☆ Inflammation and swelling of left side or starting in left side; tearing, gnawing pain; worse at night	**Mercurius bin iod. 3X**	*3 hourly*
☆ Painful inflammation, very sensitive to external impressions, touch and cold air; splinter like pain	**Hepar sulph. 30 or 200**	*4 hourly*
❏ Swelling which is painful on touch with drawing pain; sticking on swallowing and cough	**Silicea 30 or 200**	*4 hourly*
● Intercurrent remedy	**Sulphur 200 or 1M**	*weekly (3)*
Biochemic remedy	**Calcarea sulph. 6X**	*4 hourly*

Symptoms	Remedy	Frequency And Doses

MASTURBATION
Male

Fulfilment of sexual desire by artificial means is called masturbation. The after effects are very serious.

❑ Habit of masturbation during sleep; superiority complex — **Platina 1M** — *fortnightly (3)*

☆ Excessive desire to masturbate; after self-abuse, depression of spirits; fatigue with nervous weakness. Sexual power diminished — **Calcarea carb. 200 or 1M** — *weekly (3)*

❑ Weakness from masturbation due to excessive semen loss; pale, sickly expression; face pale and sallow; eyes sunken and surrounded by blue and dark margins; perspiration profuse and debilitating; sweats easily on least exertion — **China off. 6 or 30** — *4 hourly*

❑ Patient feels fatigued or un-refreshed in the morning on waking; constipated and chilly patient — **Nux vomica 200 or 1M** — *6 hourly*

☆ Chronic cases of masturbation. Face sunken; guilty look, abashed facial expression; loss of memory and sadness; hypochondriasis; nocturnal emissions; backache; legs weak — **Staphysagria 200 or 1M** — *weekly (3)*

● Intercurrent remedy; sexual thoughts and inclination to masturbate — **Sulphur 200 or 1M** — *fortnightly (3)*

● Bad effects of masturbation; impotency and unsteady gait; cannot stand erect, legs weak; drowsiness. Intellectual faculties greatly impaired. Memory absolutely lost — **Kali brom. 30** — *4 hourly*

❑ Weakness and weariness; nervous debility and trembling. Distressed by the culpability of his habit of masturbation — **Phosphorus 200 or 1M** — *weekly (3)*

☆ Uncontrolable desire for self-abuse; bad effects and weakness of pre-pubic masturbation. Patient grows too fast and too tall — **Phosphoric acid. 6 or 30** — *4 hourly*

Symptoms	Remedy	Frequency And Doses
❏ Bad effects of masturbation; tired and heavy feeling all over the body, especially of limbs. Brain fag, mentally and physically exhausted	Picric-acid. 30	4 hourly
Biochemic remedies	Calcarea phos. 30X and Natrum mur. 12X	4 hourly

MASTURBATION
Female

Symptoms	Remedy	Frequency And Doses
☆ Masturbation; resulting in leucorrhoea and hysterical disturbances; shy and timid patient	Pulsatilla 200 or 1M	weekly (3)
☆ Habit of masturbation due to excessive sexual desire	Origanum 30 or 200	6 hourly
☆ Habit of masturbation due to itching of vulva and vagina	Caladium s. 30 or 200	2 hours
❏ To remove the bad effects of excessive masturbation; sexual melancholia; guilty look on face	Staphysagria 3o or 200	4 hourly
❏ Sexual melancholia due to habit of masturbation; voluptuous crawling extending up in abdomen; superiority complex	Platina 200 or 1M	weekly (3)
❏ Habit of masturbation due to pruritus of vulva; worse at night; better during menstruation	Zincum met. 30	4 hourly
❏ Habit of masturbation due to pruritus of vulva; vagina dry and sore; sadness in mind	Natrum mur. 30 or 200	4 hourly
● Masturbation due to itching of clitoris; sexual thoughts	Sulphur 200 or 1M	4 hourly (3)
Biochemic remedies	Calcarea phos. 30X and Natrum mur. 12X	4 hourly

Other Important Remedies:

Acid-phos., Phosphorus, Lachesis, Gelsemium, and Tuberculinum, etc..

Symptoms	Remedy	Frequency And Doses

MEASLES

It is a viral, infectious disease with symptoms of acute coryza, watering of eyes, sore throat, cough, chilly feeling, fever and rash. As the rash appears the fever may rise upto 105°F with lachrymation and photophobia. The symptoms may last from 4-8 days. Pneumonia and capillary bronchitis may occur if the case is not managed properly.

Symptoms	Remedy	Frequency And Doses
❏ Prophylactic remedy	**Morbillinum 200**	*10 min. (3)*
☆ High fever with catarrh; conjunctiva red; dry cough; rash with burning. Restlessness and anxiety	**Aconite 30 or 200**	*3 hourly*
☆ Profuse lachrymation; thirstlessness with dryness of mouth; better in open cold air	**Pulsatilla 30 or 200**	*4 hourly (3)*
☆ Fever with restlessness; triangular tip of tongue red; better by movements	**Rhus tox. 30 or 200**	*4 hourly*
❏ Rattling in the chest, dyspnoea, loose cough with difficult expectoration; tongue whitish coated	**Antim-tart. 30 or 200**	*10 min. (3)*
☆ Rash bright red; skin hot and dry; congestion and rush of blood towards head; sore throat	**Belladonna 30**	*3 hourly*
☆ Dry, hard cough with stitching pain in chest. Drowsy, mild delirium; tongue coated, lips dry; stools constipated. Thirst for large quantities of water; worse by movements	**Bryonia 30 or 200**	*4 hourly (3)*
❏ High fever; kicks the coverings; eyes sore, tearful and irritable; loss of thirst; better by cold	**Apis mel. 30 or 200**	*4 hourly (3)*
❏ Hot, burning tears from eyes with photophobia; bland discharge from nose and throbbing headache	**Euphrasia 30**	*4 hourly*
☆ Chill and heat alternate; restlessness, drowsy and stupid; better passing urine	**Gelsemium 30**	*4 hourly*
❏ Croupy cough with rattling in the chest. Oversensitive to touch, cold, air, etc.	**Hepar sulph. 30/or 200**	*3 hourly*

Symptoms	Remedy	Frequency And Doses
❑ Measles with purulent, stringy, ropy discharge from eyes and ears	**Kali bich. 30**	*4 hourly*
❑ Exhaustive, dry cough with desire to vomit. Tightness in chest cannot lie on left side; craves for icy, cold drinks	**Phosphorus 30 or 200**	*4 hourly (3)*
Biochemic Remedies	**Ferrum phos. 6X** and **Kali mur. 6X**	*3 hourly*

MENINGITIS

The inflammation of the membranes of the brain or spinal cord is called meningitis. It may be due to trauma or various kinds of infections due to micro - organisms like meningococci, pneumococci, staphylococci; various kinds of bacillus, tubercle and viral infections and syphilitic origin, etc.. The onset is usually sudden with severe headache and high fever, vomiting and rigors may be in the beginning, on 2nd or 3rd day along with high fever, backache, pain in limbs and intense headache is present and often the stiffness of neck passes on to rigidity with dilation of pupils and intolerable headache, delirium, photophobia and restlessness, etc., develops. The symptoms gradually move towards fatal end.

❑ Head, neck or spine bends backwards in cerebro-spinal meningitis	**Cicuta v. 30**	*4 hourly*

In homoeopathy constitutional treatment gives good results: **Aconitum nap., Apis mel., Arnica mont., Belladonna, Bryonia, Calcarea carb., Cuprum met., Eupatorium perf., Glonoine, Helleborus, Natrum-sulph., Sulphur, Syphilinum, Tuberculinum, Zincum** met., etc., are the main remedies.

The treatment of the sick should be timely and hospitalization should be preferred.

MENOPAUSE
Change of Life

● Aversion to bathing; tiresome, loosing weight; hot and itchy feeling	**Sulphur 200**	*4 hourly (3)*
☆ Melancholic, irritable and talkative patient. Burning sensation all over the body. Cannot bear touch even of clothes. Dark coloured haemorrhage. Distressing headache, palpitation and haemorrhoids. Worse after sleep	**Lachesis 200 or 1M**	*weekly (3)*

Symptoms	Remedy	Frequency And Doses
❑ Weeping disposition; changeable temper. Hot perspiration in close and warm room; loss of thirst; desire for open, cold air	**Pulsatilla 200 or 1M**	*weekly (3)*
❑ Tired feeling due to over work; pale, flabby, relaxed and chilly patient	**Calcarea carb. 200 or 1M**	*weekly (3)*
❑ Tall, thin, easily depressed patient; dislikes sympathy. Bearing down pains, haemorrhage with prolapsus of uterus; leucorrhoea with dyspepsia or constipation. Hot flushes; tendency to faint	**Sepia 200 or 1M**	*weekly (3)*
❑ Small bones painful in morning with acidity; dirty coated tongue; filthy taste and bad breath; pallor and chilliness; worse in cold wet weather. Facial neuralgia due to suppression of leucorrhoea; better sea side	**Medorrhinum 200 or 1M**	*weekly (3)*
❑ Rheumatism of muscles of the back and soreness of neck. Violent headache, patient feels as if the top of head is torn off	**Actaea racemosa 30**	*4 hourly*
☆ Physical symptoms disappear as mental symptoms develop. Arrogant and proud patient; contempt for others. Excessive bleeding of dark clotted blood with pain in ovaries. Nymphomania	**Platina 200 or 1M**	*weekly (3)*
Biochemic remedy	**Kali phos. 6X**	*4 hourly*

MENSTRUATION
Affections Of
Including Dysmenorrhoea, Etc.

☆ Dark; clotted; copious or scanty menses; during day time only; 1st menses delayed and painful; intermittent and irregular; changing moods; likes open air	**Pulsatilla 30 or 200**	*4 hourly*

Symptoms	Remedy	Frequency And Doses
☆ Early and profuse; copious; during night, on lying down; frequently; intermittent; painful	Kreosote 30 or 200	3 hourly (3)
❑ Menses dark; acrid, excoriating; during night only, after lying down	Bovista 30 or 200	4 hourly
❑ Copious and dark; worse after injury	Hamamellis 30	3 hourly (3)
❑ Dark; clotted, painful and frequent, due to displaced uterus; during night only	Trillium p. Q or 6	3 hourly
● Copious; gushing and frequent; worse after exertion, every 2 weeks or every few days; lasting for a week or more	Medorrhinum 200 or 1M	monthly (3)
❑ Copious; offensive, clotted and painful, due to uterine fibroid; difficult to wash	Platina 200 or 1M	3 hourly (3)
❑ Menses bright red; copious, clotted, painful and frequent; worse during menopause; walking ameliorates; history of abortion	Sabina 30 or 200	6 hourly
❑ Menses bright red, mingled with dark clots; offensive	Belladonna 30	4 hourly
❑ Menses bright red, gushing; nausea or vomiting, clean tongue	Ipecac 30	4 hourly
☆ Menses bright red, copious and frequent	Millefolium Q or 30	4 hourly
❑ Menses bright red; vicarious; patient desires icy cold water	Phosphorus 30 or 200	4 hourly (3)
❑ Menses acrid; excoriating; copious after miscarriage; frequent; intermittent	China 6 or 30	4 hourly
❑ Menses copious; continues upto next period; dark and clotted; irregular	Secale cor. 30	4 hourly
❑ Menses profuse and early; copious with dark clots and abdominal distention	Nux vomica 30 or 200	6 hourly
❑ Early and excessive; bright red, long lasting with backache; copious; worse after exertion; early in young girls lasting for long; late in adults	Calc-phos. 12X or 30	3 hourly (3)
● Copious; lasting a week or more, frequent, every 2 weeks; intermittent	Sulphur 200 or 1M	4 hourly (3)

Symptoms	Remedy	Frequency And Doses
❏ Amenorrhoea; dark clotted blood; copious, frequent, delayed, first menses delayed; exhausting, pale, thin blood	**Ferrum met. 3X or 6**	*4 hourly*
☆ Irregular; painful, delayed or frequent; worse after exertion	**Sepia 30 or 200**	*3 hourly (3)*
☆ Early; profuse and frequent; every 2 weeks; during lactation; lasting a week or more; returns after excitement; suppressed after working in water or becoming wet	**Calcarea carb. 200 or 1M**	*3 hourly (3)*
❏ Menses copious; dark, frequent, intermittent and irregular; during day time only; offensive, painful and thick	**Lilium tig. 30 or 200**	*4 hourly (3)*
❏ Menstrual flow suppressed after fright or shock; in plethoric young girls; menses profuse with nose bleed; late; marked fear and restlessness	**Aconite 30 or 200**	*3 hourly*
❏ Menses frequent and copious; offensive; passive bleeding	**Helonias Q or 6**	*4 hourly*
☆ All complaints better during menstruation; copious or scanty; painful for very short period only; dark, lumpy and black	**Lachesis 200 or 1M**	*3 hourly (3)*
❏ Copious; worse after injury or coition; bruised pains	**Arnica 200 or 1M**	*3 hourly (3)*
❏ Menses copious; late or suppressed; worse while sitting; feels better after flow starts	**Zincum met. 30 or 200**	*3 hourly (3)*
❏ Dark; clotted, stringy, offensive, painful and frequent; worse from least movements	**Crocus sat. Q or 6**	*4 hourly*
☆ Delayed; especially first menses; irregular, painful, pale and scanty; stools constipated	**Graphites 30 or 200**	*3 hourly (3)*
❏ Delayed and painful; flow aggravates the complaints; neuralgic, rheumatic pain; scanty or suppressed due to emotions or fever	**Actaea race. 30 or 200**	*4 hourly (3)*
☆ Delayed; scanty; stopped due to cold; putting hands in cold water, due to cold;	**Conium mac. 200 or 1M**	*3 hourly (3)*

Symptoms	Remedy	Frequency And Doses
breasts become enlarged, sore and painful during menstrual cycle		
❑ Delayed or stopped; by putting hands in cold water; suppressed after drinking milk	**Lac-def. 200**	*3 hourly (3)*
❑ Early or delayed; exhausting, scanty or profuse; stools hard and constipated; haemorrhage between periods	**Thlaspi b-p. Q or 6**	*4 hourly*
❑ Copious; alternate periods more profuse; frequent and painful; very slight (Ist day-only), second day with vomiting; menstrual colic with large clots	**Cyclamen 30**	*4 hourly*
❑ Painful and scanty; increases while sitting and less while walking	**Alumina 30 or 0/5** (50 millesimal)	*4 hourly*
☆ Menses with neuralgic pain; dysmen-orrhoea with pains flying to other parts of the oody	**Caulophyllum 30 or 200**	*4 hourly (3)*
❑ Early; dark and stringy with neuralgic pain; better after flow starts; menstrual colic; membranous dysmenorrhoea	**Magnesia phos. 12X or 30**	*3 hourly*
❑ Menses lasts for long; thick and dark; irregular	**Nux mosch. 200**	*3 hourly (3)*
❑ Early and profuse; menses returns after over exertion; long walk, passing hard stools, etc.; discharge of blood between periods	**Ambra gr. 200**	*3 hourly (3)*
❑ Painful; only for one day or one hour; late and scanty; Amenorrhoea with ophthalmia	**Euphrasia 30 or 200**	*4 hourly*
❑ Menses appears only for one day; scanty, pain in stomach and small of back during menstruation	**Baryta carb. 200**	*4 hourly (3)*
❑ Clotted; stringy, passive and bright red; profuse after miscarriage; worse after slightest provocation	**Ustilago Q or 6**	*4 hourly*
❑ Early and profuse; suppressed after bathing in river or swimming pool; tongue thickly whitish coated	**Antim-crud. 200**	*4 hourly (3)*

Symptoms	Remedy	Frequency And Doses
☆ Suppressed with colic; better bending double and by hard pressure	Colocynth. 200	3 hourly (3)
❑ Acrid, early, profuse and prolonged; suppressed after getting feet wet	Rhus tox. 200 or 1M	3 hourly (3)
❑ Early and profuse; epistaxis instead of menses; worse by motion	Bryonia 30 or 200	4 hourly
❑ Totally exhausted during menstruation, can hardly speak; lasting for long, though not profuse	Carbo an. 200	3 hourly (3)
❑ Menses early or late; scanty or profuse; pale with soreness about genitals; pain from back passes down through left labium	Kali carb. 200 or 1M	3 hourly (3)
❑ Gushing, exhausting with colic as from sharp stones rubbing together; irregular and painful	Cocculus ind. 30 or 200	4 hourly
❑ Scanty; early or delayed; clots of black blood; menstrual flow aggravates all the complaints	Thuja oc. 200 or 1M	3 hourly (3)
❑ Frequent; early or delayed; during day time only; no menses at night; scanty and offensive	Causticum 200 or 1M	3 hourly (3)
❑ Frequent and gushing; membranous; painful and stringy; breasts swollen and painful before menses and better afterwards; excessive menstruation; discharge of bloody mucous after menses at the time of new moon	Lac-can. 200 or 1M	3 hourly (3)
❑ Menses during lactation period; while nursing the child	Silicea 200 or 1M	3 hourly (3)
☆ Membranous; early and profuse, with griping in abdomen; nausea and pain in stomach extending to small of back	Borax 30	4 hourly
❑ Early with thick and strong odour; offensive; premature and too copious	Carbo veg. 30 or 200	3 hourly (3)

Symptoms	Remedy	Frequency And Doses
● Menses offensive; vicarious; mammae swollen and painful	**Psorinum 200 or 1M**	*monthly (3)*
❑ Menses painful; suppressed; colic before the appearance of discharge	**Verat-vir. 30 or 200**	*4 hourly (3)*
❑ Dysmenorrhoea; menses usually delayed	**Pneumococcus 30 or 200**	*3 hourly (3)*

MENTAL DERANGEMENT
(See Insanity And Mania Also)

Symptoms	Remedy	Frequency And Doses
❑ Never laughs or smiles; variable mood. Suicidal tendency after seeing a knife or blood	**Alumina 200 or 1M**	*10 min. (3)*
❑ Feels happy at others misfortune; fastidious; oversensitive to disorders; wants things in proper order	**Arsenic alb. 200 or 1M**	*10 min. (3)*
❑ Lively music make the patient sad; complaints due to head injury	**Natrum sulph. 200 or 1M**	*10 min. (3)*
❑ Child weeps without tears; violent outbursts of passion; dwells on sexual matters; guilty look	**Staphysagria 200 or 1M**	*10 min. (3)*
❑ Music causes weeping and trembling; feels as if soul and body were separate	**Thuja oc. 200 or 1M**	*10 min. (3)*
❑ Irritable; always talks about business	**Bryonia 200 or 1M**	*10 min. (3)*
❑ Mild, gentle yielding, weeping; easily discouraged; religious melancholy; loss of thirst; likes cold, open air	**Pulsatilla 200 or 1M**	*10 min. (3)*
❑ Ever changing moods; sighing and sobbing; complaints after disappointments	**Ignatia 1M or 10M**	*10 min. (3)*
❑ Lack of natural affection; aversion to loved ones, even to husband and children	**Sepia 200 or 1M**	*10 min. (3)*
❑ Suicidal thoughts with no love of life; feeling of worthlessness	**Aurum met. 200 or 1M**	*10 min. (3)*

Symptoms	Remedy	Frequency And Doses
❑ Rapid alternation of mental condition; hysterical laughter and pleasant mania	Crocus sat. 200 or 1M	10 min. (3)
❑ Anxiety and inferiority complex; fear of being alone; spells or writes wrong words	Lycopodium 200 or 1M	10 min. (3)
❑ Mania due to suppressed neuralgia; dreams of impending evil	Actaea race. 200 or 1M	10 min. (3)
● Intercurrent remedy	Sulphur 200 or 1M	fortnightly (3)
Biochemic remedy	Kali phos. 6X	4 hourly

METRITIS
Inflammation Of The Uterus

❑ Due to excessive blood loss from uterus; restlessness and exhaustion	Arsenic alb. 30	4 hourly (6)
☆ After miscarriage; oversensitive to least jar; face flushed	Belladonna 30 or 200	4 hourly
☆ After premature labor or abortion. Pain from sacrum to pubis and from below upwards shooting up to the vagina	Sabina 30 or 200	4 hourly (3)
❑ With throbbing pain and over-sensitivity to pain; pressure, cold, etc.	Hepar sulph. 30	4 hourly
❑ With burning pain and swelling; puerperal metritis with cystits	Cantharis 30	4 hourly

Other Important Remedies:

Hydrastis c., Lac can., Lachesis, Aur-mur., Lilium tig. and Nux vomica, etc..

METRORRHAGIA
(See Miscarriage Also)

Uterine haemorrhage other than at the menstrual periods.

☆ Caused by a fall; blood blackish; occuring	Hamamellis Q or 30	3 hourly

Symptoms	Remedy	Frequency And Doses
between menstrual periods; soreness in abdomen		
❑ After miscarriage, haemorrhage in spells, coagulated; fits because of severe pains	**Chamomilla 30 or 200**	*3 hourly (3)*
☆ Due to threatened abortion in the 3rd month; sudden, while there is no other health problem	**Kreosote 30 or 200**	*3 hourly (3)*
❑ Due to prolapsus of uterus; after coition; due to mechanical injury	**Arnica 30 or 200**	*3 hourly (3)*
❑ Chronic haemorrhage; worse before or after an abortion	**Lycopodium 30 or 200**	*4 hourly (3)*
❑ In chilly, fat and flabby patients; threatened abortion	**Calcarea carb. 200 or 1M**	*4 hourly (3)*
❑ Blood bright red; continues for long; nausea or vomiting with clean tongue	**Ipecac Q or 30**	*4 hourly*
❑ With induration of uterus; labor like pains; followed by great exhaustion	**Carbo an. 30**	*4 hourly*
☆ Painful; due to over-exertion; profuse bleeding, like muddy water	**Acid-nit. 30 or 200**	*4 hourly (3)*
❑ During pregnancy; thirstlessness, hot feeling and stinging pain	**Apis mel. 30 or 200**	*4 hourly (3)*
☆ During pregnancy; due to lack of sleep; clotted blood with spasmodic colic	**Cocculus ind. 30**	*4 hourly*
☆ Blood profuse; thin, blackish, prolonged, continuous oozing of watery blood	**Secale cor. 30 or 200**	*4 hourly (3)*
Biochemic remedies	**Calcarea phos. 6X and Ferrum phos. 3X**	*4 hourly*

MIASMS

There are three miasms in homoeopathy which are the root cause for every chronic disease. They are **Psora, Syphilis** and **Sycosis**. We are not giving the details here as the subject is very wide and requires a separate book.

MIGRAINE
(See Headache Also)

As migraine is very troublesome disease, so we are giving the symptoms in detail.

Symptoms	Remedy	Frequency And Doses
☆ From mental work; cold, uncovering head, pressure, sitting upright or sun-stroke	Glonoinum 30	3 hourly
☆ For nervous; gastric, bilious individuals. Migraine due to mental over-exertion in teachers and students. Right sided, especially Sunday migraine, blurred vision, hemiopia; blindness; often burning pain in entire gastro - intestinal tract with violent acid vomiting at the height of the attack; worse hot weather, spring and fall; better after vomiting or sufficient night sleep	Iris v. 200 or above	10 min. (3)
❑ For irritable hypochondriacs of bad temper; cholerics, neuropathics; from abuse of alcohol, coffee, spices, tobacco, vexation and worry, mental over exertion, business worries, sexual excesses, sedentary habits and cold dry air and winds	Nux vomica 30 or 200	4 hourly
☆ For pronounced vasomotor individuals (irritable and full of fear) during pre-climacteric and menopausal stage. Tired expression, head congestion, circumscribed red cheeks; pain above right eye, throbbing, stitching, rhythmic pain, often every 8 days; early morning, beginning in nape, extending upwards, locating in region of eye; rising and falling with the sun; sensation of severe congestion	Sanguinaria c. 200	10 min. (3)
❑ For weak, fat and irritable patients; often apathetic, changing moods, strange changes of character (egocenteric); memory weak, due to disturbance during climacteric period, results of tobacco abuse.	Sepia 200	10 min. (3)

Symptoms	Remedy	Frequency And Doses
Persons with shallow complexion, yellow saddle across the nose; pain located on left temple; throbbing, stitching pains		
☆ For neuropathic persons, full of fear caused by noises, change of weather or worms; with pale face; located above left eye; especially left pupil (ciliary neuralgia); sharp, shooting, tearing, stitching, periodical pain from occiput to left eye; slowly rising in intensity with sun. Bile vomiting at height of attack slowly improving with setting sun. Feeling as if head were open along sagittal suture	**Spigelia 200 or 1M**	*10 min. (3)*
☆ Left sided; worse during and after sleep; before menstruation; heat; during menopause	**Lachesis 200 or 1M**	*10 min. (3)*
● Intercurrent remedy	**Bacillinum 200 or 1M**	*fortnightly (3)*

Other Important Remedies:

Belladonna, Bryonia alb., Carbo veg., Natrum mur., Syphilinum, Sulphur, Thuja oc., Phosphorus and Medorrhinum, etc..

MORNING SICKNESS
Vomiting, etc., During Pregnancy
(See Travel Sickness and Vomiting, Etc., Also)

☆ Persistent vomiting with gastric disturbances; nausea, bitter taste and constipation	**Symph-race. 30**	*4 hourly*
☆ Worse after lying down; tongue clean; nausea; mouth moist with saliva	**Ipecac 30**	*3 hourly*
❑ Flatulence and coated tongue; vomiting; worse morning and after eating	**Nux vomica 30**	*4 hourly*
❑ Worse sight of water; water is thrown up as soon as it gets warm in the stomach	**Phosphorus 30 or 200**	*10 min. (3)*
☆ Obstinate vomiting; constant nausea and	**Lac vac-def. 30**	*4 hourly*

Symptoms	Remedy	Frequency And Doses
vomiting with restlessness	**Arsenic alb. 30 or 200**	*4 hourly (3)*
☆ With frequent and unquenchable thirst; restlessness; vomiting worse after eating or drinking	**Lobelia inf. 6 or 30**	*4 hourly*
❑ Extreme nausea and vomiting; faintness and weakness at epigastrium		
Biochemic remedies	**Ferrum phos. 6X, Natrum mur. 12X** and **Natrum phos. 6X**	*4 hourly*

MOUTH ULCERS
(See Aphthae Also)

☆ Small ulcers of the aphthous type; bleed if touched; mouth hot and tender	**Borax 6 or 30**	*4 hourly*
☆ Excessive salivation; spongy gums which bleed easily; sweetish metallic taste in the mouth; thirst with moist mouth	**Merc-sol. 6 or 30**	*4 hourly*
☆ Aphthae with rush of blood towards head	**Belladonna 30**	*4 hourly*
❑ Small blisters or extremely sensitive ulcers; better holding cold fluids in the mouth	**Natrum sulph. 12X or 30**	*4 hourly*
❑ Ulcers are accompanied by sharp splinter like pains; acrid and offensive salivation	**Nitric acid. 30**	*4 hourly*
Biochemic remedies	**Ferrum phos. 6X, Kali mur. 6X** and **Natrum phos. 6X**	*4 hourly*

MUMPS
(See Fever Also)

☆ When affected lesion is hard and painful; skin pale; shooting pain into ears on swallowing	**Phytolacca d. 30 or 200**	*4 hourly (6)*

Symptoms	Remedy	Frequency And Doses
☆ When ear is effected and painful; worse by heat, better open cold air; loss of thirst	Pulsatilla 30 or 200	4 hourly (6)
☆ *Preventive remedy*; also to start the treatment	Parotidinum 200 or 1M	1 dose
☆ ·Swelling and inflammation with fever; restlessness; triangular tip of tongue red	Rhus tox. 30 or 200	4 hourly (6)
❑ Flushed face and neck with sweating	Pilocar-mur. 3X or 6	4 hourly
❑ Sudden onset; after exposure to dry cold winds; fever with anxiety and fear	Aconite 30 or 200	4 hourly
☆ Swelling bright red and hot; stitching pain extending into ears; face flushed	Belladonna 30 or 200	4 hourly
☆ Swelling pale; tongue flabby, moist with marks of teeth; excessive salivation with thirst	Merc-sol. 30 or 200	4 hourly (6)
❑ Associated with fever; measles, small pox, etc.; unbearable pain; anxiety, restlessness and unquenchable thirst, drinks little at a time but frequently	Arsenic alb. 30 or 200	4 hourly (3)
☆ When swelling becomes of purplish colour; intense swelling, very painful	Lachesis 30 or 200	4 hourly (3)
❑ ·When swelling becomes harder; patient desires fresh air, fanning	Carbo veg. 30	4 hourly
Biochemic remedies	Ferrum phos. 6X and Kali mur. 6X	4 hourly

MYOPIA
Shortness of Sight

It is a condition in which in consequence of an error in refraction or of elongation of the globe of the eye parallel rays are focussed in front of the retina.

Important Remedies:

Conium mac., Lilium tig., Phosphorus, Phosphoric acid., Physostigma, Pulsatilla, Calcarea carb., China off., Nitric acid., Agaricus m., Carbo- sulph., etc..

NAILS
Affections Of

Symptoms	Remedy	Frequency And Doses
❏ Nails uneven; corrugated and spotted	**Calcarea carb. 200 or 1M**	*weekly (6)*
☆ Finger or toe nails become thick; brittle, black, and fall off	**Graphites 30 or 200**	*6 hourly*
❏ Nails grow too fast; deformed, uneven, become brittle, and break easily	**Acid-fluor. 30 or 200**	*6 hourly*
☆ Nails become waxy; distorted, soft and brittle	**Thuja oc. 200 or 1M**	*weekly (6)*
❏ Nails become shrivelled and brittle	**Ambra gr. 30 or 200**	*6 hourly*
❏ Nails become discoloured and distorted	**Natrum ars. 30 or 200**	*6 hourly*
❏ Nails become loose; painful, over sensitive	**Hepar sulph. 30 or 200**	*4 hourly*
❏ Root of nails painful; general weakness and anaemia	**Calcarea phos. 6X or 30**	*4 hourly*
❏ Nails and hair unhealthy; sensitive to least touch	**Magnesia carb. 30**	*6 hourly*
☆ Finger nails painful with swelling and pain of phalanges	**Myristica seb. 3X or 6**	*3 hourly*
❏ Nails painful; grows into the flesh	**Magnetis pol-australis 30**	*6 hourly*
☆ Nails grow slowly; better in humid climate	**Causticum 30 or 200**	*6 hourly*
❏ Cold and blue nails; painful, chilblains of toes	**Acid-nitric. 30 or 200**	*6 hourly*
☆ Crippled nails; white spots on nails, ingrowing toe nails; affections of finger nails	**Silicea 12X or 30**	*6 hourly*
❏ Falling of nails; vesicular eruption between finger and toes	**Helleborus 30 or 200**	*6 hourly*
Biochemic remedies	**Natrum mur. 12X** and **Silicea 30X**	*4 hourly*

Symptoms	Remedy	Frequency And Doses

NAUSEA

Symptoms	Remedy	Frequency And Doses
❑ Relieved by eating; especially in pale, anaemic women	**Lactic-acid. 30**	*3 hourly*
☆ Nausea; worse at smell or sight of food, lying on side, in morning before eating	**Sepia 30 or 200**	*3 hourly (3)*
☆ Nausea with vertigo; when closing eyes, least motion, due to spondilosis	**Theridion 30**	*3 hourly*
☆ Deathly nausea; worse opening the eyes; least motion, smell of tobacco smoke	**Tabacum 30 or 200**	*3 hourly (3)*
❑ On looking upward with thirstlessness; worse in a warm room; better in cold, open air	**Pulsatilla 30 or 200**	*3 hourly*
❑ After abdominal operation; patient craves for tobacco	**Staphysagria 30 or 200**	*3 hourly (3)*
☆ Nausea with vomiting; worse after eating or drinking; due to food poisoning; restlessness	**Arsenic alb. 30**	*3 hourly*
❑ During pregnancy, worse in the morning, with weak digestion	**Carbo veg. 30**	*3 hourly*
❑ Nausea with vomiting in the morning; after eating; wants to vomit but can not	**Nux vomica 30**	*3 hourly*
☆ Constant nausea with clean and moist tongue	**Ipecac 30**	*3 hourly*
Biochemic remedy	**Silicea 30X**	*3 hourly*

In acute stage above remedies can be given 1/2 hourly.

NEPHRITIS
Inflammation Of The Kidneys
(See Kidney Affections Also)

Symptoms	Remedy	Frequency And Doses
❑ Nephritis due to any acute disease with constant tenesmus	**Terebinth. Q,** *5-6 drops*	*3 hourly*

Symptoms	Remedy	Frequency And Doses
☆ Acute nephritis with threatening uraemia. Albumin and renal elements in the urine. In heart diseases, the kidneys previously working well suddenly becomes affected	**Eel serum 30**	*4 hourly*
❑ In initial stage; with sharp cutting pains in the region of kidney after exposure	**Aconite nap. 30 or 200**	*2 hourly*
● With soreness in the region of kidney (intercurrent remedy)	**Medorrhinum 200 or 1M**	*fortnightly (3)*
❑ Shooting pains; extending to the bladder with heat and distension in the region of the kidneys; urine red in colour	**Belladonna 30 or 200**	*3 hourly*
☆ With burning; dragging, aching, and smarting pain as if from excoriation extending from the region of kidneys towards the groin; difficult urination	**Cannabis sat. 200 or 1M**	*10 min. (3)*
☆ With cutting pain; tenesmus, and severe burning; urine comes in drops mixed with blood or complete suppression of urine	**Cantharis 30 or 200**	*4 hourly (3)*
❑ With sharp, stitching pains; involuntary urination during coughing or sneezing, etc.	**Kali carb. 30 or 200**	*4 hourly (3)*
☆ Region of kidney tender; pain radiating from kidneys to abdomen, bladder, and lower extremities. Urine contains albumin, mucous and phosphoric acid	**Solidago Q** *4-5 drops*	*4 hourly*
❑ Due to mechanical injuries; such as continuous or severe concussions	**Arnica 30 or 200**	*4 hourly*
☆ Excessive nausea with extreme distension of abdomen; scanty, painful urination. Urine bright red; contains decomposed blood, albumin and sugar	**Colchicum 30**	*4 hourly*
❑ In chronic cases when there is induration of the glands; patient oversensitive to pain and cold, etc.	**Hepar sulph. 30 or higher**	*4 hourly*
❑ When there is diarrhoea and tenesmus with induration of glands; urine dark, scanty, bloody and albuminous	**Mercurius viv. 30**	*4 hourly*

Symptoms	Remedy	Frequency And Doses
❏ When the complication is after suppression of haemorrhoidal discharge; sedentary habits and excess of stimulants; constipation; drawing up of testes and spermatic cord	Nux vomica 30	4 hourly
☆ Due to suppression of menses; urine dribbles while coughing or sneezing; worse after lying down	Pulsatilla 30	4 hourly
☆ Due to loss of sleep; night watching; in nursing women	Cocculus ind. 30	4 hourly
❏ With excessive thirst; restlessness and exhaustion; urine contains albumin, epithelial cells, fibrin, pus and blood, etc.	Arsenic alb. 30	4 hourly
Biochemic remedies	Ferrum phos. 6X and Kali mur. 6X	4 hourly

NERVOUSNESS
(See Anxiety Also)

☆ With anxiety; better after eating	Anacardium or. 30 or 200	4 hourly
❏ With acute anxiety; extreme impatience, fears; intolerance of pain, music and least noise; confusion of mind; thoughts and ideas chase one another	Aconite 30 or 200	3 hourly
☆ Due to worries about coming events; fear of heights, of crowds, of closed places, of water; examination funk, etc.	Argentum nit. 30 or 200	3 hourly (3)
❏ Due to after effects of grief or worry; patient unhappy, inclined to tears, hopeless; jumps at least noise; critical to others, forgetful; very sympathetic	Causticum 200	3 hourly (3)
❏ With bad temperament; extreme restlessness; nothing pleases, intolerance to everything	Chamomilla 200	3 hourly (3)

Symptoms	Remedy	Frequency And Doses
☆ Unable to cope with life; depression, after influenza; mind seems paralysed; listless, indolent; fear of falling; tremulous, shaky, and apprehensive	Gelsemium 30 or 200	4 hourly
☆ After sudden shock or stress; depressed and irritable; moods alternate; dwells on sorrows in secret; cannot forget past events; involuntary tears; sighing; cannot bear pain	Ignatia 200 or 1M	3 hourly (3)
❑ Due to prolonged strain; lassitude and depression; averse to meet people	Kali phos. 6 or 30	4 hourly
❑ With indigestion; chilly, tense, active person; frustrated; quarrelsome, critical, hypersensitive; wants to throw things	Nux vomica 30	6 hourly
❑ Weepy; mild and touchy patient; effects of bad news, anxiety, emotional upset; desires company	Pulsatilla 200	4 hourly (3)
Biochemic remedy	Kali phos. 6X	4 hourly

NEURALGIA
Facial
Nerve Pain

Symptoms	Remedy	Frequency And Doses
❑ Sudden onset; after exposure to dry cold winds	Aconite nap. 30 or 200	3 hourly
❑ Periodic attacks; burning pain; worse around the eyes and temples; worse by cold; better by warmth	Arsenic alb. 30 or 200	3 hourly
☆ Facial neuralgia; darting pain in the cheek - bones, nose, jaws, temples or in the neck; rush of blood towards head	Belladonna 30	3 hourly

Symptoms	Remedy	Frequency And Doses
❑ Periodical attacks; extreme sensitivity and soreness of the skin; due to fluid loss	China off. 30	3 hourly
☆ Violent; unbearable darting pain, more towards left side of the face, extends to the head and temples; worse by touch	Chamomilla 200 or 1M	10 min. (3)
❑ Pain towards right side of the face; worse in the evening 4-8 p.m. and warmth	Lycopodium 30 or 200	10 min. (3)
☆ Facial neuralgia with coldness and torpor in the affected side of the face; loss of thirst; worse in the evening	Pulsatilla 30 or 200	4 hourly
☆ Shooting pain along the nerve; better by heat and pressure	Magnesia phos. 6X or 30	3 hourly
❑ Pain improves only with heat of stove	Mezereum 30	4 hourly (3)
☆ Left sided neuralgia; burning, stitching, intolerable pain	Spigelia 30 or 200	4 hourly
● Pain worse during night (intercurrent remedy)	Syphilinum 200 or 1M	weekly (3)
Biochemic remedy	Ferrum phos. 6X and Magnesia phos. 6X	4 hourly

Other remedies which covers the pain in general are also useful and can be given according to the symptoms.

NEURITIS
Inflammation Of Nerves

❑ Head remedy; due to injury of nerves	Hypericum 30 or 200	4 hourly
❑ Sudden onset with anxiety and fear; worse noise or light	Aconite 30 or 200	2 hourly
❑ Due to exposure to sun or heat; better by motion and uncovering the head	Glonoine 3X or 6	2 hourly

Symptoms	Remedy	Frequency And Doses
❏ Better by pressure and warmth; worse in and by cold	**Magnesia phos. 6X or 30**	*4 hourly*
❏ Due to congestion; rush of blood towards head; face flushed	**Belladonna 30**	*3 hourly*
❏ Due to uterine disorders; reflex symptoms	**Cimicifuga 30**	*4 hourly*
❏ Interstitial neuritis; sensitive to air and touch	**Ranun-bulb. 30**	*4 hourly*

NIGHTMARE

❏ Patient cries in sleep as if frightened and grasps his mother/guardian	**Borax 30 or 200**	*4 hourly*
❏ Patient awakes frequently at night, chews and swallows; profuse sweat on head	**Calcarea carb. 200 or 1M**	*weekly (3)*
❏ Patient starts weeping all of a sudden during sleep due to fearful dreams	**Chamomilla 200**	*4 hourly*
❏ Patient shrieks and trembles in sleep due to nightmare	**Kali brom. 30 or 200**	*4 hourly*
● Patient speaks during sleep	**Sulphur 200 or 1M**	*weekly (3)*
❏ Nightmare with dreams of quarrelling with dead persons	**Cedron 200**	*weekly (3)*
❏ Nightmare with a feeling as if a stone is lying upon him (in dream)	**Kali carb. 200 or 1M**	*weekly (3)*
❏ Nightmare when the patient lies with the eyes half closed	**Opium 200 or 1M**	*weekly (3)*
❏ Nightmare, with unability to move	**Rhus tox. 200 or 1M**	*weekly (3)*
Biochemic remedies	**Ferrum phos. 6X, Kali phos. 6X** and **Mag. phos. 6X**	*4 hourly*

Symptoms	Remedy	Frequency And Doses

NOSE
Affections Of

Symptoms	Remedy	Frequency And Doses
❑ Pain and swelling of nasal bones; caries and ulceration. Fetid smell from nose; yellow-green fetid pus-like discharge from the nose	**Mercurius sol. 30**	*4 hourly*
❑ Tip of nose shiny red; tickling in nostrils	**Capsicum 30**	*4 hourly*
❑ Nose hard and red; nostrils sore, scurfy and ulcerated	**Kali carb. 30 or 200**	*4 hourly (3)*
❑ Nose stuffed up; obstructed; very dry; discharging yellow mucous; with plug clinkers in nostrils as if nose would burst; nose feels heavy; septum ulcerated	**Kali bich. 30**	*4 hourly*
❑ Itching of nose; patient rubs and picks the nose all the time	**Cina 30 or 200**	*4 hourly*
❑ Burning in nose; sniffling and chronic cold affecting posterior nose	**Cistus can. 30**	*4 hourly*
● Swelling and inflammation of nose; alae red and scabby nose; ulceration in nostrils	**Sulphur 30 or 200**	*4 hourly (3)*
❑ Fissures in nose; ulceration in nostrils; warts and pimples on nose	**Causticum 30 or 200**	*4 hourly (3)*
❑ Numbness of nose; caries of nasal bones, syphilitic ozaena	**Asafoetida 30**	*4 hourly*
❑ Painful downward pressure of nose; tip swollen, red and shiny	**Borax 30**	*4 hourly*
❑ Eruptions on nose; nostrils red, excoriation of nostrils	**Mezereum 30**	*4 hourly*
❑ Ulcerated, painful and swollen nose; knobby tip of nose; caries; fetid discharge	**Aurum met. 30 or 200**	*4 hourly (3)*
❑ Discharging green mucous; nasal bones sore; pressing pain at root of nose	**Pulsatilla 30 or 200**	*4 hourly*
● Violent sneezing; when well selected remedy fails	**Opium 30 or 200**	*4 hourly (3)*

Symptoms	Remedy	Frequency And Doses
❑ Large pedunculated nasal polypus	**Calcarea phos. 12X or 30**	*4 hourly*
❑ Epithelioma or polypus of nose; soreness and bleeding from nose	**Conium mac. 30 or 200**	*4 hourly*

NOSE BLEED
(See Epistaxis)

NYMPHOMANIA
(See Masturbation Female Also)

Extreme uncontrollable sexual desire in women.

Symptoms	Remedy	Frequency And Doses
❑ Coition creates more desire for sex; worse during menstruation	**Tarentula h. 200 or 1M**	*weekly (3)*
❑ Worse before and during menses; unable to control herself	**Veratrum-alb. 30**	*4 hourly*
❑ Worse before menses and during pregnancy; easily influenced for coition	**Phosphorus 200**	*weekly (3)*
☆ In young girls; forced to masturbate due to excessive desire of sex	**Origanum 30**	*4 hourly*
☆ During menses or after suppression of menses; excessive sexual urge	**Platina 200 or 1M**	*weekly (3)*
☆ Clitoris erects after masturbation with excessive desire; worse before menses	**Calc-phos. 12X or 30**	*4 hourly*
☆ Swelling and irritation of vulva with excessive desire; sexual mania	**Cantharis 30 or above**	*4 hourly*
❑ When there is intolerance of the weight of the clothings around waist; loquacious and jealous women; especially at the time of change of life (menopause)	**Lachesis 200 or 1M**	*weekly (3)*

Symptoms	Remedy	Frequency And Doses
❑ Excessive desire with ailments of uterus; prolapsus and pulsation in neck of uterus	Lilium tig. 30 or 200	4 hourly (3)
❑ Excessive sexual excitement with enlarged and indurated uterus; least touch causes violent sexual excitement	Murex 200 or 1M	4 hourly (3)
❑ Nymphomania; libidinous thoughts and lascivious dreams; sexual passion	Salix nig. Q or 30	4 hourly
❑ Insatiable excitement with great violence; fear of dark	Stramonium 200 or 1M	4 hourly (3)
Biochemic remedy	Calcarea phos. 200X	4 hourly

OBESITY
Corpulence
(See Fatness Also)

Symptoms	Remedy	Frequency And Doses
❑ Tongue thickly whitish coated; patient feels exhausted in warm weather	**Antim-crud. 200**	6 hourly
❑ With unusual tallness in children; chilly patients	**Silicea 30X or 30**	4 hourly
❑ When the tongue is constantly whitish coated; with liver disorders	**Kali mur. 30X or 6**	4 hourly
☆ Fat, flabby and chilly patients. Profuse sweat on head; worse at night, by exertion; easily fatigued; feet are cold and damp; craving for eggs; sensitive to cold and damp climate	**Calcarea carb. 200 or 1M**	4 hourly
❑ Especially for fatty women approaching menopause; sensitive to cold weather; liver and spleen enlarged	**Calcarea ars. 200**	6 hourly
☆ Obese patients who suffer from constipation; flatulence; goitre or thyroid enlargements	**Fucus ves. Q,** *10-20 drops*	4 hourly
● Intercurrent remedy; specially when obesity is due to thyroid disturbances	**Thyroidinum 200 or 1M**	weekly (3)
☆ Obese, chilly, constipated patients, specially in women when there is history of delayed menstruation; prone to skin ailments; feels cold; easily chilled and easily overheated	**Graphites 200 or 1M**	weekly (6)
❑ For fatty women; feels completely exhausted, (whether they do anything or not)	**Lac-def. 200**	weekly (6)
❑ To reduce weight (flesh and fat); to make the muscles hard and firm	**Calotropis 30 or 200**	6 hourly

Symptoms	Remedy	Frequency And Doses
☆ To absorb abnormal tissues, new growths and fat	**Phytolacca berry Q,** *10 drops*	*4 hourly*
❏ Obese patients with weak heart; sensitive to cold; aversion to water; habits of uncleanliness; prone to colds	**Ammon-carb. 200**	*6 hourly*

Other Important Remedies:

Ammon-brom., Capsicum, Ferrum met., Iodothyroidinum, Kali brom., Kali carb., and Medorrhinum, etc..

OBSTRUCTIONS TO CURE
(See Different Ailments)

The bad effects are often the effects of addictions, alcoholism, excessive medication, burns, cauterisation, use of chloroform; epidemic diseases like measles, small pox, whooping cough, typhoid fever, etc., eating food cooked in aluminium vessels, intake of waxy kind of foods, old injuries, grief, mental shock, freight and diabetes, etc., and these are considered great obstructions to cure a case. In homoeopathy there are certain medicines which according to law of similia are curative to remove the diseased conditions of above mentioned poisonings or bad effects due to acute miasmatic flare up of chronic ailments and other reasons (For proper management to cure a case read Dr. Sandhu's 'Practical Management of the Sick').

OCCUPATIONAL AILMENTS

The important remedies which have special affinity on ailments due to occupational disturbances or causative factors have been given here.

Symptoms	Remedy	Frequency And Doses
❏ Actors; auctioneers/clergy-man/orator's sore-throat	**Arum triph. 30**	*4 hourly*
❏ Studious persons or writers (book worms) - cough; gastric complaints due to worry or sedentary life	**Nux vomica 30**	*6 hourly*
❏ Studious persons or girls and boy's headache	**Calcarea phos. 6X or 30**	*6 hourly*
❏ Teachers/businessman's - brain fag and headache	**Picric-acid. 30**	*6 hourly*

Symptoms	Remedy	Frequency And Doses
☐ Weakness due to physical and mental strain	Coca Q, 5-10 drops or Kali Phos. 6X	4 hourly
☐ Clergyman's - hoarseness; Washer woman's - toothache	Phosphorus 30 or 200	4 hourly (3)
☐ Emigrants; compositors - constipation	Platina 200 or 1M	4 hourly (3)
☐ Foundryman's - diseases of optic nerve and retina	Mercurius sol. 30	4 hourly
☐ Miners - asthma due to inhalation of coal-dust	Natrum ars. 30	4 hourly
☐ Nurses - exhausted by long nursing and loss of sleep	Cocculus ind. 30	6 hourly
☐ Sailors - asthma better going to the sea	Bromium 30	4 hourly
☐ Servant girls - coming to cities from the country side becomes anaemic	Pulsatilla 30	6 hourly
☐ Singers/speakers - nervousness	Gelsemium 30	4 hourly
☐ Stonemasons - chest affections; cough, asthma, bronchitis, etc. (use with care)	Silicea 6X or 30	6 hourly
☐ Tender feet- of sales girls	Squilla 30	6 hourly
☐ Washer women's remedy	Sepia 200	6 hourly
☐ Tailor's remedy	Ruta g. 30	6 hourly
☐ Dyer's and Painters remedy	Plumbum met. 30	6 hourly
☐ Weaver's remedy	Gossypium 30	6 hourly

OEDEMA
Dropsical Swelling
(See Ascites, Laryngitis, Pleurisy, Kidney and Heart Diseases Also)

Oedema means retention of fluid (water and sodium salts) in the sub-cutaneous tissues. It can be due to various reasons and ailments (for treatment please refer to specific ailments).

Important Remedies:

Apis mel., Arsenic alb., China off., Convallaria, Helleborus, Liatris spi. and Mercurius sol., etc.. Salt should be restricted. Skimmed milk should be used freely. Rest and warmth are essential. The diet should be light and easily digestable. Vegetarian diet is good.

Symptoms	Remedy	Frequency And Doses

OPPOSITE CHARACTERISTIC SYMPTOMS

❑ **A.** The edges of teeth decay — **Staphysagria., Merc-sol.**
   B. The roots of teeth decay — **Thuja, Mezereum**

❑ **A.** Dry mouth without thirst — **Pulsatilla**
   B. Moist mouth with thirst — **Merc-sol.**

❑ **A.** Diseases begin on the left and go to the right side — **Lachesis**
   B. Diseases begin on the right and go to the left side — **Lycopodium**

❑ **A.** Cough aggravates going from warm to cold air — **Phosphorus**
   B. Cough aggravates coming into a warm room from open air — **Bryonia alb.**

❑ **A.** Acrid coryza with bland lachrymation — **Allium cepa**
   B. Acrid lachrymation with bland coryza — **Euphrasia**

❑ **A.** Pain aggravates by motion — **Bryonia alb.**
   B. Pain ameliorates by motion — **Rhus tox.**

❑ **A.** Cough aggravates by cold drinks — **Spongia tosta**
   B. Cough ameliorates by cold drinks — **Cuprum met.**

❑ **A.** Toothache (pain) ameliorates by heat — **Magnesia phos.**
   B. Toothache ameliorates by cold water — **Coffea, Natrum s., Bismuth**

❑ **A.** Colic ameliorates from bending double — **Colocynth.**
   B. Colic ameliorates on bending backwards — **Dioscorea v.**

❑ **A.** Cough aggravates on expiration — **Aconitum n., Causticum**
   B. Cough aggravates on inspiration — **Spongia tosta**

❑ **A.** Sweats as soon as one closes his eyes to sleep — **Conium, China off.**
   B. Sweats when one wakes up — **Sambucus nig.**

❑ **A.** Constipation before and during menstruation — **Silicea**
   B. Diarrhoea before and during menstruation — **Bovista, Veratrum album, Ammon-carb**

❑ **A.** Child is good whole day; restless, screaming and troubles - whole night — **Psorinum, Jalapa**
   B. Child cries whole day, sleeps whole night — **Lycopodium**

Symptoms	Remedy	Frequency And Doses

ORCHITIS
(See Hydrocele Also)

Inflammation of the testicles.

Symptoms	Remedy	Frequency And Doses
☆ Acute; due to exposure to dry cold winds	Aconite 30 or 200	4 hourly
☆ With pain and swelling of lower part of the right testicle	Argentum nit. 30 or 200	4 hourly (3)
❑ With squeezed pain in the testicles; testes hard and inflammed	Baptisia 30 or 200	4 hourly
☆ Pain comes and goes suddenly; face flushed	Belladonna 30	4 hourly
❑ Bruised pain, swelling of the right half of the scrotum and testicle. Testicles very hard	Clematis 30	4 hourly
☆ Orchitis due to contusion; testicles hard and enlarged	Conium 200 or 1M	10 min. (3)
❑ Swelling and hardness of testicles and scrotum with shining redness; dragging pain in testicles and spinal cord	Merc-sol. 30 or 200	4 hourly (3)
❑ Pain and inflammation of testicles with painful drawing of the spermatic cord	Nitric acid. 30 or 200	4 hourly (3)
☆ Chronic orchitis; testicles feel crushed; worse during thunder storm	Rhododendron 200 or 1M	10 min. (3)
☆ Complaints after suppression of gonorrhoea with pain in spermatic cord	Spongia tosta 30 or 200	4 hourly (3)
Biochemic remedies	Ferrum phos. 6X and Kali mur. 6X	4 hourly

Other Important Remedies:

Nux vomica, Phytolacca, Lycopodium, Pulsatilla, Arnica, Aurum mur-nat. and Aurum met., etc..

Symptoms	Remedy	Frequency And Doses

OSTEOMYELITIS

Inflammation of the bone marrow and adjacent bone and epiphysial cartilage.

The Important Remedies:

Arnica mont., Alumina silicat., Hypericum, Silicea, Medorrhinum, Bryonia alb., Plumbum met., Cicuta v., Cuprum ars., Strychninum phos., etc..

OTORRHOEA
(Discharge From The Ears)

Symptoms	Remedy	Frequency And Doses
❑ Redness and swelling of both ears; after scarlatina; violent pain in left ear when chewing	Apis mel. 30 or 200	4 hourly (3)
❑ Otorrhoea with profuse, ichorous and foul discharge; accompanied by burning and itching in canal and crawling sensations in ears	Arsenic alb. 30 or 200	4 hourly (3)
❑ Otorrhoea with offensive discharge and diseased bones (caries, etc.)	Asafoetida 30 or 200	4 hourly (3)
❑ Acute; when acute symptoms arise in chronic disease	Belladonna 30	4 hourly
❑ Sub-acute otitis with much purulent and offensive discharge; fear of downward motion due to cerebral anaemia	Borax 30	4 hourly
❑ Watery, bad-smelling, thick discharge; fetid pus from ears; inner swelling of ears; swelling begins at the ear and extends half way up to the cheek	Cistus can. 30	4 hourly
❑ With catarrhal deafness and pain from throat into middle ear; patient feels chilly loss of thirst; better by pasing urine	Gelsemium 30	4 hourly
❑ With thick, mucous discharge; dropping down of mucous from the posterior nares into the throat; stools constipated	Hydrastis can. 30	4 hourly

Symptoms	Remedy	Frequency And Doses
☆ Discharge of thick, yellow, fetid pus; itching deep in ear, with stinging pain; sharp stitching pain dart from ear to throat	**Kali bich. 30 or 200**	*4 hourly*
❑ Irritating, offensive discharge; accompanied by boring, tearing pain in the temporal bone	**Kali iod. 30 or 200**	*6 hourly*
☆ With excoriation and ulceration of meatus; sensitive to cold; abundant secretion; flow of pus and blood from the ears; tonsillitis or diseased parotids; pulsative roaring in the affected ear	**Mercurius sol. 30 or 200**	*4 hourly*
☆ Offensive, purulent otorrhoea; difficult hearing; better while riding in a carriage	**Nitric acid. 30 or 200**	*6 hourly*
● Offensive, purulent otorrhoea; yellow fetid discharge; forming crusts and intolerable itching	**Psorinum 200 or 1M**	*weekly (3)*
❑ Offensive, watery, curdy otorrhoea; with soreness of inner nose and crusts on upper lip; itching in eustachian tube and in ears	**Silicea 30 or 200**	*6 hourly*
☆ Otitis media with rupture of tympanum; pouring out of pus which at first may be fair but afterwards becomes offensive, smelling like fish brine	**Tellurium 30**	*4 hourly*
❑ Watery, purulent otorrhoea; smelling like putrid meat; inner ear feels swollen with increased loss of hearing	**Thuja oc. 200 or 1M**	*weekly (3)*
❑ Otorrhoea of fetid pus; frequent, acute stitches in right ear, near tympanum;	**Zincum met. 30 or 200**	*6 hourly*
☆ With intense, shooting pain, stinking pus; patient oversensitive to touch, pain and colds, etc.	**Hepar sulph. 30**	*4 hourly*
☆ With pain and greenish pus; better open, cold air	**Pulsatilla 30 or 200**	*4 hourly (3)*
❑ Chronic, offensive discharge from ears; syphilitic origin	**Aurum ars. 30 or 200**	*10 min. (3)*
Biochemic remedies	**Calcarea phos. 6X, Kali mur. 6X** and **Silicea 30X**	*4 hourly*

Symptoms	Remedy	Frequency And Doses

OVARIES
Affections Of

Symptoms	Remedy	Frequency And Doses
❑ Ovarian complaints after exposure to dry, cold winds; anxiety and fear	**Aconite nap. 30 or 200**	*4 hourly*
❑ Stage of suppuration; frequent chill; throbbing and pricking pain	**Hepar sulph. 30 or 200**	*4 hourly (6)*
☆ Burning in ovarian region; constant urging to pass urine	**Cantharis 30**	*4 hourly (6)*
❑ Ovarian neuralgia; intense pain, causing Patient to draw up double; restlessness	**Colocynth. 30 or 200**	*4 hourly (3)*
❑ Stitching pain in ovaries on deep inspiration; worse from least motion; constipation and excessive thirst	**Bryonia 30 or 200**	*6 hourly*
☆ Throbbing pain; appear and disappear suddenly; great bearing down with feeling as if everything would protrude from vulva; worse slightest jar	**Belladonna 30**	*4 hourly*
☆ Burning, lancinating pain as if coals were burning in the part; relieved by hot application; restlessness	**Arsenic alb. 30 or 200**	*4 hourly (3)*
☆ Ovary swollen, especially right; stinging, burning pain; worse by coughing; loss of thirst and scanty urine	**Apis mel. 30 or 200**	*4 hourly (3)*
☆ Chronic ovaritis; lancinating pain; soreness and swelling of breast before menses; intermittent flow of urine	**Conium mac. 200 or 1M**	*weekly (3)*
☆ Ovarian neuralgia, inflammation and induration; the left ovary is attacked first and then the right one. Pain relieved by a discharge from uterus.Neuralgic pain (left ovary) with tenderness; worse pressure even of the clothes	**Lachesis 30 or 200**	*6 hourly (3)*
❑ Swelling and induration of left ovary with	**Graphites 30 or 200**	*6 hourly (3)*

Symptoms	Remedy	Frequency And Doses
stony hardness; violent pain on touch; stools constipated		
❏ Ovary swollen with a diffused agonizing soreness over whole abdomen	**Hamamelis virg. Q or 30**	*4 hourly*
❏ Induration and swelling of ovary with thick, yellow, burning leucorrhoea; patient feels better after eating	**Iodium 30 or 200**	*4 hourly*
❏ Stitching pain in the left ovary; thirst with moist mouth; sweating which do not ameliorate	**Merc-sol. 30 or 200**	*4 hourly (3)*
❏ Ovaritis due to suppression of menses after getting feet wet; chilliness and loss of thirst; patient feels better in open cold air	**Pulsatilla 30 or 200**	*4 hourly (3)*
☆ Ovaritis due to masturbation; face shows guilt	**Staphysagria 30 or 200**	*4 hourly (6)*

PAIN

(See Arthritis, Neuralgia And Neuritis, Etc., Also)

Symptoms	Remedy	Frequency And Doses

For pain see the relevant ailment and select the remedy accordingly. We are not giving the details in this chapter as we have given the same in different ailments.

Symptoms	Remedy	Frequency And Doses
☐ Burning pain as a result of insect bite; loss of thirst	**Apis mel 30**	*4 hourly (6)*
☐ Burning pain; especially while passing urine	**Cantharis 30**	*4 hourly*
☐ Shooting pain with any movement and in cold damp weather	**Actaea rac. 30**	*4 hourly*
Biochemic remedy	**Mag-phos. 6X**	*4 hourly*

PALPITATION

(See Heart Ailments Also)

Symptoms	Remedy	Frequency And Doses
☐ Violent palpitation in heart region	**Aethusa cy. 30**	*4 hourly*
☐ Palpitation with nausea, headache and nervous excitement	**Bromium 30**	*4 hourly*
☐ In patients subject to piles; dyspepsia or flatulence	**Collinsonia 30 or 200**	*4 hourly (3)*
☆ Palpitation with constriciton of chest/heart	**Cactus g. Q or 30**	*3 hourly*
☆ Palpitation; worse by exertion or excitement	**Crataegus ox. Q or 30**	*3 hourly*

The above two remedies act as a heart tonic and can be given alternately.

Other Important Remedies:

Aconite, Arsenic alb., Carbo veg., Phosphorus, Sulphur, Gelsemium and Argent-nit., etc..

Symptoms	Remedy	Frequency And Doses

PANCREAS
Affections Of

Symptoms	Remedy	Frequency And Doses
❑ Inflammation and catarrh of pancreas with rush of blood towards head	Belladonna 30	3 hourly
❑ Pancreas enlarged; especially for scrofulous affections	Calcarea iod. 30	4 hourly
❑ Pancreas contracted; excessive vomiting and indigestion; loosing weight and flesh while food intake is good	Iodium 30	4 hourly
☆ Fatty degeneration; indigestion and craving for icy cold drinks	Phosphorus 30 or 200	10 min. (3)
❑ Pancreas inflammed; burning sensation. Vomiting of sweetish matter and indigestion	Iris v. 30	4 hourly
Biochemic remedy	Kali phos. 6X	4 hourly

PARALYSIS
Of Different Body Parts

Symptoms	Remedy	Frequency And Doses
☆ With insensibility; especially of brain; after effects of fear, accidents, etc.	Opium 1M or above	10 min. (3)
❑ Paralysis of eye-lids; larynx; muscles refuse to obey	Gelsemium 200	10 min. (3)
❑ Paralysis of arms; great weakness and weariness; ill effects of grief or fright	Natrum mur. 200	10 min. (3)
☆ Paralysis of single parts; bladder, larynx, pharynx or tongue, etc.	Causticum 30 or 200	4 hourly (6)
❑ Paralysis of bowels; suddenness of symptoms	Phosphorus 200	10 min. (3)
❑ Paralysis of brain; left sided; patient can not bear anything tight anywhere on body	Lachesis 200	10 min (3)

Symptoms	Remedy	Frequency And Doses
❑ Paralysis of eye-lids and face; extreme prostration	Cadmium sulph. 200	10 min. (3)
❑ Paralysis of eye muscles; left side of face; heat in the face	Senega 30	4 hourly
❑ Facial paralysis, sticking pain in extremities; drags feet while walking and trembles	Nux vomica 30 or 200	6 hourly
❑ Paralysis of legs, ascending; great weakness; tired, heavy feeling all over the body	Acid-picric. 30	4 hourly
❑ Paralysis of extremities with heaviness and loss of sensation; restlessness	Rhus tox. 200 or 1M	4 hourly
❑ One sided paralysed while convulsions in the other side; fear of dark	Stramonium 200 or 1M	4 hourly
☆ Paralysis of wrist or single muscles that withers; beginning in extensor	Plumbum met. 30 or 200	6 hourly
☆ Paralysis in old patients; prone to cold; childish behaviour	Baryta carb. 200 or 1M	10 min. (3)
❑ Paralysis from below upward; especially in old bachelors or maids	Conium mac. 200 or 1M	10 min. (3)
❑ Painless paralysis of limbs; lungs	Laurocerasus 30 or 200	4 hourly (3)
Biochemic remedies	Calcarea phos. 6X, Kali phos. 6X and Mag. phos. 6X	4 hourly

PECULIAR SYMPTOMS

We have given peculiar symptoms in different ailments so we are not repeating them here.

❑ Bed feels too hard	Arnica 30 or 200	4 hourly
❑ Feels better when thinking of his/her complaints	Camphor 30	4 hourly
❑ Every symptomis worse after taking coffee	Causticum 200 or 1M	weekly (3)
❑ Desire to eat coal	Cicuta v. 30 or 200	6 hourly
❑ Talking excessively; changing topics	Lachesis 200 or 1M	weekly (3)

Symptoms	Remedy	Frequency And Doses
❑ Feeling of hollowness in head, chest or abdomen	**Cocculus ind. 30**	*4 hourly*
❑ Fan like motion of the alae nasi	**Lycopodium 30 or 200**	*4 hourly*
❑ Feels better when constipated	**Calcarea carb. 200**	*weekly (3)*
❑ Feels better after violent exertion; dancing, etc.	**Sepia 200 or 1M**	*weekly (3)*
❑ Always feels better just before a severe attack of any ailment	**Psorinum 200 or 1M**	*fortnightly (3)*

PEPTIC ULCER
Including Gastric And Duodenal Ulcers

Ulceration of gastro - intestinal tract is due to the biochemical reaction of hydrochloric acid and pepsin. It is more common in persons who leads a stressful life and also smokers. The complication is worse after taking Aspirin and strong allopathic drugs. Pain in epigastrium is the main symptom. Frequent repeatition of medicine is dangerous in chronic cases.

Symptoms	Remedy	Frequency
❑ Extreme thirst; with extreme irritability of the stomach; extreme soreness with burning heat; pain with unbearable anxiety	**Arsenic alb. 30 or 200**	*4 hourly (3)*
❑ Stinging, ulcerative pain below left short ribs; worse by touch and deep inspiration; griping with burning, warmth in epigastrium; craving for sweets which aggravate the complaints	**Argentum nit. 30 or 200**	*4 hourly (3)*
❑ Sensitiveness of epigastric region; acidity when lying on back and walking; burning; every sort of food disagrees; acid dyspepsia with heart burn; burning in the stomach sometimes extends into small of back with excessive distention by gas	**Carbo veg. 30 or 200**	*4 hourly (3)*
❑ Stomach and abdomen enormously distended and tense after every meal. Rumbling in abdomen after eating with uneasiness and thin stools	**Acid-nit. 30 or 200**	*6 hourly (3)*

Symptoms	Remedy	Frequency And Doses
❑ Craving for acids and spicy food; empty eructations; vomiting like coffee ground, mixed with dark, acid matter; worse in hot weather	**Phosphorus 30 or 200**	*4 hourly (3)*
❑ Gastric ulceration with haemorrhage; pain worse when food passes pyloric outlet. Painful sinking sensation across epigastrium	**Ornithogalum Q,** *5-7 drops*	*4 hourly*
Biochemic remedy	**Natrum phos. 6X**	*4 hourly*

Other Important Remedies:

Colchicum, Staphysagria, Syphilinum, Pyrogenium and other constitutional remedies. Alkaline mixtures, milk, etc. are helpful to neutralise the acid. In complicated cases expert opinion should be preferred. The treatment should be by experienced physician only.

PERIODICITY
Periodical Appearance Of Symptoms

The remedies which have special periodic affinity have been given here. We have given the detailed description of such remedies in different ailments, we are giving only the main remedies here.

❑ Annually	**Tarentula h.**
❑ Every spring	**Crotalus h.**
❑ Eighth day	**Iris v.**
❑ Regularly	**Rhus tox.**
❑ Whole night	**Syphilinum**
❑ Whole day	**Medorrhinum**
❑ Worse every winter; skin cracked	**Petroleum**
❑ Cough every morning	**Alumina**
❑ Diarrhoea on rising; 9 a.m.	**Natrum sulph.**
❑ Diarrhoea at 5 a.m.; morning aggravation	**Sulphur**
❑ Worse after midnight; fourth day	**Arsenic alb.**
❑ Worse 2-4 a.m.	**Kali carb.**
❑ Worse 3-5 a.m.; same hour	**Kali bich.**

Symptoms	Remedy	Frequency And Doses
❏ Worse, 8-11 a.m.	**Natrum mur.**	
❏ Worse, 6-7 p.m.; profuse urination	**Bryonia alb.**	
❏ Complaints return at regular intervals; evening; warmth	**Pulsatilla**	
❏ Complaints return at regular intervals; third day, twenty-first day; fever	**China sulph.**	
❏ Complaints return at regular intervals; seventh day; morning	**Sulphur**	
❏ Complaints return at regular intervals; tenth day	**Phosphorus**	
❏ Complaints return at regular intervals; fourteenth day; after sleep	**Lachesis**	
❏ Complaints return at regular intervals; twenty eighth day	**Nux vomica**	

PERITONITIS
(See Fever Also)

Inflammation of the serous membrane lining of the abdomen.

❏ Due to exposure to dry cold winds; high fever with peritoneal pain	**Aconite 30 or 200**	*4 hourly*
❏ With intense swelling and pain of abdomen; worse by touch or pressure; local congestion	**Belladonna 30**	*4 hourly*
❏ Peritonitis with fever and burning sensation; worse by motion; excessive thirst for large quantities of water at long intervals	**Bryonia alb. 30 or 200**	*6 hourly*
❏ When simple fever converts into typhoid fever; tongue dry - triangular tip red, restlessness; better by movements	**Rhus tox. 30 or 200**	*4 hourly*

Symptoms	Remedy	Frequency And Doses
❑ In suppurative stage with intense sweat which do not relieve; fever with loose stools	**Mercurius sol. 30**	*4 hourly*
❑ When patient can not bear even slightest touch or pressure even of clothes on abdomen	**Lachesis 30 or 200**	*4 hourly (3)*
❑ With extreme coldness of the body; cramps in the extremities and desire for cold drinks; vomiting and fever	**Veratrum alb. 30**	*4 hourly*
Biochemic remedy	**Ferrum phos. 6X**	*3 hourly*

PHARYNGITIS
(See Other Throat Troubles Also)

Symptoms	Remedy	Frequency And Doses
❑ Pharyngitis with small pin head like ulcers that bleed easily	**Belladonna 30**	*3 hourly*
❑ With chronic catarrh of pharynx; sore throat	**Silicea 12X or 30**	*4 hourly*
☆ With tough, stringy, whitish mucous	**Kali bich. 30**	*4 hourly*
☆ When there is paralysis of muscles of pharynx	**Lachesis 30**	*4 hourly*
☆ With whitish spots on ulcers in throat	**Phytolacca d. 30**	*4 hourly*
❑ With dryness of throat; thirst more; stools constipated	**Natrum mur. 30**	*4 hourly*
Biochemic remedies	**Kali mur. 6X** and **Ferrum phos. 6X**	*4 hourly*

PHIMOSIS

Narrowness of the opening of the prepuce; preventing its bringing drawn back over the glans is called Phimosis.

The Important Remedies:

Acid-nitric., Aconite, Apis mel., Belladonna, Hepar sulph., Mercurius sol., Sulphur, Medorrhinum and Tuberculinum, etc.

Symptoms	Remedy	Frequency And Doses

PILES - DRY
Haemorrhoids

Symptoms	Remedy	Frequency And Doses
● Head remedy for bleeding or blind piles; itching and burning in the anus	**Sulphur 200 or 1M**	*fortnightly (3)*
☆ Haemorrhoids; with pain in lumbo-sacral region; anus feels as if full with sticks or as if a bug is crawling	**Aesculus h. 6 or 30**	*4 hourly*
❏ Haemorrhoids; like onions, purplish in colour; hammering and throbbing in the anus	**Lachesis 30 or 200**	*4 hourly (6)*
☆ Constipation, due to sedentary life. Frequent urging to pass stool with itching and stitching in the rectum; beating or pressing pain after passing stools; worse taking alcoholic drinks; after mental exertion or after eating	**Nux vomica 30**	*4 hourly*
❏ Haemorrhoids with biting sensation; soreness in the anus; fissures or ulceration in the anus. Anus moist due to constant oozing	**Paeonia Q or 6**	*4 hourly*
❏ Haemorrhoids with prolapsus ani. Protrusion of rectum after passing stools	**Podophyllum 30 or 200**	*4 hourly*
☆ Deep or superficial fissures in the anus. Pain after passing stools as if splinters of glass were sticking in the anus and rectum. Heat and pain in the anus is so severe that patient can't keep still. Constriction of the orifice	**Ratanhia 6 or 30**	*4 hourly*
❏ Haemorrhoids protrude like bunches of grapes after every stool; cold water relieves	**Aloe soc. 6 or 30**	*4 hourly*
❏ Mucous piles (mucous coming from the anus); tongue whitish coated	**Antimonium crud. 30 or 200**	*weekly (3)*
☆ Haemorrhoids with stinging and burning pain; better by cold applications	**Apis mel. 30 or 200**	*4 hourly (3)*
❏ Haemorrhoids with burning pain; better by warm applications	**Arsenic alb. 30**	*4 hourly*

Symptoms	Remedy	Frequency And Doses
☆ Haemorrhoids; or any other trouble in anus or rectum makes walking intolerably painful	Causticum 30 or 200	4 hourly (3)
❑ Haemorrhoids with sensation as if red, hot iron were being thrushed into the rectum; better by applying cold water	Kali carb. 30 or 200	4 hourly (3)
❑ Swelling and protrusion of haemorrhoids with bleeding; even while stools are not constipated. Patient is much troubled by wind formation. Haemorrhoids with extreme sensitivity to touch, even contact of cloth is intolerable	Acid-mur. 30 or 200	4 hourly
❑ Anus moist, fissured and painful; surrounded with flat warts. Violent contraction with burning and pricking in anus followed by tearing pains	Thuja oc. 200 or 1M	weekly (6)
❑ Haemorrhoids come out every time patient urinates	Baryta carb. 200 or 1M	weekly (3)
Biochemic remedy	Calcarea fluor. 12X	4 hourly

PIMPLES
(See Acne)

PLEURISY

The treatment should be under experienced physician only, the repeation should be with great care.

☆ With high fever, due to exposure to dry cold wind	Aconite nap. 30 or 200	4 hourly
☆ With stitching pains in the chest; worse by movements; better by warmth and rest	Bryonia 30 or 200	4 hourly (3)
☆ With constriction of the chest; loss of thirst; worse by heat	Apis mel. 30	4 hourly (3)
❑ With stitching pain in the chest; worse bending forward; phlegm tastes sweet and attracts flies	Stannum met. 30 or 200	4 hourly (3)

Symptoms	Remedy	Frequency And Doses
● With stitching pain in the chest; worse lying on back and in the morning	**Sulphur 30 or 200**	*1 dose*
☆ With stitching pain in the chest; worse lying on left side; craving for cold water	**Phosphorus 30 or 200**	*4 hourly (3)*
❑ With stitching pain in the chest; worse while walking and warmth	**Kali iod. 30**	*4 hourly (3)*
Biochemic remedies	**Ferrum phos. 6X, Kali mur. 6X** and **Calcarea phos. 12X**	*4 hourly*

Other Important Remedies:

Arrenie iod., Tuberculinum, Natrum sulph. and Acalyxha ind., etc..

PNEUMONIA

❑ Due to exposure to dry cold winds; with high fever, anxiety and restlessness; expectoration bright red	**Aconite nap. 30 or 200**	*3 hourly*
☆ When bronchitis turns into pneumonia; weak feeling in the chest; tongue whitish coated	**Antim-tart. 30 or 200**	*10 min. (3)*
☆ Tongue clean; spasmodic cough with vomiting; broncho-pneumonia	**Ipecac 30**	*3 hourly*
❑ Due to excessive bile formation; chronic cough or whooping cough after measles	**Chelidonium 6 or 30**	*3 hourly*
☆ Expectoration copious; offensive, tenacious, pus like, blood streaked; coldness of chest and wandering, stitching pains; worse 3-4 a.m.	**Kali carb. 30 or 200**	*4 hourly (3)*
☆ Expectoration rusty; when croupous exudation takes place; excessive thirst and constipation; worse by motion	**Bryonia alb. 30 or 200**	*4 hourly (3)*
❑ When destruction of lung tissues starts; patient wants fresh air, fanning even though the body is cold	**Carbo veg. 30 or 200**	*3 hourly (3)*
❑ When hepatization takes place	**Iodium 30**	*3 hourly*

Symptoms	Remedy	Frequency And Doses
❏ With weak feeling in the chest; phlegm sweetish in taste and attracts flies	**Stannum met. 30 or 200**	*3 hourly*
❏ When breathing becomes difficult due to extreme hepatization; marked dyspnoea	**Lycopodium 30 or 200**	*4 hourly (3)*
❏ When some spots remain into the lungs after recovery; loss of thirst; patient feels better in open, cool air	**Pulsatilla 30**	*4 hourly (3)*
Biochemic remedies	**Ferrum phos. 6X** and **Kali sulph. 6X**	*4 hourly*

The treatment should be under experienced physician only.

POISONING
(See Allergies And Food Poisoning Also)

❏ By charcoal fumes	**Ammon-carb. 3 or 6**	*1/2 hourly*
❏ Atomic radiation	**Phosphorus 6 or 30**	*1/2 hourly*
❏ Chloroform	**Acetic acid. 30 or 200**	*1/2 hourly*
❏ Food; ptomaine poisoning; eating over ripen fruits	**Arsenic alb. 30**	*1/2 hourly*

Other Important Remedies:

Carbo veg., Verat-alb., Rhus tox., Croton tig. and Merc-sol., etc..

POLYPUS
Ear

❏ Polypus in the left ear; sensitive to air; tearing pain from zygoma into the ear	**Lachesis 30 or 200**	*4 hourly (3)*
❏ Patient prone to ear polypus; post nasal catarrh and constipation	**Hydrastis can 30**	*4 hourly*
● Polypus in the middle ear; chronic otitis	**Thuja oc. 200 or 1M**	*weekly (3)*
❏ Polypus in the external meatus	**Mercurius cor. 30**	*4 hourly*
Biochemic remedy	**Kali sulph. 6X**	*4 hourly*

Symptoms	Remedy	Frequency And Doses

POLYPUS
Nasal

Symptoms	Remedy	Frequency And Doses
☆ Head remedy; putrid or loss of smell; profuse mucous from nose; nasal obstruction	**Lemna min. Q or 30**	*4 hourly*
☆ Blockage of nose the side patient lies on; worse in wet weather	**Teucrium m-v. 30**	*4 hourly*
☆ Nasal polyp bleeds easily; frequent sneezing; imaginary foul smell; craving for cold drinks	**Phosphorus 200**	*weekly (3)*
❏ Nasal polyp with loss of smell; swelling at root of nose. Patient susceptible to cold; worse change of weather; right sided headache	**Sanguinaria c. 30 or 200**	*4 hourly (3)*
❏ Mucous polyp which bleeds easily; alternately fluent, dry or acrid coryza; chilly patient	**Calcarea carb. 200 or 1M**	*weekly (3)*
❏ Blockage of nose; nostrils inflammed; chilly patient, prone to cold; perforation of septum	**Silicea 6X or 30**	*4 hourly*
Biochemic remedy	**Calcarea phos. 6X or 12X**	*4 hourly*

POLYPUS
Uterus

Symptoms	Remedy	Frequency And Doses
☆ Polypus in uterus or vagina; worse in wet weather	**Teucrium m-v. 30**	*4 hourly*
❏ Uterine polypus protrudes while passing stools	**Conium mac. 200 or 1M**	*10 min. (3)*
● In fat and flabby patients; susceptible to colds	**Calcarea carb. 200 or 1M**	*weekly (3)*
❏ When the polypus bleeds easily	**Phosphorus 30 or 200**	*weekly (3)*
Biochemic remedy	**Calcarea phos. 6X**	*4 hourly*

PRE AND POST OPERATIVE CARE

Symptoms	Remedy	Frequency And Doses
❏ Before the operation; to take care for the shock, after effects, etc.	Arnica 200 or 1M	1 dose
❏ For surgical shock	Strontia-carb. 30 or 200	10 min. (3)
❏ Bad effects of anaesthesia with chloroform	Chloroform 200	10 min. (3)
❏ If Chloroform fails	Phosphorus 200	10 min. (3)
❏ Bad effects of anaesthesia with ether	Antimonium tart. 200	10 min. (3)
❏ Post operative - retention of urine	Causticum 30 or 200	1/2 hourly (3)
❏ For nerves injury; removal of nails, amputation or circumcision	Hypericum 200	10 min. (3)
❏ If Hypericum fails	Allium cepa 30	3 hourly
❏ After tonsilectomy	Calendula 30	3 hourly (6)
❏ To check bleeding after operation	Phosphorus 30 or 200	1 dose
❏ After operation; when haemorrhage is bright red	Millefoliun Q or 30	3 hourly

PREGNANCY
Ailments During

❏ Affections of ears during pregnancy	Capsicum 30	4 hourly (3)
❏ Shivers during first stage of pregnancy; nervousness	Cimicifuga 30	4 hourly (3)
❏ Sufferings due to mechanical pressure; bruised pains	Arnica 30 or 200	4 hourly (3)
❏ Rush of blood to head; loss of consciousness	Glonoine 30	4 hourly (3)
❏ Piles and constipation during pregnancy	Collinsonia 30 or 200	4 hourly (3)
❏ Cramps in toes and soles of feet with chilliness during pregnancy	Calcarea carb. 200	10 min. (3)
❏ Cramps in abdomen and legs during pregnancy	Viburnum op. 30	4 hourly
❏ During pregnancy sight of water makes to vomit	Phosphorus 30 or 200	10 min. (3)

Symptoms	Remedy	Frequency And Doses
❑ During pregnancy swelling and stiffness of hands and feet	Sanguinaria c. 30 or 200	4 hourly (3)
❑ Sensation as if os uteri is opening	Lachesis 200	1 dose (SOS)
❑ Toothache during pregnancy	Sepia 30 or 200	4 hourly (3)
❑ During labor patient becomes blind	Cuprum met. 200 or 1M	10 min. (3)
❑ During labor suffocating spells and convulsions	Hyoscyamus 200	1/2 hourly (3)
❑ Inability to walk during pregnancy	Bellis p. 30	4 hourly
❑ For obstinate vomiting of pregnancy	Cuprum ars. 30	4 hourly (3)

PRICKLY HEAT

Symptoms	Remedy	Frequency And Doses
☆ Prickly heat with much itching; recurrent summer boils	Syzygium jam. Q or 30	4 hourly
☆ Boils; bruised sensation, sore (one after another); crop like	Arnica 30 or 200	4 hourly
● Eruptions coming up in crops; one heal another comes, mature slowly	Sulphur 30 or 200	4 hourly
☆ Rashes; reddish, hot and rush of blood towards head	Belladonna 30	4 hourly
❑ Eruptions with burning and stinging; loss of thirst; worse heat	Apis mel. 30	4 hourly
❑ Rash or eruptions with burning and soreness; burning in urine	Cantharis 30	4 hourly
❑ Eruptions with burning and intense itching; stools constipated	Graphites 30	4 hourly
❑ Purple coloured eruptions with small vesicles around	Lachesis 30 or 200	4 hourly (3)
☆ Coppery or red coloured eruptions turning blue on getting cold; itching worse at night	Syphilinum 200	10 min. (3)
☆ Dry, scaly eruptions; dirty looking; intense itching; worse by warmth of bed	Psorinum 200	4 hourly (3)

Symptoms	Remedy	Frequency And Doses
❑ Dry eruptions; excessive thirst and constipation	**Natrum mur. 30**	*4 hourly*
❑ Eruptions with itching; worse at night, warmth and sweating	**Mercurius sol. 30**	*4 hourly*
❑ Eruptions with itching; worse warmth; stools very hard and constipated	**Alumina 30** or 0/5 onwards (50 millesimal)	*4 hourly*
❑ Itching, renewing constantly	**Sepia 30**	*4 hourly*
❑ Eruptions over whole body; worse in humid climate and washing	**Dulcamara 200**	*10 min. (3)*
❑ Eruptions only on covered parts of the body	**Thuja oc. 200** or **1M**	*4 hourly (3)*
Biochemic remedy	**Natrum mur. 12X**	*4 hourly*

PROPHYLACTICS
Preventive Remedies

❑ Cholera	**Cuprum met. 30** morning and night	*once in 3 days (6)*
❑ Conjunctivitis	**Belladonna 30** *morning and night*	*once in 3 day (6)*
❑ Chicken pox	**Variolinum 200**	*10 min. (3)*
❑ In **Variolinum** fails	**Antimonium tart. 200**	*10 min. (3)*
❑ Gastroenteritis	**Arsenic alb. 200**	*10 min. (3)*
❑ Flue	**Influenzinum 30 or 200** **Ist day,** from next day **Arsenic alb. 6**	*10 min. (3)* *morning and night (12)*
❑ Infective hepatitis	**Ferrum phos. 12X,** **Chelidonium 6**	4 hourly and *6 hourly (12)*
❑ Jaundice	**Merc-sol. 200,** *10 min.* **(3) Ist day,** **from** next day, **Kali mur. 6X**	*4 hourly*
❑ Malaria	**Malaria off. 200** or **1M**	*10 min. (3)*
❑ If **Malaria off.** fails	**Natrum mur. 200**	*weekly (3)*

Symptoms	Remedy	Frequency And Doses
❏ Measles	**Pulsatilla 30 or 200**	*once in 2-3 days (6)*
❏ Brain fever	**Belladonna 200**	*weekly (3)*
❏ Tetanus	**Ledum pal 200** and **Hypericum 200,** *alternate 3 hourly (3 each)*	
❏ Cataract	**Calcarea fluor. 12X,** 4 hourly, and **Natrum mur. 6X + Calcarea phos. 6X + Kali phos. 6X** (*2 tablets each, morning and evening*)	
❏ Cold	**Aconite 6 or 30,** In the beginning 1/2 hourly and afterward, 6 hourly, **Ferrum phos. 6X**	*2 hourly*
❏ Diphtheria	**Diphtherinum 200 or 1M**	*1 dose*
❏ Filaria	**Capsicum 30,** 6 hourly for 3-4 days, and later **Calc. fluor. 30X** *6 hourly*	
❏ Mumps	**Parotidinum 200** and **Pilocarpus 6**	*1 dose* *6 hourly (6)*
❏ Plague	**Tarentula h. 30 or 200**	*4 hourly (3)*
❏ Polio	**Lathyrus sat. 200** one dose in the first month, next month **1M** and in the 3rd month **10M** should be given	
❏ Meningitis	**Belladonna 30** **Ferrum phos. 12X**	*3 hourly (6)* *3 hourly*
❏ Small pox	**Variolinum 200**	*10 min. (3)*
❏ Tonsillitis	**Baryta carb. 200 or 1M**	*fortnightly (6)*
❏ Tuberculosis	**Tuberculinum k. 10M** 1st month, **50M** - 2nd month and **CM** - 3rd month	*(1 dose each)*
❏ Typhoid fever	**Typhoidinum 200 or 1M**	*10 min. (3)*
❏ Whooping cough	**Pertussin 200 or 1M**	*10 min. (3)*

Symptoms	Remedy	Frequency And Doses

PROLAPSUS
Rectum

Protrusion of the mucous membrane of the rectum through the anus.

Symptoms	Remedy	Frequency And Doses
☆ Before or while passing stools; constipation and diarrhoea alternates	Podophyllum 10M or 50M	fortnightly (3)
❏ While passing urine; due to piles, specially in children	Acid-mur. 30	4 hourly
❏ With hardness, distension and swelling of the abdomen	Mercurius sol. 30	4 hourly
❏ In persons leading sedentary life and taking stimulating diet and drinks	Nux vomica 30 or 200	6 hourly
● Intercurrent remedy	Sulphur 200 or 1M	10 min. (3)
❏ In persons suffering from piles; after passing stools; low backache	Aesculus hip. 30	4 hourly
☆ Diarrhoea followed by prolapsus of rectum	Belladonna 30	4 hourly
☆ In children who are constipated and prone to colds	Hydrastis can. 30	4 hourly
❏ Prolapsus rectum; worse when stools are soft	Ignatia 200 or 1M	10 min. (3)
Biochemic remedy	Calcarea fluor. 12X	4 hourly

Other Important Remedies:

Lycopodium, Calcarea carb. and Tuberculinum, etc..

PROLAPSUS
Uterus

This is a condition in which the womb falls from its natural position on account of the relaxed state of its ligaments; a consequence of severe labor, and enlarged or inflammed state of the womb. The organ comes down until it appears at the orifice of the vagina, and may even protrude.

In recent cases rest in the recumbent position will allow the parts to recover to their original state themselves. In older cases support must be used, and some form of pessary should be applied.

Symptoms	Remedy	Frequency And Doses
☆ Feeling of weight in the uterus; pressure, bearing down sensation; sinking feeling at epigastrium	**Sepia 30 or 200**	*4 hourly (3)*
☆ If Sepia fails; patient feels that contents of pelvis will come out through the vagina, supports vulva with hand. Constant desire to urinate	**Lilium tig. 30 or 200**	*4 hourly (3)*
❏ Due to concussion; bruised feeling	**Arnica 200 or 1M**	*10 min. (3)*
❏ When the ligaments of uterus are relaxed because of heavy uterus	**Fraxinus a. Q,** *5-10 drops*	*4 hourly*
❏ Patient feels worse during menstrual period; after lifting heavy weight. Depression or suicidal thoughts	**Aurum met. 200 or 1M**	*10 min. (3)*
☆ Associated with prolapsus of rectum; due to weakness	**Podophyllum 30 or 200**	*6 hourly*
❏ In weepy, timid patients; worse after lying down; patient feels better in cool, open air	**Pulsatilla 30 or 200**	*6 hourly*
❏ Bearing down sensation; pain in left ovarian region; cannot bear tight clothings around waist	**Lachesis 30 or 200**	*4 hourly (3)*
❏ Bearing down sensation; profuse and offensive menses; worse jar	**Belladonna 30**	*4 hourly*
❏ Menses early and scanty; bearing down sensation; worse during inter-course	**Pneumococcin. 30 or 200**	*4 hourly (3)*
Biochemic remedies	**Calcarea fluor. 12X** and **Calcarea phos. 3X**	*4 hourly*

Other Important Remedies:

Aloe s., Agaricus m., Aesculus hip., Argentum met., Helonias, Murex and Syphilinum, etc.. Physical exercises/preferably Yogic exercises) are helpful which can be learned under expert guidence.

Symptoms	Remedy	Frequency And Doses

PROSTATE GLAND
Ailments Of

☆ Head remedy; for inflammation and enlargement of prostate gland	**Sabal ser. Q,** *5-10 drops*	*4 hourly*
● Patient can pass urine easily only while standing; especially for old bachelors	**Conium mac. 200 or 1M**	*weekly (3)*
❑ Though the urge to pass urine is great but urine dribbles in small quantity only	**Staphysagria 30 or 200**	*4 hourly (3)*
❑ Great tenesmus with enlarged prostate; loss of thirst with dryness of mouth	**Pulsatilla 30 or 200**	*4 hourly (3)*
● In old age; childish behaviour, shy nature	**Baryta carb. 200 or 1M**	*weekly (3)*
❑ Cancer of prostate gland	**Cistus can. 30 or 200**	*4 hourly*
❑ Cancer of prostate gland, when urine dribbles after lying down	**Kreosote 30 or 200**	*3 hourly (3)*
● Intercurrent remedy	**Sulphur 200 or 1M**	*fortnightly (3)*

PRURITUS
Itching Of Genital Organs
(See Itching Also)

❑ Pimples on vulva; itching when patient becomes warm in bed	**Aethusa cy. 30**	*4 hourly*
❑ Itching of orifice of urethra; pruritus vaginae, anus, scrotum and shoulder	**Alumen 30**	*4 hourly*
☆ Itching on scrotum; itching on pudenda; swelling of labia; pruritus vulva during pregnancy	**Ambra gr. 30**	*4 hourly*
❑ Itching and burning of anus; itching of genitals	**Ammonium carb. 30**	*4 hourly*
❑ Itching with soreness if scratched; itching of penis; of tip of glans; biting, itching as from salt on left side of scrotum	**Antim-crud. 30**	*4 hourly*

Symptoms	Remedy	Frequency And Doses
❏ Itching of pudenda; pustules on external genitals	**Antim-tart. 30**	4 hourly
❏ Itching and stitches in internal or external vulva	**Calcarea carb. 30 or 200**	4 hourly (3)
✩ Pruritus vulvae; especially from masturbation, with strong sexual desire, during climaxis	**Cantharis 30**	4 hourly
❏ Crawling and itching in rectum and on perineum; sticking and itching in anus; itching and creeping in scrotum and glans	**Chelidonium 30**	4 hourly
❏ Pruritus vulva; accompanied by haemorrhoids; obstinate constipation during dysmenorrhoea or in pregnancy; worse when lying down	**Collinsonia 30 or 200**	4 hourly (3)
❏ Violent itching of pudenda and even within vagina; worse just after menstruation	**Conium mac. 30 or 200**	4 hourly (3)
✩ Itching on glans and scrotum; worse while walking; intense itching of female genitals; worse at night; better by very gentle scratching	**Croton tig. 30**	4 hourly
❏ Itching of mons veneris	**Euphorbium 30**	4 hourly
❏ Pruritus recti; the worms creep at night out of the anus	**Ferrum met. 30**	4 hourly
❏ Pruritus ani; itching within and around anus, on perineum	**Fluoric acid. 30**	4 hourly
❏ Pruritus ani with moisture and tendency to form little vesicles; itching in vulva; worse just before menses	**Graphites 30 or 200**	4 hourly (3)
❏ Itching at anus; which feels sore as if raw; pruritus of female genital parts	**Hamamelis 30**	4 hourly
❏ Pruritus vulvae; puffed, hot, redness and itching; labia swollen and covered with a curdy, white deposit	**Helonias 30**	4 hourly

Symptoms	Remedy	Frequency And Doses
❏ Itching of penis at fraenum preputii; smarting; itching of vulva; little injuries suppurate	**Hepar sulph. 30**	*4 hourly*
❏ Pruritus vulvae; with profuse leucorrhoea and sexual excitement	**Hydrastis can. 30**	*4 hourly*
❏ Irresistible nocturnal itching; compelling one to scratch and thus causing insomnia	**Iodium 30**	*4 hourly*
❏ Itching in region of mons veneris	**Kali carb. 30**	*4 hourly*
☆ Itching; soreness and smarting between labia and vulva	**Kreosotum 30**	*4 hourly*
☆ Itching of anus; worse after sleep	**Lachesis 30**	*4 hourly*
❏ Slight excoriation and itching of the external labia; feels at times as if caused by something alive in it	**Lac caninum 30**	*4 hourly*
❏ Itching in vagina with feeling of fullness in parts; stinging in left ovarian region	**Lilium tig. 30**	*4 hourly*
❏ Biting, itching when becoming warm during the day; itching, eruption at anus, painful to touch; itching of inner surface of prepuce	**Lycopodium 30**	*4 hourly*
❏ Itching on genitals and scrotum; extending to anus; worse while sitting; better by exercise and motion	**Magnesia mur. 30**	*4 hourly*
❏ Itching of scrotum which is not relieved by scratching	**Muriatic acid. 30**	*4 hourly*
❏ Itching, soreness and moisture between scrotum and thighs; leucorrhoea causes itching with yellow complexion; itching of female external parts with falling off of the hair	**Natrum mur. 12X or 30**	*4 hourly*
❏ Falling off of the hair from genitals; itching, swelling and burning of vulva and vagina	**Nitric-acid. 30**	*4 hourly*

Symptoms	Remedy	Frequency And Doses
❑ Itching between scrotum and thighs; on perineum; soreness and moisture on female genitals with violent itching	**Petroleum 30**	*4 hourly*
❑ Itching inside the uterus; pruritus vulvae	**Platina 200**	*4 hourly (3)*
● Due to amenorrhoea; during pregnancy; pimples, itch violently; about nipples, oozing out of fluid; worse in bed and from warmth; scratches until it bleeds, which gives relief	**Psorinum 200**	*4 hourly (3)*
❑ Itching and burning on inner and upper side of prepuce; worse at night, from delayed menses; better from washing with cold water	**Pulsatilla 30 or 200**	*4 hourly (3)*
❑ Worse by cold; better by warmth, more formication than burning	**Rumex c. 30**	*4 hourly*
❑ In newly-married with frequent urging to urinate; stinging and itching of vulva	**Staphysagria 30 or 200**	*4 hourly (3)*
● Itching with burning; worse evenings and in bed; worse after scratching	**Sulphur 30 or 200**	*4 hourly (3)*
❑ Intense itching of vulva and vagina; worse night with dryness and heat of the parts	**Tarentula hisp. 30**	*4 hourly (3)*
❑ Patient cannot sleep on account of the intense itching of the anus; causing him to toss and roll at night; at times due to pin worms	**Teucrium m-v. 30**	*4 hourly*
❑ Excessive itching during menses; inducing masturbation, with fidgety feet	**Zincum met. 30**	*4 hourly*
Biochemic remedy	**Biocombination No. 20**	*4 hourly*

PSORIASIS

A condition characterized by the eruption of circumscribed, discrete and confluent, reddish, silvery-scaled maculopapules; the lesions occur pre-eminently on the elbows, knees, scalp, and trunk; and microscopically show characteristic parakeratosis and elongation of rete ridges.

Symptoms	Remedy	Frequency And Doses
● Head remedy (to start the treatment); aversion to take bath; in deep thinking, stoop shouldered patients	**Sulphur 10M or 50M**	*monthly (3)*
● Intercurrent remedy; in obstinate and chronic cases	**Carcinocin 1M or 10M**	*monthly (3)*
❏ In cautious, constipated and indecisive individuals; little injury suppurates	**Graphites 200 or 1M**	*10 min. (3)*
❏ Individuals over sensitive to cold and other changes; desire for warmth	**Hepar sulph. 200 or 1M**	*10 min. (3)*
❏ With extensive thickening and exfoliation of the skin	**Hydrocotyle a. 200**	*6 hourly*
● Worse cold application and better by warmth; burning sensation	**Arsenic a. 0/7 or above**	*6 hourly*
● In chronic cases when well selected remedy fails; burning and itching	**Radium brom. 200 or above**	*fortnightly (3)*
Biochemic remedies		
— In allergic conditions	**Natrum mur. 12X** and **Natrum sulph. 12X**	*4 hourly*
— With thickening of scab formation	**Calcarea fluor. 12X** and **Kali sulph. 6X**	*4 hourly*

Other Important Remedies:

Nitric acid., Psorinum, Syphilinum, Sepia, Medorrhinum, Petroleum, Thuja oc., Thyroidinum, Arsenic brom., Kali ars., Natrum mur. and Ocimun sanc., etc..

PTERYGIUM

It is a vascular, triangular thickening of a portion of the conjunctiva with its apex resting on the edge of the cornea. The most frequent location of a pterygium is over the internal rectus muscle. Pterygium grows very slowly and has a tendency to spread over the cornea, though rarely seen to grow beyond the centre of the pupil.

Constitutional treatment in Homoeopathy is quite satisfactory.

❏ Head remedy	**Zincum sulph. 1M and above**	*fortnightly (6)*
❏ If caused by exposure to cold and wet; chilly, fat and flabby patient	**Calcarea carb. 200 or 1M**	*weekly (6)*

Symptoms	Remedy	Frequency And Doses
❑ With scrofula and glandular enlargements	**Chimaphila 30**	*4 hourly*
❑ Smarting and stinging pains at inner canthus; profuse lachrymation and marked photophobia; worse in cold air and at night; better in warm room	**Zincum met. 30**	*4 hourly*

Other Important Remedies:

Amm-brom., Arg-nit., Arsenic alb., Lachesis, Nux-m., Psorinum, Ratan., Spigelia, Staphysagria, Sulphur, and Tellurium, etc..

PULSE
Affections Of

Symptoms	Remedy	Frequency And Doses
❑ Fast and thready; in cases of internal haemorrhage, chilly feeling and restlessness	**Arsenic alb. 30 or 200**	*1/2 hourly (3)*
❑ Bounding pulse; after waking	**Petroleum 30 or 200**	*6 hourly*
❑ Improportionate with temperature	**Pyrogenium 200 or 1M**	*10 min. (3)*
❑ Excited and frequent pulse; chilly feeling; every fourth or fifth beat intermittent	**Nux vomica 30 or 200**	*4 hourly*
❑ Frequent; while in bed	**Sulphuric acid. 30**	*4 hourly*
❑ Fast; after midnight	**Acid-benz. 30**	*4 hourly*
❑ Fast; after eating	**Lycopodium 200 or 1M**	*10 min. (3)*
❑ Frequent; during rest	**Magnesia mur. 200**	*10 min. (3)*
❑ Frequent; after passing stool	**Conium mac. 200**	*10 min. (3)*
❑ Heavy and slow; body icy cold; in exhaustive diseases	**Veratrum v. 30**	*1/2 hourly*
❑ Every other beat intermittent	**Spigelia 200**	*6 hourly*
❑ Every third beat intermittent; irregular, after exertion, lying on left side; excessive thirst and constipation	**Natrum mur. 30 or 200**	*4 hourly*

Symptoms	Remedy	Frequency And Doses
❏ Every third or fourth beat intermittent	Nitric acid. 200	10 min. (3)
❏ Every third or fourth beat intermittent	Cimicifuga 30	4 hourly
❏ Every sixth or seventh beat intermittent	Acid-mur. 30	4 hourly
❏ Every tenth beat intermittent; worse exertion, apprehension	Gelsemium 30	4 hourly
❏ Tenth to thirtieth beat intermittent	Cina 200 or 1M	10 min. (3)
❏ Slow; in the evening; stools constipated	Graphites 30 or 200	6 hourly

PYORRHOEA

● Head remedy	Calendula 30	4 hourly
☆ Spongy gums with moist mouth; bad odour with excessive saliva and thirst	Merc-sol. 30	4 hourly
❏ Boils on gums; painful inflammation, sensitive to cool air	Silicea 12X or 30	4 hourly
❏ Profuse salivation; toothache, better while eating; worse cold air and contact	Plantago 30	4 hourly
❏ Rapid decay of teeth with bleeding of spongy gums; offensive smell from mouth	Kreosotum 30	4 hourly
☆ A good remedy for Pyorrhoea	Calcarea ren. 30	4 hourly
❏ Suppuration of gums with pus formation	Gun powder 3X or 6	4 hourly
☆ Gums retracted; bleeds easily	Carbo veg. 3X or 6	4 hourly
Biochemic remedy	Silicea 12X or 30X	4 hourly

For External Use (to massage the gums):

Calendula Q, Echinacea Q and Arnica Q + Glycerine in 1: 9.

RENAL CALCULI
Kidney Stone

The formation of an urinary stone usually takes place in the kidney and from there it passes down the ureter into the bladder, causing severe pain during its travel along the ureter. This severe pain is known as Renal Colic. But when the size of a stone is big it remains in the kidney, causing severe or less pain or no pain at all. Hereditary gout or rheumatism plays important role in the formation of Renal Calculi.

Symptoms	Remedy	Frequency And Doses
☆ During acute stage; when the pain is unbearable	**Aconite 200 or 1M and Chamomilla 200 or 1M** *alternate, every 15 minutes (3 doses each)*	
❑ Ineffectual urging to pass urine; renal colic extending to genitals with dribbling urine; itching in urethra and neck of bladder while passing urine; chilly feeling	**Nux vomica 200**	*4 hourly (3)*
☆ Can pass urine after long effort only; flow of urine feeble; red sand in the urine; burning, cutting pain before and during passing urine in the back part of kidney; better after passing urine; worse right side	**Lycopodium 200 or 1M**	*10 min. (3)*
☆ Digging, tearing or pulsative pain in region of one kidney or both; worse from deep pressure; extending from kidney to bladder and urethra with urging to urinate; worse left side. Backache with severe prostration	**Berberis vulg. Q or above**	*4 hourly*
❑ Urine bloody red or brownish red with white and mealy sediment. Urine looks like lime-water after keeping for sometime; burning in urethra during urination	**Calcarea carb. 200**	*6 hourly (3)*
❑ To expel renal calculi or vesical calculi and to stop the formation of stones	**Calcarea renalis 3X or 30**	*4 hourly*

Symptoms	Remedy	Frequency And Doses
☆ Severe pain is experienced near the neck of bladder soon after emission of urine	**Sarsaparilla Q or 30**	*4 hourly*
❑ Agonizing pain in back and hips from passage of calculi. Brick-dust sediment in urine	**Arnica 30 or 200**	*4 hourly*
❑ Kidney pain penetrates chest. Dark brown sediment in urine; foul smell	**Benzoic acid. 30**	*4 hourly*
❑ Passage of calculi with twisting, crampy pain; better bending backwards	**Dioscorea 30**	*4 hourly*
☆ Calculi consisting of calcium oxalate. Red sand, or sediment in urine. Urine is cold when it is passed; intolerable; smell strong like horse urine	**Nitric-acid. 30 or 200**	*4 hourly (3)*
☆ Can pass urine better by getting down on hands on knees; Urine contains much viscid, thick, whitish mucous or deposit of red sand; smells strongly like ammonia	**Pariera br. Q,** *5-10 drops*	*4 hourly (3)*
❑ Turbid urine with red, sandy or brick-coloured sediment	**Sepia 30 or 200**	*4 hourly (3)*
❑ Renal colic; deathly nausea - which disturbs greatly	**Tabacum 30**	*4 hourly*
❑ Calculi in bladder; flow of urine stops suddenly; urine ropy and bloody. Painful urination with burning sensation	**Uva ursi 30**	*4 hourly*
☆ Sharp, tearing pain; burning with urination; inflammation of urinary passage	**Cantharis 30**	*4 hourly*
❑ Can pass urine with difficulty; passes urine comfortably by leaning back	**Zincum met. 200**	*10 min. (3)*
❑ Can pass urine better while lying down; cant' hold urine; dribbles after lying down	**Kreosote 30**	*4 hourly*

Biochemic remedy

— For pain	**Magnesia phos. 6X**	*1/2 hourly*
— To dessolve the stone	**Silicea 12X or 30X** and **Calc-phos. 30X**	*4 hourly*

RESTLESSNESS
(See Anxiety Also)

Symptoms	Remedy	Frequency And Doses
☆ Sudden with anxiety and acute imagination; after exposure to dry, cold wind	**Aconite nap. 200 or 1M**	*10 min. (3)*
☆ With debility and exhaustion; unquenchable thirst-drinks less at a time but frequently	**Arsenic alb. 30 or 200**	*4 hourly (3)*
☆ With great apprehension at night; restlessness, keep tossing in bed	**Rhus tox. 200 or 1M**	*4 hourly (6)*
Biochemic remedy	**Kali phos. 6X**	*4 hourly*

RETINA
Ailments Of

Symptoms	Remedy	Frequency And Doses
❑ Detachment of retina; exudation in the retina; retina is inflammed. Pain and soreness in the head and around the eyes; sadness	**Naphthaline 30 or 200**	*10 min. (3)*
❑ When the eyes are sensitive to light, patient sees ring shaped halo around the light; inflammation of the retina; craving for cold drinks	**Phosphorus 200 or 1M**	*weekly (3)*
❑ Inflammation of retina; severe, sharp pain through the eye; worse by motion	**Bryonia 30 or 200**	*4 hourly*
❑ Upper half of vision seems as if covered by a black body; lower half visible; retinal infiltration; deposits on the retina	**Aurum met. 200 or 1M**	*weekly (3)*
❑ Fluid beneath the retina. Passive pain in the lower part of the ball with flushed face and head. Stinging pain through the eye. Oedematous swelling of the lids	**Apis mel. 200**	*weekly (3)*

Separation of the retina from the choroid is usually the result of an exudation of serum, but may occur from any other exudation or haemorrhage under the retina, or from tumor also.

Symptoms	Remedy	Frequency And Doses
❏ Inflammation of retina with restlessness, especially after midnight with thirst for small quantities of water. Urine scanty and albuminous	Arsenic alb. 30	4 hourly
❏ Inflammation of retina during pregnancy; sudden dimness of vision; detachment of retina due to injury or myopia	Gelsemium 30	4 hourly
❏ Haemorrhages into the retina with inflammation	Lachesis 30 or 200	10 min. (3)
❏ Blood in retina in cases of snake poisoning; inflammation of the retina	Crotalus h. 200	10 min. (3)
❏ Sudden sensitiveness to light; aching pain in eyes and the retina	Belladonna 30	3 hourly
❏ Retina over sensitive to the light; pain deep in the eye	Conium mac. 200	10 min. (3)
❏ Detachment of retina due to injury. Retinal haemorrhage	Arnica m. 200 or 1M	10 min. (3)

Other Important Remedies:

Digitalis, Rhus tox. and Syphilinum, Ruta and Hypericum, etc..

RHEUMATISM
(See Arthritis)

RICKETS

Its character consists essentially of an irritation of the osteo-plastic tissue in consequence of which there is an over-growth of the same, with less earthy salts than are required for the formation of healthy bone.

❏ Abnormal cravings; loose or hard constipated stools with much straining; absence of sweat; dry, lustreless hair; slow in walking, speaking and cutting teeth;	Alumina 30	4 hourly

Symptoms	Remedy	Frequency And Doses
large head; open fontanelles; bathed in cold sweat; voracious appetite		
❏ Curvature of the lumbar vertebrae; squinting; enlarged pupils; pain in the throat when swallowing; thick, protruding belly	**Belladonna 30**	*4 hourly*
❏ Slow, difficult teething; profuse sweating about the head; fontanelles open; abdomen enlarged; whitish, frothy diarrhoea; curvature of the spine and deformities of the extremities	**Calcarea carb. 200 or 1M**	*weekly (6)*
❏ The fontanelles remain widely open; the diarrhoea and the emaciation of the child; general weakness	**Calcarea phos. 12X or 30**	*4 hourly*
❏ When the thighs are notably emaciated, and the disease is in its early stages; with slight pliability of the bones	**Natrum mur. 12X or 30**	*4 hourly*

Other Important Remedies:

Phosphorus, Asafoetida, Aurum mur., Hepar sulph., Iodium, Sulphur, Fluor-ac., Lact-ac., Lycopodium, Merc-sol., Mezereum., Phosphoric ac., Sepia, Silicea, Staphysagria., Symphytum, Theridion, etc..

RIGHT SIDED REMEDIES

The Important Remedies:

Anacardium, Apis mel., Bryonia, Causticum, Chelidonium, Cinnaberis, Conium mac., Dolichos, Equisetum, Ferrum phos., Iodium, Kali carb., Lithium carb., Lycopodium, Magnesia phos., Merc-sol., Phytolacca, Podophyllum, Rhus tox., Sanguinaria c. and Tarantula h., etc..

RINGWORM

☆ Head remedy	**Bacillinum 200 or 1M**	*weekly (3)*

Symptoms	Remedy	Frequency And Doses
☆ When accompanied with acidity, indigestion and retching; loss of appetite; aversion to take bath	Sulphur 200	10 min. (3)
☆ With offensive, garlic like odour of the body and sweat	Tellurium 30	4 hourly
☆ Ringworm on face; isolated spots on upper parts of the body; better by warmth or warm applications	Sepia 200	weekly (3)
● With intense itching; scratches till it bleeds which ameliorates; foul smell from effected lesions	Psorinum 200 or 1M	weekly (3)
❏ Ringworm on scalp; hair falls in patches; skin dry and rough; restlessness; thirst unquenchable	Arsenic alb. 30	4 hourly
❏ Ringworm with fetid sweat; worse in warm damp weather	Dulcamara 30 or 200	6 hourly (3)
Biochemic remedy	Natrum mur. 12X or 30X	4 hourly

Other Important Remedies:

Tuberculinum k., Calcarea carb., Hydrastis can., Acid-chryso., Natrum carb. and Clematis, etc..

SADNESS
(See Suicidal Disposition Also)

Symptoms	Remedy	Frequency And Doses
❏ Sadness with weeping moods, due to grief	**Causticum 200 or 1M**	*3 hourly (3)*
❏ Sadness; in morning, after sleep, after walking; in sun	**Lachesis 200 or 1M**	*3 hourly (3)*
❏ Sadness; twilight, at night, in darkness, causeless	**Phosphorus 200 or 1M**	*3 hourly (3)*
❏ Sadness; evening, with suicidal thoughts	**Aurum met. 200 or 1M**	*3 hourly (3)*
❏ Sadness; while in bed, night, after grief, during heat, cannot weep	**Natrum mur. 200 or 1M**	*3 hourly (3)*
❏ Sadness; when alone, with restlessness	**Arsenic alb. 200 or 1M**	*3 hourly (3)*
❏ Sadness; from anger, in warm room	**Pulsatilla 200 or 1M**	*3 hourly (3)*
❏ Sadness; after eating; irritable	**Nux vomica 200 or 1M**	*3 hourly (3)*
❏ Sadness; due to suppressed eruptions, morning	**Sulphur 200 or 1M**	*3 hourly (3)*
❏ Sadness; while at home, during rest	**Rhus tox. 200 or 1M**	*3 hourly (3)*
❏ Sadness; with impotency, melancholic	**Kali br. 200 or 1M**	*3 hourly (3)*
❏ Sadness; from itching; hopelessness	**Psorinum 200 or 1M**	*3 hourly (3)*
❏ Sadness; from disappointed love; after mortification, with sighing	**Ignatia 200 or 1M**	*3 hourly (3)*
❏ Sadness; from masturbation; loss of vital fluids	**Acid-phos. 30 or 200**	*3 hourly (3)*
❏ Sadness; from delayed menses, nervous exhaustion	**Kali phos. 6X or 30**	*3 hourly (3)*
❏ Sadness; every fourteenth day, periodical; during perspiration; lack of interest	**Conium mac. 200 or 1M**	*3 hourly (3)*

Symptoms	Remedy	Frequency And Doses
❏ Sadness; during pregnancy; superiority complex	**Platina 200 or 1M**	*4 hourly (3)*
Biochemic remedy	**Natrum mur. 30X**	*4 hourly*

SALIVATION

Though the remedies can not be given for salivation only, but they can be helpful when abnormal salivation is associated with other complaints.

❏ Constant spitting due to accumulation of saliva in mouth	**Ammon-carb. 30**	*4 hourly*
❏ Saliva acrid; excessive	**Arum triph. 30**	*4 hourly*
❏ Saliva soapy; frothy	**Bryonia 30**	*4 hourly*
❏ Saliva profuse; swallows constantly; tongue clean	**Ipecac 30**	*4 hourly*
❏ Saliva roapy; profuse; drips from mouth while talking	**Iris v. 30**	*4 hourly*
❏ Saliva profuse; foul and bloody	**Nitric-acid. 30**	*4 hourly*
❏ Saliva sweetish; watery, frothy, cotton like; bad taste; worse morning; thirstlessness	**Pulsatilla 30**	*4 hourly*
Biochemic remedy	**Natrum mur. 12X**	*4 hourly*

Other Important Remedies:

Alumina, Bromium, Chamomilla, Graphites, Hepar sulph., Nux vomica, Sepia, Ignatia, Jaborandi, Lac can., Sulphur, Stannum met., Rhus tox., Merc-sol., Kreosote and Silicea, etc..

SCABIES

This is a parasitic infection of various layers of epithelium of the skin. The symptoms start with itching and inflammation/eruptions on the skin. The infection affects the skin of the body, starting usually from folds, eruptions on fingers and toes.

☆ Head remedy; itching with burning or soreness after scratching	**Sulphur 2X or 6**	*4 hourly*
☆ Pustular eruptions; specially on bends of	**Mercurius sol. 30**	*4 hourly*

Symptoms	Remedy	Frequency And Doses
elbows; itching worse from heat and at night	(Sulphur 30 and Mercurius sol. 30 *can be given alternately*)	
❏ With soreness in folds of skin; involuntary urination while coughing or walking; better in humid climate	Causticum 30 or 200	*4 hourly*
❏ Eruptions in bends of knees; pustular with burning and itching; better by warmth	Arsenic alb. 30 or 200	*4 hourly (3)*
❏ Bluish, pustular eruptions; patient feels worse after sleep	Lachesis 30 or 200	*4 hourly (3)*
❏ Chronic cases; when itch returns in every spring; burning in the food pipe	Acid-sulph. 30	*4 hourly*
❏ Itch of genital organs; numbness of skin; numbness of arms	Ambra gr. 30	*4 hourly*
❏ Itching; small reddish eruptions; worse by cold and after rest	Rhus tox. 30	*4 hourly*
● Chronic cases; itching and soreness; intercurrent remedy	Psorinum 0/6 and above	*4 hourly*
❏ Pustular, painful eruptions; sensitive to touch; chilly patient	Hepar sulph. 30	*4 hourly*
❏ Intense itching; scratches till it bleeds; itching worse from warmth of bed	Mezereum 30	*4 hourly*
☆ Scabies with honey like discharge; stools constipated	Graphites 30	*4 hourly*

For External Use:

Sulphur Q mixed in oil or Benzyl benzoate solution should be used and clothes of the patient should be washed in boiling water for 3 - 4 days regularly.

SCARLET FEVER
(See Fever Also)

☆ Head remedy	Belladonna 30	*3 hourly*

Symptoms	Remedy	Frequency And Doses
❑ Lack of proper eruptions; turning into malignant scarlatina; threatening paralysis of brain. Body red; malignancy with swollen throat	**Ammon-carb. 30**	*3 hourly*
❑ With pains alternating from side to side	**Lac-can. 30 or 200**	*3 hourly (3)*
❑ Cases of blood poisoning; pulse rapid and feeble; prostration	**Mur-acid. 30**	*3 hourly*
● In obstinate cases - intercurrent remedy	**Psorinum 200**	*3 hourly (3)*
❑ Fever with restlessness; triangular tip of tongue red and dry	**Rhus tox. 30**	*3 hourly*

Biochemic remedy

With hot dry skin	**Ferrum phos. 6X**	*3 hourly*

SCIATICA
(See Arthritis, Slipped Disc, Lumbago, Etc., Also)

Symptoms	Remedy	Frequency And Doses
❑ Feels as if tendons in left hip were too short; limps while walking due to this tension; worse while sitting. Pain better while lying down	**Ammonium mur. 200**	*4 hourly*
❑ Pain worse at night; from least jar; from hanging limb down and warmth	**Belladonna 30 or 200**	*3 hourly*
❑ Violent drawing, tearing pains; numb feeling with pain in affected parts; worse in bed at night and by motion	**Chamomilla 200 or 1M**	*4 hourly*
✰ Tearing pains; shoot down from hip to thigh, leg and feet; shooting pain like lightning down the whole limbs; sudden pain; worse by touch, cold and motion; better during rest, pressure and warmth	**Colocynth 200 or 1M**	*3 hourly*
✰ Shooting pains in course of left sciatic nerve, gnawing in hip-bone; legs feels tired	**Eupatorium perf. 200 or 1M**	*3 hourly*

Symptoms	Remedy	Frequency And Doses
❑ Due to injury to nerve; excruciating pain	**Hypericum 30 or 200**	*4 hourly*
☆ Pain runs upwards. Affected limb cooler than rest of the body. Pain worse in bed when getting warm; better by cold compresses	**Ledum pal. 200 or 1M**	*4 hourly*
❑ Pain like electric shocks; shooting; on outer side of thigh; desire to move, but movement aggravates pain.	**Phytolacca 30 or 200**	*4 hourly*
☆ Caused by exposure to wet, straining while lifting; with numbness; worse during rest; better by heat and rubbing. Pain worse in damp cold weather and at night	**Rhus tox. 200 or 1M**	*6 hourly*
❑ Deep seated pain. Worse during rest, after injuries, contusions, etc.	**Ruta g. 30 or 200**	*4 hourly*
❑ Worse exposure to cold or even to air; better by covering	**Stillingia 30 or 200**	*4 hourly*
❑ Due to over exertion; bed feels very hard	**Arnica mont. 30 or 200**	*4 hourly*
❑ Pain start from small of back; extend down lower limbs and keep them in constant uneasiness; worse by cold; chilly patient	**Calcarea carb. 200 or 1M**	*10 min. (3)*
❑ Tendons of knees feel too short; stiff and contracted; constant desire to move the foot; worse in open air; better by warmth	**Causticum 30 or 200**	*4 hourly*
❑ Frequent shooting pain; radiate downwards; better stretching the limb and by moving	**Dioscorea 30**	*4 hourly*
☆ Numbness alternating with pain; intense darting, burning pain along posterior sciatic nerve; worse by motion	**Gnaphalium 200 or 1M**	*4 hourly*
❑ Pain worse motion; exposure to air; patient over sensitive to cold, etc.	**Hepar sulph. 30 or 200**	*4 hourly*
❑ Tearing pain in hip-joint and knee; worse at night. Profuse sweat which do not relieve	**Merc-sol. 30 or 200**	*4 hourly*

Symptoms	Remedy	Frequency And Doses
❑ Left-sided sciatica; worse on beginning to move; relieved by gentle motion; better by rubbing and from pressure. Worse in the evening, night and in a warm room; better in open air	**Pulsatilla 200**	*4 hourly*
☆ Weakness and lameness of extremities; bruised feeling in muscles of thighs; worse standing and walking; radiates downwards	**Kalmia lat. 200**	*4 hourly*
☆ Pain worse at night; specially towards morning; gnawing pain in periosteum of left leg	**Kali iod. 200 or 1M** or even higher	*weekly (6)*
Biochemic remedies	**Magnesia phos. 6X** and **Calcarea phos. 6X**	*4 hourly*

SCARS
(See Beauty Tips And Keloids)

SCURVY

A form of haemorrhagic diathesis due to deficient and improper diet. Mucous membrane of the mouth becomes sore, inflamed, and dry; or becomes the seat of shallow ulcers, or the gums become spongy and bleed. This last is one of the chief symptoms of the disease called scurvy.

❑ In cases of scurvy or sore mouth; where the gums are tender and bleed easily	**Mercurius sol. 30**	*4 hourly*
❑ For sore mouth; caused by mercury or pyorrhoea	**Carbo veg. 3X or 30**	*4 hourly*
❑ Great debility; low feverish state, burning in ulcers and anxiety	**Arsenic alb. 30**	*4 hourly*
Biochemic remedies	**Kali mur. 6X** and **Natrum phos. 6X**	*4 hourly*

Symptoms	Remedy	Frequency And Doses

SEMINAL EMISSION
Ejaculation
(See Spermatorrhoea Also)

❑ Ejaculation; bloody at night	**Mercurius sol. 200**	4 hourly (3)
❑ Ejaculation; cold during coition	**Natrum mur. 200 or 1M**	weekly (3)
❑ Ejaculation; difficult, very quick	**Zincum met. 200 or 1M**	weekly (3)
❑ Ejaculation; failling during coition	**Graphites 200 or 1M**	weekly (3)
❑ Ejaculation; frothy	**Mur-acid. 200 or 1M**	weekly (3)
❑ Ejaculation; erection before, painful	**Sulphur 200 or 1M**	weekly (3)
❑ Ejaculation; very late, early	**Calcarea carb. 200 or 1M**	weekly (3)
❑ Ejaculation; lemon-coloured	**Hura b. 30 or 200**	weekly (3)
❑ Ejaculation; milky with strong odour	**Lachesis 200 or 1M**	weekly (3)
❑ Ejaculation; odour abnormal or odourless	**Selenium 30 or 200**	weekly (3)
❑ Ejaculation; like stale urine	**Natrum phos. 200**	weekly (3)
❑ Ejaculation; reddish-brown	**Fluoric acid. 200 or 1M**	weekly (3)
❑ Ejaculation; sticky	**Staphysagria 200 or 1M**	weekly (3)
❑ Ejaculation; sudden	**Phosphorus 200 or 1M**	weekly (3)

SENSATIONS

Feeling the translation into consciousness of the effects of a stimulus exciting any of the sense organs.

❑ Tingling sensations; stitching and stabbing; numbness	**Aconite nap. 30 or 200**	4 hourly
❑ Sensation as if bugs are crawling over bed; bed feels too hard; moving of the brain in skull; anxiety and restlessness	**Arsenic alb. 30 or 200**	4 hourly (3)

Symptoms	Remedy	Frequency And Doses
❑ Sensation as if dogs and cats are running across the room	**Aethusa cyn. 200 or 1M**	*weekly (3)*
❑ Sensation as if he is not fit for this world	**Aurum met. 200 or 1M**	*weekly (3)*
❑ Sensation as if a rat is running up leg	**Ailanthus gl. 30 or 200**	*weekly (3)*
❑ Sensation of falling	**Belladonna 200**	*weekly (3)*
❑ Sensation of bugs running over lips	**Borax 200 or 1M**	*weekly (3)*
❑ Sensation as if he/she is 'scattered about'	**Baptisia 30 or 200**	*4 hourly (3)*
❑ Sensation of water in the chest; red hot iron at vertex; shortening of right limb; an opening in stomach through which air passes; falling out of bed; as if something were alive in the head	**Crotalus casc. 200**	*4 hourly (3)*
❑ Sensation of being transparent; gradual swelling; a dual existence; as if time and space extended	**Cannabis ind. 200 or 1M**	*4 hourly (3)*
❑ Sensation of ants running through the whole body	**Cistus can. 30 or 200**	*4 hourly (3)*
❑ Sensation of heart being stopped	**Cicuta v. 30 or 200**	*4 hourly (3)*
❑ Sensation as if the room were too small	**Cyclamen 30 or 200**	*4 hourly (3)*
❑ Sensation as if a black cloud enveloped the patient	**Cimicifuga 30 or 200**	*4 hourly (3)*
❑ Sensation as if worms were crawling in the stomach	**Cocculus ind. 200**	*4 hourly (3)*
❑ Sensation as if mouse is running up legs and arms	**Calcarea phos. 30 or 200**	*4 hourly (3)*
❑ Sensation of shiverings better by moving	**Drosera. 200 or 1M**	*4 hourly (3)*
❑ Sensation of as if someone is following; hammering	**Lachesis. 200 or 1M**	*4 hourly (3)*
❑ Sensation of shivering worse by moving	**Nux vomica. 200**	*4 hourly (3)*
❑ Sensation of suffocation	**Viburnum opulus. 200**	*4 hourly (3)*
❑ Sensation of arms and legs crowding the patient; covering the whole bed	**Pyrogenium 200 or 1M**	*4 hourly (3)*

Symptoms	Remedy	Frequency And Doses
❑ Sensation of cold water in the body	**Ranun-bulb. 30 or 200**	*4 hourly (3)*
❑ Sensation of insects crawling over surface of the body	**Phosphorus 200**	*4 hourly (3)*
❑ Sensation of something alive in the body; as if legs were made of wood; body were brittle	**Thuja oc. 200 or 1M**	*4 hourly (3)*
❑ Sensation as if someone else is in bed	**Petroleum 200 or 1M**	*4 hourly (3)*
❑ Sensation of bed being too small	**Sulphur 200 or 1M**	*4 hourly (3)*
❑ Sensation as if patient is in a strange place	**Opium 200 or 1M**	*4 hourly (3)*
❑ Sensation as if tongue were scalded	**Platinum 200 or 1M**	*4 hourly (3)*
❑ Sensation as if cold water ran down outside the oesophagus	**Veratrum alb. 200 or 1M**	*4 hourly (3)*
❑ Sensation as if damp clothing was on arms and legs	**Veratrum vir. 200 or 1M**	*4 hourly (3)*
❑ Sensation as if bag of water turns when turning over in bed	**Ornithogalum 200 or 1M**	*4 hourly (3)*
❑ Sensation as if drunk; skull would split	**Mezereum 200 or 1M**	*4 hourly (3)*
❑ Sensation as if hot water poured from breast into abdomen	**Sanguinaria c. 200 or 1M**	*4 hourly (3)*
❑ Sensation as if dogs gnawed flesh and bones	**Nitric-acid. 200 or 1M**	*4 hourly (3)*
❑ Sensation as if spiders crawled over hand	**Viscum alb. 30 or 200**	*4 hourly (3)*
❑ Sensation as if things and people are black	**Stramonium 200 or 1M**	*4 hourly (3)*

SEPTICAEMIA
Blood Poisoning

☆ When due to injuries; veins become darker in colour and fever goes upto 97° to 105°F. Infection spreading from uterus; after child birth	**Echinacea Q or 30**	*2 hourly*

Symptoms	Remedy	Frequency And Doses
☆ Muscular soreness; restlessness; great debility and prostration. Particularly in long continued fever like typhoid, etc.	**Baptisia 6 or 30**	*4 hourly*
❑ Patient over sensitive to touch; can not even tolerate touch of clothes; worse after sleep. Bruised, lacerated wounds, gangrene and carbuncles, etc. with high fever	**Lachesis 30 or 200**	*4 hourly (3)*
❑ Due to bruises; bed feels very hard; restlessness and bruised pain	**Arnica 200 or 1M**	*4 hourly (3)*
☆ Septic fever; pulse fast, out of all proportion to the temperature; discharges offensive	**Pyrogenium 200**	*10 min. (3)*
❑ Septic fever with excessive thirst for little water at a time at short intervals; anxiety and restlessness; burning sensation; putrid discharge	**Arsenic alb. 30**	*3 hourly*
❑ Septicaemia after surgical operations; loss of vital fluids, coldness of body and desire for fanning	**Carbo veg. 30**	*3 hourly*
Biochemic remedy	**Kali phos. 6X**	*4 hourly*

SEXUAL DESIRE
Female
(See Masturbation And Nymphomania Also)

☆ Nymphomania; unbearable sexual desire especially in young unmarried girls. Wishes to embrace everybody	**Platina 200 or 1M**	*10 min. (3)*
☆ If Platina does not relieve the above symptoms; exposes the genital organs, sexual desire unbearable; easily influenced	**Phosphorus 200 or 1M**	*10 min. (3)*
❑ Patient exposes her genitals; indecent, obscene and talks nonsense	**Hyoscyamus 200**	*10 min. (3)*

Symptoms	Remedy	Frequency And Doses
❑ Least touch of the genital organs produces excessive sexual desire	**Murex 30 or 200**	*4 hourly*
❑ Itching of genitals; restlessness, sexual excitement; excessive desire to embrace	**Agaricus mus. 30 or 200**	*4 hourly*
☆ Worms in vagina cause itching; excessive sexual excitement due to scratching the genital organs	**Caladium s. 30 or 200**	*4 hourly*
❑ Excessive sexual excitement during menstrual periods	**Stramonium 200 or 1M**	*10 min. (3)*
❑ Leucorrhoea with increased sexual desire	**Sepia 200**	*10 min. (3)*
❑ Timid, weepy, thirstless and chilly women, likes consolation, open air and to be embraced	**Pulsatilla 200**	*10 min. (3)*
❑ Aversion to coition due to dryness of vagina	**Natrum mur. 200**	*4 hourly (3)*

SEXUAL DESIRE
Male

❑ Desire diminished or completely lost	**Lycopodium 200 or 1M**	*weekly (3)*
❑ Desire diminished after excessive indulgence in sex	**Staphysagria 200 or 1M**	*weekly (3)*
❑ Desire excessive; disturbing sleep	**Cantharis 200 or 1M**	*weekly (3)*
❑ Excessive desire; easily excited	**Zincum met. 200 or 1M**	*weekly (3)*
❑ Excessive desire; without erections	**Caladium 200 or 1M**	*weekly (3)*
❑ Excessive desire; fear of water	**Lyssin 200 or 1M**	*weekly (3)*
❑ Excessive desire; can not control; trembles	**Platina 200 or 1M**	*weekly (3)*
❑ Sexual desire with violent erections	**Fluoric-acid. 200 or 1M**	*weekly (3)*
❑ Sexual desire excessive in the morning	**Antim-crud. 200 or 1M**	*weekly (3)*
❑ Excessive desire in children or in old	**Baryta-crab. 200 or 1M**	*weekly (3)*
❑ Excessive sexual desire in patient of chorea	**Verat-v. 200 or 1M**	*weekly (3)*

Symptoms	Remedy	Frequency And Doses
❑ Sexual desire even after excess of coition	**Phosphoric-ac. 200 or 1M**	*weekly (3)*
❑ Desire more during delirium; fear of dark	**Stramonium 200 or 1M**	*weekly (3)*
❑ Increased sexual desire at sight of erotic things	**Tarentula h. 200 or 1M**	*weekly (3)*

SINUSITIS
(See Cold, Catarrh, Etc., Also)

The inflammation of the para-nasal sinuses is called sinusitis. It may be maxillary sinusitis, frontal sinusitis or ethmoiditis according to the location of the particular sinus lesion involved. The condition may be acute or chronic.

Symptoms	Remedy	Frequency And Doses
❑ Right sided frontal sinusitis; discharge thick, yellowish; worse by cold, damp and exertion	**Penicillinum 30 or 200**	*6 hourly*
❑ Sinusitis after mastoid operation	**Hekla lava 3X or 6X**	*4 hourly*
☆ In acute or chronic sinusitis; catarrh with stringy discharge	**Kali bich. 30**	*4 hourly*
❑ Tearing pain in head; from root of nose, extending to forehead with nausea; dryness of mucous passages	**Natrum mur. 30**	*4 hourly*
☆ Pain begins at the back of the head and settles over the eyes; worse under a fan	**Silicea 1M**	*weekly (6)*
❑ Chronic cold with loss of smell and yellow green phlegm; better in cool, open air	**Pulsatilla 30 or 200**	*4 hourly*
● Intercurrent remedy	**Bacillinum 200 or 1M**	*fortnightly (3)*
❑ Complaints worse early morning; aversion to take bath	**Sulphur 200**	*weekly (3)*
Biochemic remedies	**Kali mur. 6X** and **Silicea 30X**	*4 hourly*

Symptoms	Remedy	Frequency And Doses

SKIN DISORDERS
(See Eczema, Psoriasis, Scabies, Abscess And Boils, etc., Also)

❑ Cracked; weeping eczema; constipation	**Graphites 30 or 0/5**	*4 hourly*
❑ Injuries tend to suppurate; patient oversensitive to touch and cold, etc.	**Hepar sulph. 30**	*6 hourly*
❑ Intolerable itching; scratching relieves but results in burning	**Sulphur 30 or 0/5**	*4 hourly*
❑ Irresistible desire to scratch and scratching brings out blood	**Arum triph. 30**	*6 hourly*
❑ When the stools and body odour is offensive alongwith skin complaints	**Pyrogenium 200**	*10 min. (3)*
Biochemic remedy	**Biocombination No.20**	*4 hourly*

SLEEP
Affections Of

❑ Aggravation of complaints during or after sleep	**Lachesis 200 or 1M**	*10 min. (3)*
❑ Aggravation of complaints due to loss of sleep; child nursing, etc.	**Cocculus ind. 30**	*4 hourly*
❑ Amelioration of complaints after good sleep	**Phosphorus 200**	*10 min. (3)*

SLEEPLESSNESS
(See Insomnia)

SLIPPED-DISC
(See Backache, Spondylosis, Etc., Also)

❑ Head remedy (to start the treatment); spine very sensitive; spasms in muscles of	**Arnica 200 or 1M**	*4 hourly (3)*

Symptoms	Remedy	Frequency And Doses
neck and back; feels bruised pain; as if 'bed too hard'; worse by movement but has to keep moving		
❏ Sudden onset of severe pain after exposure to dry cold winds; worse with every movement and at night; patient thirsty, restless, touchy and scared	**Aconite 200**	*3 hourly*
❏ Burning, stinging and stitching pain; whole back feels tired and bruised; worse by heat and least movement; patient restless, irritable, and depressed; wants to be uncovered and to be in cool air	**Apis mel. 30 or 200**	*3 hourly (3)*
❏ Violent cutting or tearing pain in neck, spine, or hips; walks restlessly to and fro in search of comfort; bed seems to be surging up and down; worse when at rest	**Belladonna 30 or 200**	*3 hourly*
❏ Pain in nape, back, and limbs; after exposure to dry cold, especially eastern winds; better from heat, least movement; great thirst for large amount of water at long intervals	**Bryonia alb. 200**	*3 hourly (3)*
✿ Drawing and tearing pain in limbs; specially at back of knee with stiffness and weakness; lower limbs very restless at night; better from warmth and moist weather, cold winds, draughts and taking coffee	**Causticum 30 or 200**	*3 hourly (3)*
❏ Pain intolerable; patient says that he would prefer death than this severe pain	**Chamomilla 30 or 200**	*1/2 hourly (3)*
❏ Wandering pain; felt specially in fingers and wrists; pain at bottom of spine when sitting; worse by cold air; patient is cross and listless	**Kali bich. 30 or 200**	*3 hourly*
✿ Stitching and cutting pain; often stabbing while at rest; pain extending up and down back and into thighs; worse by walking;	**Kali carb. 200**	*3 hourly (3)*

Symptoms	Remedy	Frequency And Doses
feels as if 'back would break'; firm pressure in small of back gives relief		
❑ Pain which shift rapidly and spread centrally; associated with great stiffness; better from cold; worse by heat and movement	**Ledum pal. 200**	*3 hourly (3)*
❑ Pain which comes on after getting wet or over-exertion; specially in lower part of back; hurts while turning in bed, muscles seem paralysed; cramps in calves or soles at night; worse by dry cold, before rain	**Nux vomica 30 or 200**	*3 hourly*
❑ Shooting pain in nape and elsewhere; neck and shoulders 'crack' on movement; legs feel heavy in daytime and ache at night	**Pulsatilla 200**	*3 hourly (3)*
☆ Pain brought on by over-exertion or exposure to cold and wet; back pain is relieved by bending body backwards; finger tips feel numb on grasping objects; pain and stiffness worse after rest and better by continued movement	**Rhus tox. 200 or 1M**	*3 hourly*
☆ Pain worse walking on uneven surface, pavements, etc. in old bachelors or maids	**Conium mac. 200**	*4 hourly (3)*
❑ Prolapsed disc; pain lumbar region; worse by coughing	**Ammon-carb. 200**	*4 hourly (3)*
❑ Feels as if walking on cotton wools due to degeneration of spinal cord; stools hard, constipated	**Alumina 200**	*4 hourly (3)*
● In fat, flabby and chilly patients; worse while bathing and exposure to cold	**Calcarea carb 200 or 1M**	*4 hourly (3)*
Biochemic remedies	**Calcarea phos. 6X, Natrum mur. 12X and Silicea 30X**	*4 hourly*

Symptoms	Remedy	Frequency And Doses

SMALL POX

This is a viral and contagious disease characterized by vesicular and pustular eruptions. The initial symptoms are low feeling, shivering, headache, and backache; cough with sore throat, hoarseness of voice and fever, etc..

Symptoms	Remedy	Frequency And Doses
☆ Preventive remedy	**Malandrinum 200**	*1 dose*
❏ Fever with restlessness and excessive thirst; fear of death and anxiety	**Aconite 30 or 200**	*3 hourly*
☆ High fever with redness of eyes and face; rush of blood towards head	**Belladonna 30**	*3 hourly*
❏ Initial stage with dullness, dizziness and drowsiness; nausea or vomiting and fever	**Gelsemium 30**	*4 hourly*
❏ High fever with burning, hot, flushed face, and thirstlessness; better by cold	**Apis mel. 30**	*4 hourly*
☆ Eruptions and fever with desire to lie down quietly; lips dry, tongue coated; stools constipated; thirst for large quantities of water at long intervals	**Bryonia alb. 30 or 200**	*4 hourly*
☆ Eruptions fail to appear causing great anxiety; anger or delirium, etc.; patient desires to run out	**Hyoscyamus 30 or 200**	*3 hourly*
❏ When pus forms in eruptions with pain; moist and swollen eruptions	**Mercurius sol. 30**	*4 hourly*
❏ Loss of strength, restlessness, and burning pain; thirst unquenchable for small quantity of water at short intervals	**Arsenic alb. 30**	*4 hourly*
☆ When typhoid like symptoms of fever appear. Redness of triangular tip of tongue; restlessness	**Rhus tox. 30 or 200**	*4 hourly*
❏ Patient collapses due to complications; desire to be fanned; body cold	**Carbo veg. 30**	*1/2 hourly*
Biochemic remedy	**Ferrum phos. 6X**	*4 hourly*

Symptoms	Remedy	Frequency And Doses

SNEEZING
(See Catarrh, Cold, Cough and Allergies Also)

☆ Due to sudden exposure to dry cold winds	**Aconite 30 or 200**	*2 hourly*
☆ With burning, excoriating discharge; anxiety and unquenchable frequent thirst	**Arsenic alb. 30**	*3 hourly*
☆ Sneezing with body pain; cold sensation up the spine; dizziness and lazyness	**Gelsemium 30**	*3 hourly*
☆ Sneezing worse entering a warm room; better open air	**Allium cepa 30**	*3 hourly*
● Intercurrent remedy	**Bacillinum 1M**	*1 dose*

SORE THROAT
(See Hoarseness Also)

☆ Due to exposure to dry cold wind; sudden with anxiety and fear	**Aconite nap. 30 or 200**	*3 hourly*
❏ Dryness and burning in throat; unquenchable thirst drinks small quantity at a time but frequently	**Arsenic alb. 30**	*3 hourly*
☆ With excess of saliva; pus formation without pain in throat	**Mercurius sol. 30**	*3 hourly*
❏ Smarting pain; worse empty swallowing; can swallow liquids only; tonsils swollen	**Baryta carb. 200 or 1m**	*10 min. (3)*
☆ Due to congestion; throat red, hot and swollen with burning	**Belladonna 30**	*3 hourly*
☆ With pus formation; shooting and piercing pain; patient oversensitive to cold, touch, etc.	**Hepar sulph. 30**	*3 hourly*
❏ With purple colour inflammation in the throat; pressure of clothes around throat intolerable	**Lachesis 30**	*4 hourly*

For External Use:

For gargling Phytolacca Q, 8-10 drops in 1/2 glass luke warm water thrice daily is very useful.

Symptoms	Remedy	Frequency And Doses

SNORING

A rough, rattling, inspiratory noise produced by vibration of the pendulous palate, or sometimes of the vocal cords during sleep is called snoring.

● Intercurrent remedy	**Bacillinum 200 or 1M**	*fortnightly (3)*
☆ Due to nasal polyp; chronic cases of atrophic rhinitis	**Lemna min. Q or 6**	*4 hourly*
☆ In cases of chronic rhinitis; nose red and swollen; acrid, corroding catarrh; bloody offensive discharge	**Hippozaeninum 30**	*4 hourly*
❑ Snoring when the patient is unconscious or in coma; breathes through mouth; stools constipated	**Opium 200**	*3 hourly (3)*
❑ During labor pains; after convulsions; weepy patients; feels better in open air	**Pulsatilla 30**	*4 hourly*
Biochemic remedy	**Silicea 12X**	*4 hourly*

SPERMATORRHOEA
Involuntary Discharge of Semen
(See Seminal Emissions Also)

☆ Due to weakness; after sexual excesses	**Acid phos. Q or 6**	*4 hourly*
☆ In unmarried persons; old bachelors	**Conium mac. 200**	*fortnightly (3)*
❑ Sexual organ cold and relaxed	**Agnus cast. Q or 30**	*4 hourly*
❑ Frequent; during sleep; seminal emissions accompanying erotic dreams	**Phosphorus 30 or 200**	*weekly (3)*
❑ Prostatic fluid dribbles out while straining to pass stools	**Calcarea silic. 30**	*6 hourly*
● Due to suppressed gonorrhoea; intercurrent remedy	**Medorrhinum 200 or 1M**	*fortnightly (3)*

Symptoms	Remedy	Frequency And Doses
❑ Emission with voluptuous dream and intense nervous thrill	**Zincum phos. 30**	*4 hourly*
● Intercurrent remedy; morning erections and pollutions; psoric patient	**Psorinum 200 or 1M**	*fortnightly (3)*

SPINE
Affections Of
(See Slipped Disc, Backache And Spondylosis Also)

Symptoms	Remedy	Frequency
❑ Pain back; with paralytic weakness	**Cocculus ind. 30 or 200**	*4 hourly*
❑ Pain back; from below up	**Conium mac. 200 or 1M**	*4 hourly*
❑ Pain back; worse by anger and indignation; nerve pain in spine; pain in left scapula when at rest; drawing sensation in right scapula	**Colocynth. 200 or 1M**	*4 hourly*
❑ Pain back; cramp like pain in region of kidneys; paralytic effects	**Causticum 200 or 1M**	*4 hourly*
❑ Pain in upper dorsal vertebrae; lumbar and sacral areas	**Cimicifuga 30 or 200**	*4 hourly*
❑ Pain in sacrum; pain due to injuries to coccyx	**Hypericum 200 or 1M**	*4 hourly*
❑ Pain across shoulders	**Cannabis ind. 200 or 1M**	*4 hourly*
❑ Pain in lumbo-sacral area; worse by slightest movement	**Bryonia alb. 200 or 1M**	*4 hourly*
❑ Pain in whole of spine or sacrum region	**Nux mosch. 30 or 200**	*4 hourly*
❑ Pain in shoulder joint	**Staphysagria 200 or 1M**	*4 hourly*
❑ Pain in coccyx when sitting	**Kali bich. 30 or 200**	*4 hourly*
❑ Pain with numbness in coccyx when sitting; pain in umbilical region goes through to back	**Platina 200 or 1M**	*4 hourly*
❑ Pain with lancinations; like needles in dorsal spine	**Croton tig. 30 or 200**	*4 hourly*

Symptoms	Remedy	Frequency And Doses
❑ Pain tearing; downwards through whole spine	**Cina 30 or 200**	*4 hourly*
❑ Pain in middle of spine	**Muriatic acid. 30 or 200**	*4 hourly*
❑ Pain better by walking and pressure against something hard; icy cold feeling between scapulae	**Sepia 200**	*4 hourly*
❑ Pain shooting up dorsal spine to occiput	**Phosphorus 200**	*4 hourly*
❑ Pain violent; with opisthotonos	**Natrum sulph. 200 or 1M**	*4 hourly*
❑ Pain better by heat; pain with chilliness along the spine	**Magnesia phos. 12X or 30**	*4 hourly*
❑ Pain worse by touch and pressure	**Kali carb. 30 or 200**	*4 hourly*
❑ Pain shooting down to gluteal muscles or hips	**Lac-can. 200**	*4 hourly*
❑ Burning pain; like hot iron thrust into the spine	**Alumina 30 or 200**	*4 hourly*
❑ Pain better by straightening and bending stiffly backwards with rectal symptoms	**Aethusa cy. 30**	*4 hourly*
❑ Rheumatic pain in shoulder	**Sanguinaria c. 30 or 200**	*4 hourly*
❑ Interscapular pain	**Cicuta v. 30 or 200**	*4 hourly*
❑ Pain better warmth; worse rest and cold	**Rhus tox. 200 or 1M**	*4 hourly*
❑ Pain between scapulae; burning pain	**Arsenic alb. 30 or 200**	*4 hourly*
● Pain in left scapulae; pain worse by lying down; better by warmth	**Tuberculinum k. 200 or 1M**	*4 hourly*
❑ Stitches in and between scapulae	**Nitric acid. 30 or 200**	*4 hourly*
Biochemic remedies	**Calcarea phos. 6X** and **Silicea 30X**	*4 hourly*

SPLEEN
Ailments Of

❑ Dropsy due to enlarged spleen; restlessness and unquenchable thirst	**Arsenic alb. 30**	*4 hourly*

Symptoms	Remedy	Frequency And Doses
❑ Spleen hard and enlarged; emaciation of body though eats well	**Iodium 30**	*4 hourly*
❑ Spleen enlarged and sore to touch; craving for cold drinks	**Phosphorus 30 or 200**	*4 hourly (3)*
❑ Spleen painful and enlarged; pain in the whole of left side; dyspnoea	**Ceanothus Q,** *5-10 drops*	*4 hourly*
❑ Sharp pain in the region of spleen; stools constipated	**Hydrastis can. Q or 30**	*4 hourly*
❑ Swelling of spleen; worse in damp places or weather, chilly feeling; digestion slow	**China off. 6 or 30**	*4 hourly*
❑ Enlargement of liver and spleen in infants	**Calcarea ars. 6**	*4 hourly*
Biochemic remedies		
Cutting pain in the region of spleen	**Calcarea phos. 6X**	*4 hourly*
Stitching pain in the region of spleen; worse by motion	**Kali phos. 6X**	*4 hourly*

SPONDYLOSIS
(See Cervical Spondylosis Also)

The term 'Spondylosis' is used for the disorder resulting from chronic disc degeneration. Degenerative changes occur in the inter-vertebral discs. This may effect one disc only or there may be involvement of several discs. The spondylosis is specially liable to interfere with the blood supply to the spinal cord and thus lead to further damages.

☆ Head remedy for cervical spondylitis. Inflammation of vertebrae; feels as if bones were scrapped with a knife; paralytic weakness of spine and general weakness; worse by exertion; loss of vital fluids; better by warmth	**Acid-phos. 30**	*4 hourly*
❑ Pain in lumbar and sacral region; pain spreading to right scapula	**Chloromycetin. 30**	*4 hourly*
❑ Pain cervical region with frontal and dorsal aching; worse in the morning and before menses	**Pneumococcus 200**	*6 hourly*

Symptoms	Remedy	Frequency And Doses
● Dorsal and lumbar spondylosis; to correct deformities of bones. Fat, flabby, weak, and chilly patient; injury of lower spine; over lifting, softening and weakness of bones	**Calc-carb. 200 or 1M**	*weekly (6)*
● Intercurrent remedy. To correct deformities of vertebrae. Burning pain; worse small of back and coccyx	**Sulphur 200 or 1M**	*weekly (3)*
❏ In delicate persons who grow very fast; waxy, anaemic, craves for salt and icy cold preparations; fear of dark; curvature of spine. Burning, shooting pain up dorsal spine to occiput. Vertigo after rising; broken pain in back; worse by exertion	**Phosphorus 30 or 200**	*4 hourly (3)*
❏ Spinal weakness; when bones become necrosed, breaks easily. Pain coccyx; fetid foot sweat; timid, chilly, over sensitive patient; to correct curvature of bones; vertigo from looking up; better by warmth	**Silicea 200 or 1M**	*weekly (3)*
☆ Pain back; between shoulders, lumbar and sacral region; history of over working; chronic bachelors/maids; weakness of body and mind; vertigo, while lying down and turning over in bed	**Conium mac. 200 or 1M**	*weekly (3)*
☆ Pain small of back and coccyx; worse by heat; stiffness and swelling of joints. Bad effects of mercury; worse by warmth; better by motion and open air	**Kali iod. 200 or 1M**	*weekly (3)*
❏ Vertigo with sensation of something rolling round in head. Pain and weakness in small of back; better by lying down, walking and pressure on back	**Sepia 30 or 200**	*4 hourly (3)*
❏ Pain and weakness small of back; burning in spine, shooting down to hips; worse by walking; 3-4 a.m.	**Kali carb. 30 or 200**	*4 hourly (3)*
☆ Back pain because of over lifting; getting wet while perspiring; small of back stiff	**Rhus tox. 200 or 1M**	*4 hourly*

Symptoms	Remedy	Frequency And Doses
and bruised. Pain better after continued motion and warmth; worse by cold and rest		
❑ Soreness and pain in lumbar region; worse rising from chair; back stiff and tense; pain shoulder blades; tearing and drawing pain; better by warmth, damp and wet weather	Causticum 30 or 200	6 hourly
☆ Pain back bones as if broken; burning pain lumbar region; vertigo; worse by motion specially when closing eyes by pressure, noise, least jar	Theridion 30	4 hourly
❑ Pain in small of back; lumbar and sacral area; cracking of cervical vertebrae; worse by walking; bruised pain in shoulder and arms; worse by loss of sleep	Cocculus ind. 30	4 hourly
❑ Pain small of back; lumbar and sacral vertebrae; mental confusion; pain ascending from nape of neck; worse after getting wet	Dulcamara 200 or 1M	10 min. (3)
❑ Pain lumbo - sacral region; worse by slightest motion; vertigo; stitching pain and stiffness in small of back	Bryonia 30 or 200	4 hourly
❑ Pain sacrum region. Vertigo when walking in open air; worse by cold; better warmth	Nux vomica 30 or 200	3 hourly
❑ Pain coccyx and sacrum when sitting; unable to stoop because of pain between scapula. Vertigo with nausea when rising from seat; better by heat	Kali bich. 30 or 200	4 hourly
☆ Pain nerves in spine; drawing pain left scapula when at rest; pain between scapulae; drawing pain in left cervical muscles. Vertigo when turning head to the left; worse after anger and indignation	Colocynth. 200 or 1M	10 min. (3)
● Backache and chilliness along spine; pain better by heat. Vertigo on moving, falls forward on closing eyes; better walking in open air	Mag-phos. 12X or 30	4 hourly

Symptoms	Remedy	Frequency And Doses
❑ Severe pain from brain to coccyx; pain worse when touched, pressure; sensation of walking or floating in the air	**Lac-can. 200**	*10 min. (3)*
❑ Back bent backwards like an arch; jerking, tearing pain in coccyx, specially during menses. Vertigo with gastralgia and muscular spasms	**Cicuta v. 30**	*4 hourly*
☆ Numbness and pain in extremities; tearing pain in sciatic nerve. Numbness alternate with pain	**Gnaphalium 200 or 1M**	*6 hourly*
❑ Neck stiff and tense with drawing pain; nape rigid; worse before storms	**Rhododendron 200 or 1M**	*10 min. (3)*
❑ Pain upper dorsal, lumbar and sacral vertebrae; spine very sensitive, stiffness and contraction of neck and back; worse moving, cold, and during menstrual period	**Ledum pal. 200 or 1M**	*10 min. (3)*
● Intolerable pain in the back; worse during day and better sea side; neck stiff	**Medorrhinum 200 or 1M**	*fortnightly (3)*
❑ With bruised pain due to carrying heavy weights; over exertion, injury of bones and sprain; worse by lying down, cold and wet	**Ruta g. 30 or 200**	*6 hourly*
❑ Soreness of coccyx; dislocated feeling in sacrum; better by lying on right side. Fear of downward motion	**Sanicula 30**	*4 hourly*
❑ Cervical spondylosis; crackling in the vertebrae	**Magnetis polus areticus 30 or 200**	*6 hourly*
❑ Spondylosis due to sexual excess; injury of back-bone	**Symphytum 6 or 30**	*4 hourly*
☆ Pain lumbar region; bruised, feels as if vertebrae are dislocated; can not walk erect because of back pain	**Arnica 200 or 1M**	*6 hourly*
❑ Pain lumbar region; stiffness of back; worse by heat, bending backwards, anger and night	**Chamomilla 200**	*6 hourly*

Symptoms	Remedy	Frequency And Doses
❏ Pain lumbar region; shooting pain in the nape and back, between shoulders and sacrum after lifting; vertigo; better in open air	**Pulsatilla 30 or 200**	*6 hourly*
● Despair of recovery; worse by cold air; better by warmth; patient puts warm clothings even in summer	**Psorinum 200 or 1M**	*weekly (3)*
● Patient feels as if bones are made of glass	**Thuja oc. 200 or 1M**	*weekly (3)*
❏ Due to concussion of spine; pain sacrum vertebrae and coccyx	**Hypericum 30 or 200**	*6 hourly*
Biochemic remedies	**Calcarea phos. 6X, Calcarea fluor. 12X** and **Magnesia phos. 6X**	*4 hourly*

SPRAINS

An injury to a joint with possible rupture of some of the ligaments or tendons, but without dislocation or fracture is called sprain.

❏ Accompanied by bruised pain	**Arnica 30 or 200**	*3 hourly*
☆ Sprains of joints of tendons; pain worse by cold; better by warmth	**Rhus tox. 200**	*3 hourly*
❏ Of wrists and ankles	**Ruta gr. 30 or 200**	*3 hourly*
Biochemic remedies	**Calcarea phos. 6X** and **Magnesia phos. 6 X**	*4 hourly*

For External Use:

Arnica and Rhus tox. Q in vegetable oils in 4:6.

SQUINT
Strabismus

The inability to bring the visual axes of both eyes to meet at a certain point, and yet one eye will follow the other in all its movements. If the squinting eye deviates inward, it is 'strabismus convergens';

Symptoms	Remedy	Frequency And Doses

if outward then it is 'divergens'; if upward then it is 'sursumvergens'; and if downward then it is 'deorsumvergens'.

The use of homoeopathic remedies has in the early stages of some cases relieved the tendency to permanent strabismus. In obstinate cases surgery is necessary.

Symptoms	Remedy	Frequency And Doses
❑ In convergent strabismus occurring in children, particularly if spasmodic in nature, or caused from convulsions	Cicuta vir. 30	4 hourly
❑ Convergent strabismus; periodic, and resulting from spasm of the internal recti	Jaborandi 30	4 hourly
❑ Due to worms	Cina 30 or 200	4 hourly
Biochemic remedy	Magnesia phos. 6X	4 hourly

Other Important Remedies:

Cyclamen, Spigelia, Agaricus m., Belladonna, Gelsemium, Hyoscyamus, Nux vomica, Stramonium and Psorinum, etc..

STAMMERING

Mispronunciation or transposition of certain consonants, especially l, r, and s, etc., is called Stammering. Chronic cases are hard to cure.

Symptoms	Remedy	Frequency And Doses
❑ Head remedy; often pronounces words wrong, and transposes letters and syllables; stuttering in words rich in consonants; lisping; paretic state of tongue and lips	Causticum 30	4 hourly
❑ Trembling, heaviness and paralytic weakness of tongue; stammering speech	Belladonna 30	4 hourly
❑ Patient becomes angry when not understood; stammering speech	Bufo rana 30	6 hourly
❑ Difficulty in pronouncing some letters or particular words; 2nd or 3rd word is particularly difficult to pronounce	Lachesis 30 or 200	3 hourly
❑ Rapid and stammering speech	Merc-sol. 30	4 hourly

Symptoms	Remedy	Frequency And Doses
❑ Stammering; weak speech	**Secale cor. 30**	*4 hourly*
❑ Repeats the first syllable of the first word several times; after that speaks plainly	**Spigelia 30**	*4 hourly*
❑ Stammering, speech being difficult and unintelligible	**Stramonium 200**	*6 hourly*

STERILITY

The inability of the female to conceive, due to inadequacy in structure or function of the genital organs is called Sterility.

❑ Without any structural changes	**Mandragora 30**	*4 hourly*
☆ When conception doesn't take place due to white, thick mucilaginous, acid reacting mucous (leucorrhoea), destroying the self mobility of the spermatozoa; feels as if warm water was flowing from the vagina. Menses early, painful, profuse or prolonged. Chronic cases of cervix erosion	**Borax 30**	*4 hourly*
☆ Biochemic remedy for similar symptoms	**Natrum phos. 6X**	*4 hourly*
❑ To arouse the activity of the ovaries and pleasurable feeling, specially in tall, slender and oversensitive women	**Phosphorus 200**	*fortnightly (3)*
❑ Inflammation and induration of the ovaries; albumen like sharp, excoriating, acid reacting discharge; throbbing, tearing, and burning pain in uterus and the ovaries. Sex desire prostrated. Pain and swellings of the breast before and after menses. Dizziness on turning the head to the side	**Conium mac. 200**	*fortnightly (3)*
❑ In cases of dysmenorrhoea and severe uterine haemorrhage. Neck of the bladder feels as if swollen with intense desire to pass urine	**Mitchella Q,** *5-7 drops*	*4 hourly*

Symptoms	Remedy	Frequency And Doses
☆ Cases of scanty and delayed menstruation associated with severe backache and pain in the sacral region; uterine atony	**Gossypium Q,** *5-10 drops*	*4 hourly*
● Perspiration, sleeplessness and general weakness after every sexual intercourse. Menses early, profuse and long lasting; profuse, acrid, creamy, leucorrhoea continuing day and night. Fat and flabby patient	**Calcarea carb. 200 or 1M**	*fortnightly (3)*
❑ Menses scanty, pale, late, and often missing for months. Constipation; skin unhealthy, slow to heal, tendency to eczema, cracking of corners of mouth and eye-lids	**Plumbum met. 30**	6 hourly
❑ Colic like pain; during menstruation radiating towards groins and anus. Stools constipated	**Graphites 30 or 0/5**	6 hourly
❑ History of repeated abortions. Contractions in the uterus stimulating labor	**Caulophyllum 30**	6 hourly
☆ In cases of functional weakness of the procreative organs; abortion shortly after every conception; membranous dysmenorrhoea	**Viburnum opulus Q or 6**	*4 hourly*
❑ To tone up the uterus. Backache, cutting, pressing, contracting pain partly from the uterus and partly from the ovaries; irritability of the bladder; frequent, painful, pressing pain in the neck of the bladder	**Eupatorium purp. 30**	*4 hourly*

Other Useful Remedies:

Aurum met., Pulsatilla, Sepia, Helonias, Fraxinus am., Kali carb., Aletris f., Secale cor., Lilium tig., Chamomilla, Apis mel., Platina, Hamamelis, Thyroidinum, Natrum mur., Kali brom., Baryta carb., Onosmodium, Salix nig., Staphysagria, Medorrhinum, Thuja oc., Ashoka, Sulphur, Syphilinum and Tuberculinum, etc..

Symptoms	Remedy	Frequency And Doses

STONE IN THE BLADDER

● Frequent urge to pass urine; worse at night; scanty, strong smelling, and coloured urine. Flow of urine slow due to inactive bladder — **Medorrhinum 200 or 1M** — *10 min. (3)*

❑ Catarrh of the bladder, with thick ropy mucous in urine; smells decomposed — **Hydrastis can. 30** — *4 hourly*

☆ Burning, cutting pain; frequent urge to pass urine — **Cantharis 30** — *4 hourly*

❑ Urine scanty; frequent urge; worse lying on back, tenesmus; patient feels better in open, cool air — **Pulsatilla 30** — *4 hourly*

❑ Dribbling of urine; though bladder is full of urine — **Nux vomica 30** — *4 hourly*

☆ Urge constant; immediately after a few drops of urine collects in the bladder; can not control the urge; loss of thirst — **Apis mel. 30** — *4 hourly*

STONE IN THE KIDNEY
(See Renal Calculi)

STOOLS
Affections Of
(See Constipation, Diarrhoea, Dysentery And Cholera, Etc., Also)

❑ Spasmodic pain of sphincter after stool; gelatinous stools; aversion to smell of food — **Colchicum 30** — *4 hourly*

❑ Stools passes with great pain and exertion; stools clay coloured — **Hepar sulph. 30** — *4 hourly*

❑ Stools painless, much flatulence; diarrhoeic-smell as of rotten eggs; dark brown in colour — **Psorinum 200** — *weekly (3)*

Symptoms	Remedy	Frequency And Doses
❑ Intolerable pain in rectum during and after passing stools	**Paeonia Q or 6**	*4 hourly*
❑ Pain in perineum while passing stool; must go to stool after eating; strong, long lasting odour of stools	**Sanguinaria c. 30 or 200**	*4 hourly*
❑ Stools pass only when leaning back with pain	**Medorrhinum 200 or 1M**	*weekly (3)*
❑ Stools pass only when standing; hard, constipated	**Alumina 30 or 0/5** and **above**	*4 hourly*
❑ Stool passes better when standing	**Causticum 30 or 0/5** and **above**	*6 hourly*
❑ After stool soreness and burning of perineum	**Nitric-acid. 30**	*4 hourly*
❑ After taking a drink must go to stool; thirst after passing stool	**Capsicum 30**	*4 hourly*
❑ Unability to strain due to paralytic weakness of rectal muscles; weakness and palpitation after passing stool; stools cool	**Conium mac. 30 or 200**	*4 hourly*
❑ With protrusion of stomach; black blood, partly solid, partly fluid; tongue white coated	**Antim-crud. 30 or 200**	*4 hourly*
❑ Long intervals between stools; offensive, bloody with muscular pain	**Arnica 200**	*4 hourly*
❑ With pus; loose, slimy, mushy, very hot	**Calcarea phos. 6X or 6**	*4 hourly*
❑ Involuntary, after fright; hard and dry stools	**Opium 200 or 1M**	*4 hourly (3)*
❑ Passing stools after excitement; while urinating	**Hyoscyamus 200**	*4 hourly (3)*
❑ Hurried; early morning stools	**Sulphur 200**	*4 hourly (3)*
❑ Ineffectual urging; irritability	**Nux vomica 30**	*4 hourly*
❑ Stools like coffee grounds	**Terebinth. Q or 6**	*4 hourly*
❑ Stools dry; faecal matter-light coloured	**Collinsonia Q or 30**	*4 hourly*
❑ Stools soft but difficult to expel	**Nux mosch. 30**	*4 hourly*
❑ Stools lumpy, shredy with mucous	**Graphites 30 or 1M**	*4 hourly*

Symptoms	Remedy	Frequency And Doses
❑ Stools sudden, gushing, noisy, spluttering	**Natrum sulph. 30 or 200**	*4 hourly*
❑ Stools recedes back when almost voided	**Silicea 12X or 30**	*4 hourly*
❑ Stools changes colour; not two stools alike	**Pulsatilla 30 or 200**	*4 hourly*
❑ Stools green in colour; sour smelling	**Natrum phos. 6X or 30**	*4 hourly*
❑ Even solid stools are passed unnoticed	**Aloe soc. 30**	*4 hourly*
❑ Passing stools immediately after washing the head	**Tarentula h. 200 or 1M**	*10 min. (3)*

STYE
Eyes
(See Cysts Also)

It is a small dark red boil like growth on the eye-lid with inflammation and pain. It may suppurate slowly or becomes a cyst and may re-occur repeatedly.

Symptoms	Remedy	Frequency And Doses
❑ Styes with stitching pain; worse straining eyes; burning lachrymation from eyes; better by cold application; sensation of dust particles in the eyes	**Aegle mar. Q or 30**	*4 hourly*
❑ Head remedy for styes	**Calcarea pic. 3X or 6**	*thrice daily*
☆ Stye; specially on upper eye-lid, recurrent; worse by heat; better by cold	**Pulsatilla 30 or 200**	*4 hourly*
☆ Stye; recurrent, ulcerating, do not suppurate, remains hard like a nodule, may convert into a cyst if not treated properly	**Staphysagria 30**	*4 hourly*
❑ Stye; condylomatous and hard	**Thuja oc. 200 or 1M**	*10 min. (3)*
❑ Stye; near outer canthus	**Aurum sulph. 30**	*4 hourly*
❑ Stye; recurrent, suppurating, painful; worse by cold; better by heat	**Hepar sulph. 30**	*4 hourly*
❑ Stye; eye-lids swollen	**Alumina silic. 30**	*4 hourly*
❑ Stye; pustular, suppurating; burning and redness in eyes	**Silicea 30**	*4 hourly*

Symptoms	Remedy	Frequency And Doses
❏ To dissolve cystic formations	**Thiosinamine 3X**	*3 hourly*
❏ Stye; inner canthi with watering of eyes	**Natrum mur. 30**	*4 hourly*
❏ Stye; right upper eye-lid	**Ammonium carb. 30**	*4 hourly*
❏ Stye; burning sensation; better by hot fomentation	**Arsenic alb. 30**	*4 hourly*

Biochemic remedy

For both cyst and stye	**Calcarea fluor. 12X or 30X**	*4 hourly*

SUGAR IN URINE
(See Diabetes Melitus Also)

☆ Well proven Indian drug	**Cephalandra ind. Q,** 5-10 drops	*4 hourly*
☆ Head remedy	**Syzygium j. Q,** *5-10 drops*	*4 hourly*
❏ Sugar in urine; fidgety feet	**Zincum phos. 30**	*4 hourly*
❏ Sugar in urine; urine copious; emaciation, patient ill tempered	**Tarentula h. 30 or 200**	*4 hourly (3)*
❏ With great emaciation; craves for icy cold water	**Phosphorus 30 or 200**	*4 hourly (3)*
☆ The proven Indian drug called 'Gur Mar'	**Gymnema syl. Q,** *5-10 drops* *4 hourly*	
Biochemic remedies	**Calcarea phos. 6X, Kali mur. 6X** and **Natrum mur. 6X**	

Constitutional treatment gives good results in Homoeopathy.

SUICIDAL DISPOSITION
(See Sadness Also)

❏ Suicidal disposition; by hanging; after midnight	**Arsenic alb. 200 or 1M**	*4 hourly (3)*
❏ Thoughts driving to suicide; anger	**Carbo veg. 200**	*4 hourly (3)*
❏ Desire to suicide; with an axe	**Naja trip. 200 or 1M**	*4 hourly (3)*
❏ Suicidal disposition; always talks of committing suicide but lacks courage	**Nux vomica 200**	*4 hourly (3)*

Symptoms	Remedy	Frequency And Doses
❏ Suicidal disposition; by drowning	**Rhus tox 200 or 1M**	*4 hourly (3)*
❏ Suicidal disposition; from disappointed love; desire to run away	**Hyoscyamus nig. 200 or 1M**	*4 hourly (3)*
❏ Suicidal disposition; with fear of death	**Nitric-acid. 200 or 1M**	*4 hourly (3)*
❏ Suicidal disposition; to set oneself on fire	**Hepar sulph. 200 or 1M**	*4 hourly (3)*
❏ Suicidal disposition; with a knife, during menses, by starving	**Mercurius sol. 200 or 1M**	*4 hourly (3)*
❏ Suicidal disposition; with a razor; fear of dark	**Stramonium 200 or 1M**	*4 hourly (3)*
❏ Suicidal disposition from pain; desires to throw himself from height, window	**Aurum met. 200 or 1M**	*4 hourly (3)*
❏ Suicidal disposition; during perspiration, by stabbing	**Calcarea carb. 200 or 1M**	*4 hourly (3)*
❏ Suicidal disposition; by poison	**Belladonna 200 or 1M**	*4 hourly (3)*
❏ Suicidal disposition; from sadness, due to indignation, by shooting	**Staphysagria 200 or 1M**	*4 hourly (3)*
❏ Suicidal disposition after seeing blood or a knife	**Alumina 200 or 1M**	*4 hourly (3)*
Biochemic remedy	**Kali phos. 6X or 12X**	*4 hourly*

SUN BURN

❏ With redness; heat and throbbing pain	**Belladonna 30**	*3 hourly*
❏ After a day in the sun; when a reaction is expected	**Cantharis 6 or 30**	*3 hourly*
❏ When patient is in coma; due to fatigue in sun	**Opium 200 or 1M**	*10 min. (3)*
❏ Chronic effects of sun-stroke; excessive thirst and constipation	**Natrum mur. 6X or 30**	*3 hourly*
❏ With severe headache; sinking and vomiting	**Glonoine 3X or 6**	*1/2 hourly*
❏ With cold sweating on forehead; nausea, throbbing pain and loose motions	**Veratrum alb. 30**	*1/2 hourly*

Symptoms	Remedy	Frequency And Doses

SUN STROKE
Affections Of

Symptoms	Remedy	Frequency And Doses
❏ Head exposed in sun; specially while asleep; thirst more, eyes and face red; anxiety, restlessness and fear of death	**Aconite 30 or 200**	*1/2 hourly*
❏ With severe, throbbing headache; worse jar. Rush of blood towards head	**Belladonna 30**	*1/2 hourly*
☆ Head very hot while body temperature is normal; eyes bloody red, attack sudden; stools and urine passes involuntarily	**Arnica mont. 30**	*1/2 hourly*
❏ When body becomes cold with complete prostration of vital forces. Cold sweating and cramps in muscles	**Camphora Q,** 5-10 drops	*1/2 hourly*
❏ Confusion of mind after sunstroke with prostration and trembling; dimness of vision; headache worse occiput	**Gelsemium 30**	*1/2 hourly*
☆ Intense nausea; vomiting; throbbing, violent headache; brain feels as if expanding	**Glonoine 3X or 6**	*1/2 hourly*
❏ Face dark; red and bloated; eyes almost closed; unconsciousness	**Opium 200 or 1M**	*1/2 hourly (3)*
❏ Sudden; with rapid congestion, heaviness, and fullness of head. Vomiting; cold sweat on face, hands, and feet	**Veratrum v. 30**	*1/2 hourly*
☆ Vertigo; headache, nausea, vomiting and vision loss; worse by motion, opening the eyes and noise	**Theridion 30**	*1/2 hourly*
❏ Sudden; violent congestion of head as if bandaged; bursting headache with prostration	**Cactus g. Q or 30**	*1/2 hourly*
Biochemic remedies	**Natrum mur. 6X** and **Kali phos. 6X**	*1/2 hourly*

Symptoms	Remedy	Frequency And Doses

SUN STROKE
After Effects Of

Symptoms	Remedy	Frequency And Doses
☆ Sun's heat and electrical changes in the atmosphere makes the patient worse; hammering headache; patient feels weak in summer	**Lachesis 200**	*10 min. (3)*
☆ Patient feels worse in hot weather; headache; cannot think properly while in sun	**Natrum carb. 200**	*10 min. (3)*
☆ Feels worse in sun and heat; anaemic, cachectic, faints easily in sun; excessive thirst; stools constipated	**Natrum mur. 200**	*10 min. (3)*
❑ The complaints become worse with the rising sun and patient feels energetic as the sun sinks down	**Selenium 30**	*4 hourly*
☆ Forgets the known streets and roads due to sun stroke	**Glonoine 3X or 30**	*4 hourly*
Biochemic remedy	**Natrum mur. 6X**	*4 hourly*

SUPPRESSIONS
Bad Affects Of
(See Other Relevant Ailments Also)

Symptoms	Remedy	Frequency And Doses
❑ Mania; due to suppression of eruptions	**Zincum met. 200 or 1M**	*10 min. (3)*
❑ Insanity; due to suppression of eruptions	**Sulphur 200 or 1M**	*10 min. (3)*
❑ Convulsions or cataract, etc.; after suppression of foot sweat	**Silicea 200 or 1M**	*10 min. (3)*
❑ Asthma; due to suppression of foot sweat	**Oleum an. 200**	*10 min. (3)*
❑ Gonorrhoea; after effects of	**Medorrhinum 200 or 1M**	*10 min. (3)*
❑ Haemorrhoids; due to suppression of leucorrhoea	**Ammon-mur. 30 or 200**	*4 hourly*

Symptoms	Remedy	Frequency And Doses
❏ Deafness; due to suppression of syphilis	**Kreosote 30 or 200**	*10 min. (3)*
❏ Burns; after effects of	**Causticum 30 or 200**	*weekly (3)*
❏ Itching; due to suppression of eruptions	**Arsenic alb. 30 or 200**	*4 hourly (3)*
❏ Twitchings; due to suppression of eruptions	**Zincum met. 200**	*10 min. (3)*
❏ Bad effects of insults; humiliation or indignation	**Staphysagria 200 or 1M**	*10 min. (3)*
❏ Kidney troubles; after diphtheria, scarlatina or typhoid fever	**Terebinth. Q or 30**	*4 hourly*
❏ Rheumatism; after suppression of diarrhoea	**Abrotanum 30 or 200**	*4 hourly (3)*

SWEAT
Affections Of

Symptoms	Remedy	Frequency And Doses
❏ Never sweats; stools hard and constipated	**Alumina 200 or 0/5 onwards**	*6 hourly*
❏ Sweat on uncovered parts; or on every part except face; no sweat on covered parts; smells like honey	**Thuja 200 or 1M**	*10 min. (3)*
❏ Cold, greasy sweats; while eating; complaints increase with sweats; profuse, without relief	**Mercurius sol. 30 or 200**	*4 hourly*
❏ Profuse; after acute diseases, bringing relief	**Psorinum 200 or 1M**	*4 hourly (3)*
❏ Sweat constant; gastric complaints with	**Colchicum 30 or 200**	*4 hourly*
❏ With great thirst and weakness; on being covered	**China 6 or 30**	*4 hourly*
❏ With smarting sensation in the skin	**Chamomilla 30 or 200**	*4 hourly (3)*
❏ With vomiting	**Camphora 30**	*4 hourly (3)*
❏ With palpitation; bloody sweat and hammering pain	**Lachesis 30 or 200**	*4 hourly (3)*

Symptoms	Remedy	Frequency And Doses
❏ With itching on waking; sweats, but cannot bear to be covered; on hands and feet, warm sweats; worse by heat of bed	Ledum pal. 30 or 200	4 hourly (3)
❏ Slight; over whole body; with anxiety and fear	Aconite nap. 30 or 200	4 hourly (3)
❏ Lack of sweat even in summer	Nux mosch. 30 or 200	4 hourly (3)
❏ Partial sweats; on hands with coldness, on neck and chest	Calcarea phos. 6X or 30	4 hourly
❏ Only on covered parts	Belladonna 30	4 hourly
❏ Can not bear to be uncovered while sweating	Aethusa cy. 30	4 hourly
❏ Cold sweats; on feet and legs; patient over sensitive	Hepar sulph. 30 or 200	4 hourly
❏ Cold sweats; on arms and hands; with ravenous hunger	Acid-phos. Q or 30	4 hourly
❏ Sweats cold and clammy	Veratrum vir. 30	4 hourly
❏ One sided sweat of face; worse by heat	Pulsatilla 30 or 200	4 hourly (3)
❏ Sweat sticky	Cannabis ind. 30 or 200	4 hourly (3)
❏ Sweat stains linen yellow; tubercular patient	Tuberculinum k. 200	4 hourly (3)
❏ Sweat all over after a meal; axillary sweat	Nitric-acid. 30 or 200	4 hourly (3)
❏ Feels hungry while sweating	Sanguinaria c. 30 or 200	4 hourly (3)
❏ Sweat better on walking; stains yellow	Chelidonium Q or 30	4 hourly
❏ Worse while walking in open air; odour of spice	Rhododendron 30 or 200	4 hourly
❏ On making any motion sweat disappears and heat comes on; smells like onion	Lycopodium 30 or 200	4 hourly (3)
❏ Sweat only while awake	Sepia 30 or 200	4 hourly (3)
❏ Sweat from music; enjoys music	Tarentula h. 200	4 hourly (3)
❏ Sweat on forehead; desires fanning	Carbo veg. 30 or 200	4 hourly (3)
❏ Sweat on legs	Terebinth. Q or 30	4 hourly

Symptoms	Remedy	Frequency And Doses
❑ Smells like garlic in armpits	**Sulphur 30 or 200**	*4 hourly (3)*
❑ Offensive; carrion-like	**Pyrogenium 200**	*4 hourly (3)*
❑ On painful parts	**Kali carb. 30 or 200**	*4 hourly (3)*
❑ Sweat that attracts flies	**Caladium s. 30**	*4 hourly (3)*
❑ Stains the linen; spotted, stiffening	**Selenium 30**	*4 hourly (3)*

The above rubrics if found in any ailment are very helpful for the proper selection of a homoeopathic remedy.

SYPHILIS

❑ In acute cases or in secondary stage when the chancer is hard; ulceration spreads deeply, bleeds easily; yellowish, fetid discharge; chronic nasal catarrh; acrid, greenish, offensive discharge; pain and swelling of nasal bones	**Merc-sol. 30 or 200**	*4 hourly*
❑ When Merc-sol. fails; chancer offensive, the outlines are irregular with the zig-zag edges; looks like raw flesh but is deeper then **Merc-sol.** ulcer. Chancer very sensitive to touch, filled with granulations; bleeds from slightest touch and when dressing; offensive urine	**Acid-nit. 30 or 200**	*6 hourly*
❑ When the chancer and bubo are hard since long with swelling of glands; gums swollen and tender	**Merc-bin iod. 3X or higher**	*4 hourly*
❑ Painless chancers with great swelling of inguinal glands; to prevent secondary symptoms of syphilis	**Merc-proto iod. 3X or higher**	*4 hourly*
❑ When chancer spreads rapidly, and emit acrid, corroding pus which leads to spreading of ulcers which de-generates the parts	**Merc-cor. 30 or 200**	*4 hourly*

Symptoms	Remedy	Frequency And Doses
❏ In severe cases when gummatous tumors effects the nervous tissues; the edges of chancers are hard, and emits curdy pus. Severe pain in bones; worse at night	**Kali iod. 200 or above**	*6 hourly*
❏ When the ulcers are very sensitive to touch; bleeds easily; the discharge smells like old cheese; sticking, pricking pains	**Hepar sulph. 30 or 200**	*6 hourly*
❏ When chancers are extremely sensitive to slightest touch; even cloth of bandage is intolerable; gangrenous, phagedenic chancer, surrounded by a bluish lesion	**Lachesis 30 or 200**	*6 hourly*
❏ For indolent chancer; ulcers on legs which do not heal easily; copper colour eruptions on head	**Lycopodium 30 or 200**	*6 hourly*
❏ With debility and emaciation; patient desires open air or fanning; secretions foul	**Carbo veg. 30 or 200**	*4 hourly*
● Intercurrent remedy	**Syphilinum 200 or 1M**	*fortnightly (3)*
Biochemic remedies	**Kali mur. 3X** and **Silicea 30X**	*4 hourly*

Other Important Remedies:

Anacardium or., Arsenic alb., Asafoetida, Badiaga, Carbo an., Cinnabaris, Phytolacca d. and Aurum met., etc..

TASTE

Symptoms	Remedy	Frequency And Doses
❏ Bitter for everything; except water	**Aconite 30 or 200**	*4 hourly*
❏ Bitter for everything; in tubercular patients	**Stannum met. 30 or 200**	*4 hourly*
❏ Even sweets taste bitter	**Rumex 30 or 200**	*4 hourly*
❏ Though taste in mouth is bitter; but food and drinks tastes normal	**Nux vomica 30 or 200**	*4 hourly*
❏ Sugar tastes bitter	**Sanguinaria c. 30 or 200**	*4 hourly*
❏ Plums taste bitter	**Iodium 30 or 200**	*4 hourly*
❏ Water tastes bitter	**Arsenic alb. 30 or 200**	*4 hourly*

TEARS
(See Lachrymation)

TEETH
Affections Of
(See Toothache and Pyorrhoea Also)

Symptoms	Remedy	Frequency And Doses
❏ Teeth feel too long	**Chamomilla 30 or 200**	*4 hourly*
❏ Slow dentition	**Calcarea phos. 6X or 30**	*4 hourly*
❏ Chilly feeling through teeth	**Antim-tart. 30 or 200**	*4 hourly*
❏ Loose; when chewing	**Nitric acid. 30 or 200**	*4 hourly*
❏ Irresistible desire to bite teeth together	**Phytolacca d. 30 or 200**	*4 hourly*
❏ Grinding of teeth	**Plumbum met. 30 or 200**	*4 hourly*

Symptoms	Remedy	Frequency And Doses
❑ Black eruptions on teeth	**Staphysagria 30 or 200**	*4 hourly*
❑ Tartar on teeth	**Calcarea renalis 30**	*4 hourly*
❑ Painful cutting of wisdom teeth	**Cheiranthus ch. 30**	*4 hourly*

TENNIS ELBOW

☆ Trembling of arms after exertion; aching in elbow; stiffness of arms	**Rhus Tox. 1M or 10M**	*4 hourly (3)*
❑ Stiffness all over; sharp, shooting, neuralgic pains under the skin; worse by motion	**Agaricus m. 30 or 200**	*4 hourly*
❑ Tearing pain; with a sprained and paralysed feeling; drawing in fingers and thumb	**Ambra gr. 30 or 200**	*4 hourly*
☆ Tearing in bones of arms; cramp like drawing; buised pain in bones of wrists and back of hands; wore by motion	**Ruta g. 30 or 200**	*4 hourly*
☆ Pain in elbow due to a blow	**Allium cepa 30**	*4 hourly*

TESTICLES
Affections Of

● Undescended in young boys	**Thyroidinum 1M**	*10 min. (3)*
❑ A proven remedy for undescended testicles	**Aurum mur-nat. 3X**	*4 hourly 2-3 months*

TETANUS

☆ Tetanus after punctured wounds; to prevent	**Ledum 200 or 1M**	*1/2 hourly (3)*
❑ Tetanus with deathly coldness	**Camphora 200 or 1M**	*1/2 hourly (3)*
❑ Tetanus with drawing up corners of mouth	**Strychnin. 200 or 1M**	*1/2 hourly (3)*

Symptoms	Remedy	Frequency And Doses
❏ Tetanic convulsions	Veratrum vir. 200 or 1M	1/2 hourly (3)
Biochemic remedies	Kali phos. 3X and Magnesia phos. 3X	1/2 hourly

Tetanus is a fatal disease, once the symptoms develop fully it is hard to manage. Hospitalize the patient in acute stage and give the indicated remedy in the meanwhile.

THALASSEMIA

Any of a group of inherited disorders of hemoglobin metabolism in which there is a decrease in net synthesis of a particular globin chain without change in the structure of that chain; several genetic types exists, and the corresponding clinical picture may vary from barely detectable hematologic abnormality to severe and fatal anaemia. The hemoglobin Lepore syndromes are clinically indistinguishable, but the non-α-globin chains are structurally altered.

❏ To increase the time period of successive blood-transfusion; aplastic anaemia	T.N.T. 200	weekly (12)

Constitutional homoeopathic treatment is useful in cases of Thalassqemia.

THERMAL VARIATIONS
Effects Of Hot And Cold

❏ Feels chilly after every drink	Capsicum 30 or 200	4 hourly (3)
❏ Though body is cold yet wants to be fanned	Carbo veg. 30 or 200	4 hourly (3)
❏ Feels cold yet better from cold; patient feels better putting feet in cold water; worse after getting warm in bed	Ledum pal. 30 or 200	4 hourly (3)
❏ Feels worse from cold	Sepia 30 or 200	4 hourly (3)
❏ Chilly on slightest movement; though cold, but do not feel it; better by warmth	Nux vomica. 30 or 200	4 hourly (3)
❏ Patient feels worse from draughts	Belladonna 30 or 200	4 hourly (3)
❏ Desires to be uncovered; burning of soles and palms	Sulphur 30 or 200	4 hourly (3)

Symptoms	Remedy	Frequency And Doses
❑ Burning sensations; relieved by heat; feels better after getting warmth in bed	**Arsenic alb. 30 or 200**	*4 hourly (3)*
❑ Feels externally warm; without internal heat	**Ignatia 30 or 200**	*4 hourly (3)*
❑ Patient cannot bear heat; sun	**Glonoine 30 or 200**	*4 hourly (3)*

THIRST
Absence Of

❑ With swollen throat	**Apis mel. 30 or 200**	*4 hourly*
❑ Even in high temperature	**Gelsemium 30 or 200**	*2 hourly*
❑ Even though the mouth is dry	**Pulsatilla 30 or 200**	*4 hourly*

Though we can not prescribe a remedy only on the basis of absence of thirst but it often helps to select a remedy.

THIRST
Excessive

❑ With high temperature and anxiety	**Aconite nap. 30 or 200**	*2 hourly*
❑ For cold drinks; large quantities at a time	**Bryonia 30 or 200**	*4 hourly*
❑ Due to intake of excessive salt; constipated	**Natrum mur. 30 or 200**	*4 hourly*
❑ Dry mouth and throat; desire for milk	**Rhus tox. 30 or 200**	*4 hourly*
❑ Unquenchable; drinks frequently though little at a time	**Arsenic alb. 30**	*4 hourly*
Biochemic remedies	**Kali phos. 6X** and **Natrum mur. 12X**	*4 hourly*

THROMBOSIS
Coronary
(See Coronary Thrombosis)

The formation of a thrombus (clot) is called thrombosis.

Symptoms	Remedy	Frequency And Doses

THYROTOXICOSIS

The state produced by excessive quantities of endogenous or exogenous thyroid hormone.

❏ Though eats well but looses weight	**Iodium 30 or 200**	*4 hourly*
❏ Eats well but looses weight, worse after a shock or grief	**Natrum mur. 30 or 200**	*4 hourly*
● Intercurrent remedy	**Thyroidinum 200 or 1M**	*weekly (3)*

Constitutional medicines like **Calcarea carb., Lachesis and Pulsatilla**, etc., are very useful.

TIME MODALITIES
Aggravation Of Symptoms At A Specific Time

As time modality disturbs the patient as a whole so the same is very useful for proper selection of a remedy.

❏ Worse about midnight; rest during	**Rhus tox.**
❏ Worse midnight to 3 a.m.	**Drosera**
❏ Worse 1 a.m. to 2 a.m. (mid night)	**Arsenic alb.**
❏ Worse before 3 a.m.	**Nux vomica, Thuja oc.**
❏ Worse 2 a.m. to 3 a.m.	**Kali bich.**
❏ Worse 3 a.m. to 4 a.m.	**Hypericum**
❏ Worse about 3 a.m.	**Kali carb.**
❏ Worse during day time	**Medorrhinum**
❏ Worse 10 a.m. to 11 a.m.	**Gelsemium, Natrum mur.**
❏ Worse about 11 a.m.	**Ipecac., Sulphur**
❏ Worse morning	**Ignatia**
❏ Worse about 2 p.m.	**Calc-carb.**
❏ Worse about 3 p.m.	**Belladonna**
❏ Worse about 4 p.m. (fever)	**Pulsatilla**
❏ Worse 4 p.m. to 5 p.m.	**Carbo veg.**

Symptoms	Remedy	Frequency And Doses
❑ Worse 4 p.m. to 6 p.m.	**Apis mel.**	
❑ Worse 4 p.m. to 8 p.m.	**Lycopodium**	
❑ Worse 5 p.m. to 6 p.m.	**Hepar sulph.**	
❑ Worse about 7 p.m.	**Rhus tox.**	
❑ Worse before mid night	**Aconite**	
❑ Worse at night	**Syphilinum**	
❑ Worse whole night, specially first part	**Merc-sol.**	

TOBACCO CRAVING

Symptoms	Remedy	Frequency And Doses
❑ To reduce the craving; while discontinuing its use	**Tabacum 30**	*4 hourly*
❑ Though addicted to tobacco; but cannot bear the odour of it	**Lobelia in. Q,** *5-10 drops*	*4 hourly*
❑ Great desire to smoke; tobacco heart; oppression of breathing as in asthma	**Caladium s. 30**	*4 hourly*
❑ To produce disgust for tobacco in habitual tobacco chewers	**Plantago 30**	*4 hourly*

TONGUE
Affections Of

Symptoms	Remedy	Frequency And Doses
❑ Blackish (bluish in typhoid) cracked; with thirst to sip small quantity of water frequently	**Arsenic alb. 30 or 200**	*4 hourly*
❑ Dry; with thirst for large quantity of water at a time at long intervals	**Bryonia 30 or 200**	*4 hourly*
❑ Dry; without thirst, feels better in open air	**Pulsatilla 30 or 200**	*4 hourly*
❑ White; thickly coated; gastric complaints	**Antim-crud. 30 or 200**	*4 hourly*

Symptoms	Remedy	Frequency And Doses
❏ Tip of tongue (triangular) red	**Rhus tox. 30 or 200**	*4 hourly*
❏ Flabby; moist with thirst, with imprints of teeth	**Mercurius sol. 30 or 200**	*4 hourly*
❏ Smooth as if varnished	**Pyrogenium 200 or 1M**	*10 min. (3)*
❏ With red streak in the centre	**Veratrum vir. 30 or 200**	*4 hourly*
❏ Moist; dirty yellow with imprints of teeth; stools constipated	**Hydrastis can. Q or 30**	*4 hourly*
❏ Cold; bluish	**Camphora Q or 30**	*4 hourly*
❏ Bluish black; cracked	**Bufo rana. 30 or 200**	*4 hourly*
❏ Dry; stiff, leathery	**Baptisia Q or 30**	*4 hourly*
❏ Dry; blackish; protrusion difficult; patient feels worse after sleep	**Lachesis 30 or 200**	*4 hourly*
❏ Dry; pale and clammy	**Acid-phos. 30**	*4 hourly*
❏ Dry; sticking to the roof	**Nux mos. 30 or 200**	*4 hourly*
❏ Hangs out of the mouth	**Stramonium 200 or 1M**	*10 min. (3)*
❏ White coated; with imprints of teeth; diarrhoea	**Podophyllum 30**	*4 hourly*
❏ Retraction and protrusion like snake	**Cuprum met. 30 or 200**	*10 min. (3)*
❏ Sensation of hair on tongue	**Silicea 200 or 1M**	*10 min. (3)*
❏ Clean with nausea or vomiting	**Ipecac 30**	*4 hourly*

Biochemic remedies

Greyish, white, dry or slimy	**Kali mur. 6X**	*4 hourly*
Dry, swollen, dark red, imprints of teeth	**Ferrum phos. 6X**	*4 hourly*

TONSILLITIS

Inflammation of a tonsil is called tonsillitis.

● Intercurrent remedy	**Bacillinum 1M**	*fortnightly (3)*

Symptoms	Remedy	Frequency And Doses
☆ High fever, with redness and enlarged tonsils; after exposure, throbbing pain extending to ears	**Belladonna 30**	*3 hourly*
☆ In chilly patient; over sensitive to any sort of cold; tonsils enlarged, throbbing pain, suppurative stage	**Hepar sulph. 30 or 200**	*4 hourly (3)*
☆ Empty swallowing difficult; worse by smoke	**Ignatia 200 or 1M**	*10 min. (3)*
☆ Complaints of tonsils begin in the left side; worse by heat, vinegar, sour food and better by cold	**Lachesis 30 or 200**	*4 hourly (3)*
❑ Complaints begin in the right side; extremely painful	**Lycopodium 200 or 1M**	*10 min. (3)*
☆ With fetid breath; redness and stinging pains; worse at night	**Mercurius sol. 30 or 200**	*4 hourly*
☆ Slight exposure makes the tonsils worse; tonsils inflammed	**Baryta carb. 200 or 1M**	*10 min. (3)*
☆ Tonsils red with white spots; painful	**Phytolacca d. 30**	*4 hourly*
❑ Tonsillitis; alternate side	**Lac caninum 200**	*10 min. (3)*
❑ Swallowing difficult; dry cough	**Spongia 30**	*4 hourly*
❑ Can swallow liquids only; solid food gages	**Baptisia 30**	*4 hourly*
❑ Worse by heat; and better by cold; loss of thirst; stinging pain in tonsils	**Apis mel. 200**	*10 min. (3)*
❑ Follicular tonsillitis; due to streptococcus infection; pain while swallowing extending to the ears	**Ailanthus g. 30**	*4 hourly*
❑ Swallowing difficult; patient looks prematurely old	**Zincum phos. 30 or 200**	*4 hourly*
❑ Tonsils enlarged; painful with tendency to suppurate; chilly patient	**Silicea 200 or 1M**	*10 min. (3)*
● Chronic cases; tonsils ulcerating; patient covers himself with warm clothings even in summer	**Psorinum 200 or 1M**	*10 min. (3)*

Symptoms	Remedy	Frequency And Doses
❏ With chronic hardness of parotid glands; cough; worse 3 to 4 a.m.	**Kali carb. 200**	*10 min. (3)*
❏ Better from heat or hot drinks; and worse by cold; restlessness and burning sensation	**Arsenic alb. 30**	*4 hourly*
Biochemic remedy	**Biocombination No.10**	*4 hourly*

TOOTHACHE

Symptoms	Remedy	Frequency And Doses
❏ Better by sweat; pain extends to ear, temple and cheek-bone	**Aphis chenopodi Q or 30**	*4 hourly*
☆ Better holding cold (ice) water in the mouth; worse by heat and hot fluids	**Coffea 30 or 200**	*2 hourly*
❏ With thirstlessness; better holding cold water in the mouth; worse by warmth	**Pulsatilla 30 or 200**	*2 hourly*
❏ Worse dipping hand in cold water; washer woman's toothache	**Phosphorus 30 or 200**	*10 min. (3)*
☆ Due to decayed teeth; very rapid decay of teeth; decay of milk teeth	**Kreosote 30 or 200**	*4 hourly*
☆ Pain extending to ears; sensitive to touch; teeth feel too long	**Plantago 30**	*3 hourly*
❏ Severe pain at the roots of decayed teeth; worse by pressure, mastication; pain extending to eyes; over-sensitive to touch and cold	**Staphysagria 30 or 200**	*4 hourly*
☆ Due to inflammation of decayed tooth; worse at night, cold or hot applications	**Mercurius sol. 30 or 200**	*4 hourly*
❏ Severe pain; better by cold, open air, sucking teeth	**Allium cepa. 30**	*3 hourly*
❏ Worse by eating; drinking cold water, night; carious hollow teeth	**Antim-crud. 30 or 200**	*4 hourly*
❏ Worse taking anything sweet	**Natrum carb. 30 or 200**	*4 hourly*

Symptoms	Remedy	Frequency And Doses
❑ Worse after loss of vital fluids; while nursing the child	**China off. 30 or 200**	*4 hourly*
❑ Intolerable; radiating to ears and face; worse by warmth and drinking coffee	**Chamomilla 200**	*10 min. (3)*
❑ Toothache due to pyorrhoea	**Carbo veg. 30**	*4 hourly*
❑ To check bleeding after extraction of teeth; falling of teeth, and also to reduce pain due to filling, etc.	**Arnica mont. 200**	*1/2 hourly (3)*
☆ Throbbing pain with dry mouth; gumboil	**Belladonna 30**	*4 hourly*
☆ Teeth and gums very sensitive to touch; bleed easily	**Hepar sulph. 30 or 200**	*4 hourly*
❑ Toothache relieved by heat and hot fluids; during teething in children	**Magnesia phos. 30**	*4 hourly*
Biochemic remedy	**Kali phos. 6X**	*4 hourly*

TRACHOMA
Granular Conjunctivitis
(See Conjunctivitis Also)

Known as granular conjunctivitis; it is highly communicable and is caused by a virus.

❑ Acrid discharge from eyes; worse in open air; eye-lids stick together at night	**Calcarea carb. 200**	*10 min. (3)*
❑ Cracks in the corner of eyes, profuse lachrymation; stools constipated	**Graphites 30 or 200**	*4 hourly*
❑ With ulceration of the cornea and eye-lids; patient oversensitive to open air and cold. Chronic catarrh of the conjunctiva	**Hepar sulph. 30 or 200**	*4 hourly*
❑ Eye-lids granulated; stringy, yellow discharge; worse in the evening and at night	**Kali bich. 30 or 200**	*4 hourly*
❑ With thick, yellow, bland discharge; better in open, cold air; worse by warmth	**Pulsatilla 30 or 200**	*4 hourly*

Symptoms	Remedy	Frequency And Doses
❏ Catarrhal conjunctivitis; worse in inner canthus	Zincum met. 30	4 hourly
❏ Conjunctivitis; catarrhal and purulent; granular lids	Cuprum sulph. 30	4 hourly
Biochemic remedies	Ferrum phos. 6X and Kali mur. 6X	4 hourly

TRAVEL SICKNESS

Symptoms	Remedy	Frequency And Doses
☆ With nausea while travelling by road; car, rail, sea, or air; with loathing and inclination to vomit	Cocculus ind. 30	1/2 hourly
❏ Deathly nausea; vomiting, fainting and sinking feeling; worse by smell of tobacco; sea sickness	Tabacum 30	1/2 hourly
☆ With constant nausea and clean tongue	Ipecac 30	1/2 hourly
☆ In air travel; fear of downward motion	Borax 30	1/2 hourly
❏ Nausea with accumulation of water in mouth; pain with emptiness in stomach; better eating; worse sitting up, stiffness of muscles	Nux vomica 30 or 200	1/2 hourly
❏ Nausea with splitting headache; loathing for food, etc.; ineffectual vomiting	Petroleum 30	1/2 hourly
❏ Nausea and vomiting accompanied by loss of appetite and giddiness attempting to rise; scalp sensitive to touch; air sickness	Rhus tox. 30 or 200	1/2 hourly
❏ Mountain sickness	Coca 6X or 30	2 hourly

TUBERCULOSIS

A specific disease caused by the presence of Mycobacterium tubercle bacilli; it may affect almost any tissue or organ of the body; the most common seat of the disease being the lungs; the general symptoms are those of sepsis; hectic fever, sweats, and emaciation. A rapidly fatal disease due to the general dissemination of tubercle bacilli in the blood, resulting in the formation of miliary tubercles in various organs and tissues, and producing symptoms of profound toxaemia.

Symptoms	Remedy	Frequency And Doses

In homoeopathy the treatment of tuberculosis is based on the law of similia which consists of applying drugs which will lower the resistance to tuberculosis of the normal person, if given in crude doses for a long time. The weakness of such resistance is revealed in certain constitutional characteristics much earlier than the actual development of the disease. The tubercular persons are badly effected by damp, humid climate, by over exertion, after loss of vital fluids and many other factors.

Symptoms	Remedy	Frequency And Doses
❏ Pleurisy, stitching pain, and oedema above the eye-lids; patient feels worse at 3 a.m.	Kali carb. 30 or 200	4 hourly (3)
❏ Haemoptysis; craving for icy cold drinks	Phosphorus 30 or 200	4 hourly (3)
❏ Loss of weight and emaciation; even while eating well	Iodium 30 or 200	6 hourly
❏ Pungent odour from mouth; on coughing due to lung abscess	Capsicum 30	4 hourly
Biochemic remedies	Kali phos. 6X, Natrum phos. 6X and Magnesia phos. 6X	4 hourly

Other Important Remedies:

Acalypha ind., Arsenic iod., Bacillinum, Bromium, Baryta carb., Calcarea carb., Drosera, Silicea, Sepia, Sulphur, Symphytum, Merc-sol., Theridion and Tuberculinum, etc..

TUMOURS
Affections Of

Symptoms	Remedy	Frequency And Doses
❏ Vomiting without nausea in cases of intracranial tumours	Ferrum met. 30	4 hourly
❏ Fibrous tumours of eye-lids; uterine fibroids	Teucrium m-v. 30	4 hourly
❏ Tumour on skull with morbid matter; about neck	Baryta carb. 30 or 200	4 hourly
❏ Tumour with intolerable pain	Stramonium 200 or 1M	6 hourly
❏ Painless or painful nodules under the skin all over the body; lancinating pain in tumour	Conium mac. 200 or 1M	weekly (3)

Symptoms	Remedy	Frequency And Doses
❏ Malignant tumour of uterus; bleeds easily	**Crotalus h. 200 or 1M**	*weekly (3)*
❏ Tumour on knees	**Calcarea fluor. 12X or 30**	*4 hourly*
❏ Fibroid tumour of uterus	**Ustilago Q or 30**	*4 hourly*
❏ Glandular tumour where no glands are usually found	**Lapis alb. 30**	*4 hourly*
❏ Hard tumour on skin	**Manganum aceticum 30**	*4 hourly*
❏ Tumour on forehead; tibia, and other places	**Stillingia Q or 30**	*4 hourly*
❏ Fibrous tumours of breast	**Thyroidinum 200 or 1M**	*weekly (3)*
❏ Abdominal tumour	**Kali iod. 30 or 200**	*6 hourly*
Biochemic remedies	**Calcarea phos. 6X, Calcarea fluor. 12X** and **Silicea 30X**	*4 hourly*

TYPHOID
Fever
(See Fever Also)

Ist Stage (Time of Invasion):

Usually the following medicines cover almost 90% cases and cut short the duration of treatment if given in time.

☆ Weakness; mild delirium; pain head, back, and limbs; worse by motion; tongue whitish coated; lips dry and parched; with or without thirst for water in large quantities at a time; constipation; restless sleep, full of dreams of business; urine scanty and highly coloured	**Bryonia alb. 6 or 30**	*3 hourly*
☆ Extreme muscular and nervous prostration with desire to lie down; drowsiness, general trembling, muscles refuse to obey the will; little or no thirst;	**Gelsemium 6 or 30**	*3 hourly*

Symptoms	Remedy	Frequency And Doses
stools normal; urine profuse; drooping of eye-lids		
☆ Prostration and soreness as if bruised; patient falls asleep while answering; stupid, besotted, drunken expression; tongue coated with well defined streak down the middle, at first white and soon turns brown with red edges; stools loose; body parts feel as if scattered; tosses around to get together; profuse, scanty, dark, and offensive urine	**Baptisia Q or 30**	*3 hourly*
● Diarrhoea; tongue dry as a board, red triangular at the tip; delirium and stupor with muttering; restlessness; better by motion, patient toss and changee position	**Rhus tox. 6 or 30**	*3 hourly*
❑ Chilliness yet cant' bear to be in a close warm room; tongue white, no thirst; weeps easily; menses retarded (usually for women)	**Pulsatilla 30**	*4 hourly*
❑ High fever with bright red face; chilly, desires to be covered properly; nervous, sensitive and irritable (usually for men)	**Nux vomica 6 or 30**	*4 hourly*
❑ Stupid, indifferent, apathetic condition; lies still on back; don't' want to talk; painless diarrhoea, yellowish or white, watery stools with distension of the abdomen with rumbling (usually a remedy for married man),	**Acid-phos. 6 or 30**	*4 hourly*
❑ Apathetic; depressed; sleeps while answering; stupor, bruised feeling; bed feels hard	**Arnica 6 or 30**	*3 hourly*

In Severe Cases:

● Muttering, stupor, almost complete insensibility; sleeps with mouth open; dry, red, or dark tongue, trembles and catches	**Lachesis 30**	*3 hourly*

Symptoms	Remedy	Frequency And Doses
on to the lower teeth; stools offensive; if haemorrhage, it is of dark decomposed blood, as of flakes of charred straw; can't tolerate anything about the throat or chest; sleep aggravates		
❑ Prostration; power of life greatly exhausted; restlessness and anxiety, constant movements of head and limbs, while trunk lies still due to weakness; tongue either red, dry, cracked, or black, and stiff; excessive thirst for little water at a time but at frequent intervals; burning in stomach, watery, brownish or bloody, offensive stools; worse at mid night	Arsenic alb. 30	1/2 hourly
❑ Stage of collapse; prostration, torpor, dissolution of blood, paralytic conditions; face deathly pale, sunken, cold; there may be haemorrhage from nose, mouth, or anus; abdomen distended rumbling and gurgling of wind, cadaverous involuntary diarrhoea; rattling in chest, filled with mucous; circulation weak, blood stagnates in the capillaries with cyanotic blueness of face, lips and tongue; cold sweat; desires constant fanning to get more oxygen	Carbo veg. 30 (China follows Carbo veg.)	1/2 hourly
❑ Due to weakness the patient constantly slides down in the bed; with moaning and groaning; lower jaw dropped; tongue greatly shrunken, leathery; paralysed pulse, intermitting every third beat; involuntary bloody stools	Acid-mur. 30	3 hourly
❑ Fetidness of all excretions and secretions; pulse out of all proportion to temperature; tongue red, like raw beef, fiery red	Pyrogenium 6 or 30	1/2 hourly (3)
Biochemic remedies	Ferrum phos. 6X, Kali phos. 6X and Kali mur. 12X	3 hourly

ULCERS

Affections Of
(See Abscess And Boils Also)

Symptoms	Remedy	Frequency And Doses
❑ Fistulous ulcers; with red, hard, inflamed areola, discharging more blood than pus of offensive odour	**Causticum 30**	*4 hourly*
❑ Gangrenous degeneration of ulcers	**Kreosote. 30**	*4 hourly*
❑ Gastric ulcers with haemoptysis	**Ornithogalum Q or 30**	*4 hourly*
❑ Syphilitic ulcers; worse in cold weather	**Petroleum 30 or 200**	*4 hourly*
❑ Ulcers very red; dark glistening ulcer	**Lac caninum 30 or 200**	*4 hourly*
❑ Yellowish ulcer, deep in tonsils; localised; old leg ulcer; on wrist	**Kali bich. 30 or 200**	*4 hourly*
☆ Purple coloured ulcer; with blackish patches; ulcer with feeble relaxed tissues; stagnating capillaries	**Carbo veg. 30 or 200**	*4 hourly*
☆ Ulcer dark; putrid; ulceration of mucous surface	**Baptisia 30**	*4 hourly*
❑ Ulcer with thick whitish-yellow scabs; vesicles around	**Mezereum 30**	*4 hourly*
● Ulcer with sensation of coldness; when after prolonged allopathic medication, and indicated drug do not act	**Mercurius sol. 1M or higher**	*1 dose*
☆ Ulcer without any sensation; due to intake of opium	**Opium 30 or 200**	*4 hourly*
❑ Ulcer better from cold; and worse by heat	**Ledum pal. 30 or 200**	*4 hourly*
❑ To help discharge, and healing the ulcer, of soft palate; sensitive to touch, cold, etc.	**Hepar sulph. 30**	*4 hourly*

Symptoms	Remedy	Frequency And Doses
	Lachesis 30 or 200	4 hourly (3)
☆ Ulcer very sensitive, purple coloured; cannot bear even touch of clothes	Argentum nit. 30	4 hourly
❑ Ulcer internal; due to abuse of mercury	Borax 30	4 hourly
☆ Ulcer of mouth; aphthae; slight injuries suppurate and ulcerate	Bromium 30	4 hourly
❑ Chronic stomach ulcers; foul ulcers on skin	Kali carb. 30	6 hourly
❑ Ulcer on lungs; cough or breathing complaints are worse at 3 to 4 a.m.	Silicea 12X or 30	4 hourly
❑ Ulcer of legs; about the nails and heels	Salicylic acid. 30	4 hourly
❑ Ulcer of mucous membranes; of stomach and bowels	Conium mac. 200	6 hourly
❑ Ulcer of face and lips; excessive weakness	Asafoetida 30	4 hourly
❑ Ulcer very sensitive; ulcers with high and hard edges; easy bleeding		

UNCONSCIOUSNESS
(See Collapse And Fainting Also)

Symptoms	Remedy	Frequency And Doses
❑ When new born child do not breathe, and becomes blue without any visible obstruction	Laurocerasus 6 or 30	15 min. (3)
❑ After inhaling charcoal gas	Bovista 30	15 min. (3)
❑ After drinking alcohol or inhaling coal gas	Carbo-sulph. 30	15 min. (3)
❑ Due to excessive loss of blood or vital fluids	China 30 or 200	1/2 hourly
● If syphilitic miasm is in the background (when there is organic change in heart or lungs, avoid Syphilinum)	Syphilinum 10M	1 dose
❑ If pulse and urine shows set back	Helleborus 200 or 1M	4 hourly (3)
❑ When, due to suppressed anger	Colocynth. 200 or 1M	4 hourly (3)
❑ When after fright or lightning	Phosphorus 200 or 1M	15 min. (3)

Symptoms	Remedy	Frequency And Doses
● Intercurrent remedy	**Sulphur 200**	*1 dose*
❑ When there is history of high blood pressure; depression and weakness of head	**Aurum met. 10M**	*15 min. (3)*
Biochemic remedies	**Kali mur. 6X** and **Ferrum phos. 6X**	*4 hourly*

URINE
Affections Of

❑ Burning before and after micturition	**Cantharis 30 or 200**	*4 hourly (3)*
❑ Burning in urethra when not micturating; complaints of newly married persons	**Staphysagria 30 or 200**	*4 hourly (3)*
❑ Burning, stinging pains before, during and after micturition	**Cannabis ind. 30 or 200**	*4 hourly (3)*
❑ Difficult micturition; uraemic coma	**Plumbum met. 30 or 200**	*4 hourly (3)*
❑ Urine profuse with weakness	**Calcarea phos. 6X or 30**	*4 hourly*
❑ Retention of urine with a full bladder	**Opium 30 or 200**	*4 hourly (3)*
❑ Can not pass urine; except when standing, involuntary, due to paralysis of sphincter; urine passes at every cough. Retention of urine after operation	**Causticum 30 or 200**	*4 hourly (3)*
❑ Urine alkaline and ropy; feels as some urine still remains in bladder even after passing	**Kali bich. 30 or 200**	*4 hourly*
❑ Urine dribbles while sitting; frequent urging with scanty urination and burning. Can pass urine only while standing; discharge of gas with urine	**Sarsaparilla 30 or 200**	*4 hourly (3)*
❑ Urging to pass urine; due to impending fever; pulse out of all proportion to the temperature	**Pyrogenium 200 or 1M**	*4 hourly (3)*

Symptoms	Remedy	Frequency And Doses
❑ Urine drops down vertically and patient must wait before urine starts	**Hepar sulph. 30 or 200**	*4 hourly (3)*
❑ Cannot pass urine without straining; frequent during day	**Lilium tig. 30 or 200**	*4 hourly (3)*
❑ Has to wait a long time to pass urine; frequent desire to urinate	**Lycopodium 30 or 200**	*4 hourly (3)*
❑ Can urinate only while lying down; frequent and profuse urination	**Kreosote. 30 or 200**	*4 hourly (3)*
❑ Can pass urine only while passing stools; frequent and copious	**Acid-mur. 30 or 200**	*4 hourly (3)*
❑ Pain in neck of bladder while urinating; ineffectual urging to urinate	**Nux vom. 30 or 200**	*4 hourly (3)*
❑ Involuntary urine during first sleep; red sediment in urine which adheres tightly to the vessel	**Sepia 30 or 200**	*4 hourly (3)*
❑ Passes urine when walking, coughing, sneezing; can not pass urine in presence of anyone	**Natrum mur. 12X or 30**	*4 hourly*
❑ Urine very acidic; passes in drops; thick with pus; bruised pain in urethra	**Arnica 30 or 200**	*4 hourly*
❑ Urine dribbles while sitting and walking; patient feels better in open, cold air	**Pulsatilla 30 or 200**	*4 hourly*
❑ Patient cries and screams before urination; urine hot and smarting	**Borax 30 or 200**	*4 hourly*
❑ Urine comes with tickling in urethra	**Ferrum phos. 6X or 30**	*4 hourly*
❑ Urine offensive; haematuria	**Salicylic acid. 30 or 200**	*4 hourly*
❑ Urine fetid; burning when urinating	**Baptisia. 30 or 200**	*4 hourly*
❑ Urine pungent; ammoniacal smell; urine dark brown and scanty	**Asafoetida 30 or 200**	*4 hourly*
❑ Urine gelatinous; yellowish as in jaundice	**Crotalus h. 30 or 200**	*4 hourly (3)*
❑ Urine turbid; involuntary discharge of urine due to paralysis of neck of bladder	**Dulcamara 30 or 200**	*4 hourly (3)*

Symptoms	Remedy	Frequency And Doses
❏ Urine albuminous; cloudy with sediment; smells of violets; haematuria	Terebinth. Q or 30	4 hourly
❏ Urine with red sand; milky; with sandy deposits	Lycopodium 30 or 200	4 hourly (3)
❏ Urine cold; strong smelling; patient feels cold while passing urine	Nitric-acid. 30 or 200	4 hourly (3)
❏ Urine highly coloured; flows very slowly; painful tenesmus when urinating	Medorrhinum 200 or 1M	4 hourly (3)
❏ Urine like ink; pale, like lime water; retention of urine	Chelidonium Q or 30	4 hourly
❏ Urine very yellow or dark brown; turbid when passed	Colchicum 30 or 200	4 hourly (3)
❏ Urine frequent at night, micturition stops 5-6 times before bladder is empty	Thuja oc. 200 or 1M	4 hourly (3)
❏ Itching from contact of urine; constant desire but little is passed	Merc-sol. 30 or 200	4 hourly (3)
❏ Itching during micturition; dribbling after micturition; discharge of mucous with urine	Petroleum 30 or 200	4 hourly (3)
❏ Blood in urine; persistent tenesmus of the bladder	Mercurius cor. 30	3 hourly
☆ Painful urination and constriction of urethra; accompanied by backache	Cucurbita cit. 30	3 hourly
❏ Pain in urethra when not passing urine; urine light yellow and cloudy	Natrum carb. 30	4 hourly
● Everytime patient urinates, jumps due to a sharp pain as if a sharp instrument had been struck under the great toe nail	Sulphur 30 or 200	4 hourly (3)
❏ Can pass urine only while sitting down on knees with knees wide apart	Veratrum alb. 30	4 hourly
● Intercurrent remedy for all kinds of urinary infections	Morgan pure 200 or 1002	fortnightly (3)
❏ Urinary complaints in syphilitic patient	Syphilinum 200 or 1M	weekly (3)

Symptoms	Remedy	Frequency And Doses

URTICARIA
Hives

It is an eruption or itching wheal usually of systemic origin. It may be due to a state of hypersensitivity to foods or drugs, foci of infection, physical agents (heat, cold, light, friction), or psychic stimuli.
It occurs in hypersensitive or allergic persons. Constitutional treatment is essential.

Symptoms	Remedy	Frequency And Doses
☆ After taking rich, fatty food, meat, etc.; better open, cold air; loss of thirst	**Pulsatilla 30 or 200**	*3 hourly*
❑ After taking tinned food; acid fruits, ice cream, over ripen fruits; better by heat	**Arsenic alb. 30 or 200**	*3 hourly*
❑ After taking strawberries	**Oxalic acid. 30**	*3 hourly*
❑ After taking mushrooms	**Absinthium 30**	*3 hourly*
☆ With severe burning and swelling; after taking crabs; no thirst; frequent urination	**Urtica urens Q or 30**	*3 hourly*
❑ After taking spoiled fish	**Carbo veg. 30 or 200**	*3 hourly*
❑ After taking milk	**Sepia 30 or 200**	*3 hourly*
❑ After taking Aspirin, Anacin, etc.	**Antipyrin. 30**	*3 hourly*
❑ After taking Quinine; excessive salt or after suppression of Malaria	**Natrum mur. 30 or 200**	*3 hourly*
❑ After mosquito bites; better washing with icy cold water	**Ledum pal. 30 or 200**	*3 hourly*
❑ After undressing; cold weather; better by warmth	**Rumex 30 or 200**	*3 hourly*
❑ Due to change of weather, exposure to cold wet weather; violent itching while undressing	**Dulcamara 30 or 200**	*4 hourly*
❑ Sudden; after exposure to cold dry wind with anxiety	**Aconite nap. 30 or 200**	*2 hourly*
❑ After bathing; itching on getting warm, disturbing sleep	**Bovista 30**	*2 hourly*

Symptoms	Remedy	Frequency And Doses
☆ Every spring; better by heat. Throwing off the clothes aggravates	**Rhus tox. 30 or 200**	*3 hourly*
☆ With sudden, severe swelling and burning; worse by heat; loss of thirst	**Apis mel. 30 or 200**	*3 hourly*
● In the beginning of winter; filthy smell from the body even after a bath	**Psorinum 200 or 1M**	*10 min. (3)*
❑ Due to gastric catarrh; tongue thickly whitish coated; worse by heat	**Antimonium crud. 200**	*10 min. (3)*
☆ Chronic urticaria; rashes on whole body with itching	**Astacus fl. 30**	*3 hourly*
❑ After taking alcoholic drinks; chilly patient; feels better in warmth	**Nux vomica 30 or 200**	*3 hourly*
❑ Urticaria without itching	**Uva ursi Q or 30**	*4 hourly*
❑ Due to suppression of intermittent fever	**Elaterium 30**	*3 hourly*
❑ Urticarial rash with burning; fever; worse by heat, wearing woollen clothes; better by cold	**Hygrophila spinosa 30**	*4 hourly*
Biochemic remedies	**Kali mur. 6X** and **Natrum mur. 6X**	*4 hourly*

UTERUS
Affections Of
(See Prolapse Of Uterus Also)

❑ Burning in uterus with metrorrhagia	**Terebinth. Q or 30**	*4 hourly*
❑ Cramps in uterus; labor-like pain; hysterical convulsions due to uterine irritation	**Viburnum op. 30**	*4 hourly*
❑ Bruised pain in the uterus; complaints after dilatation and curettage (D & C)	**Arnica mont. 30 or 200**	*4 hourly*

Symptoms	Remedy	Frequency And Doses
❑ Congestion in uterus; feeble contractions; habitual abortion due to uterine debility	**Caulophyllum 30 or 200**	*4 hourly*
❑ Griping and pinching in uterus; uterine haemorrhage; intolerance of pain	**Chamomilla 30 or 200**	*4 hourly*
❑ Bright and stringy haemorrhages from uterus	**Lac. caninum 200**	*4 hourly (3)*
❑ Dark and stringy haemorrhages from uterus	**Crocus sat. 30 or 200**	*4 hourly (3)*
❑ Haemorrhages profuse, bright, in gushes from uterus with nausea and clean tongue	**Ipecac. Q or 30**	*4 hourly*
❑ Severe neuralgic pains in uterus; worse by touch or jar; displacement of uterus	**Lilium tig. 30 or 200**	*4 hourly (3)*
❑ Vulva painful and itchy; excessive itching in uterus with excessive sexual urge	**Platina 200 or 1M**	*4 hourly (3)*
❑ Cancer; with profuse haemorrhages from uterus	**Iodium 30 or 200**	*4 hourly*
❑ Fibroid tumours in uterus; ill effects of suppressed sexual desire; ulcer on neck of uterus; haemorrhage after coition	**Kreosote 30 or 200**	*4 hourly (3)*
❑ Polypus and weakness of uterus; prolapsus due to weakness	**Calcarea phos. 12X or 30**	*4 hourly*
❑ Feels as if everything would fall out from uterus; haemorrhages, gushing and hot	**Belladonna 30 or 200**	*4 hourly*
❑ Uterine epilepsy and hysteria; feels better after flow from uterus starts	**Cimicifuga 30 or 200**	*4 hourly (3)*
❑ To expel remaining contents from uterus after dilatation and curettage (D & C) in post operative cases	**Pyrogenium 200 or 1M**	*4 hourly (3)*
❑ Uterine disorders of maids; unmarried old women	**Conium mac. 200 or 1M**	*4 hourly (3)*

VACCINATION
Affections Of

Symptoms	Remedy	Frequency And Doses
● Head remedy; ill effects of vaccination	**Thuja oc. 200 or 1M**	*10 min. (3)*
❑ When Thuja oc. fails to take care of ill effects of vaccination	**Antimonium tart. 200**	*1 dose*
☆ Abscesses or convulsions after vaccination	**Silicea 30 or 200**	*4 hourly (3)*
❑ Puffiness of whole body after vaccination; loss of thirst	**Apis mel. 30 or 200**	*4 hourly (3)*
☆ Fever with inflammation of vaccinated area of skin	**Belladonna 30**	*4 hourly (3)*
❑ Dry, rough skin even after years of vaccination	**Malandrinum 200**	*weekly (6)*
❑ Eczema and eruptions with itching after vaccination	**Mezereum 30**	*4 hourly*
❑ To relieve eruptions and itching from face and other parts after vaccination	**Sarsaparilla 30**	*4 hourly*
❑ Keloid or scar formation after vaccination	**Vaccininum 200**	*weekly (6)*

VARICOSE VEINS

Symptoms	Remedy	Frequency And Doses
☆ Head remedy; even for varicose ulcers	**Hamamellis 30**	*4 hourly*
❑ When affected parts are bluish and sore; stinging pain; better open, cold air	**Pulsatilla 30**	*4 hourly*
❑ With burning sensation like fire; worse mid night; better by warmth and hot	**Arsenic alb. 30**	*4 hourly*
❑ Chronic cases; worse by warmth; better by cold and while walking	**Acid-fluor. 30**	*4 hourly*

Symptoms	Remedy	Frequency And Doses

VERTIGO
(See Giddiness Also)

Symptoms	Remedy	Frequency And Doses
☆ Vertigo; worse by noise, with nausea on closing eyes; sea sickness	Theridion 30	4 hourly
❑ Vertigo; worse riding in a carriage or boat; raising eyes, with roaring in ears	Petroleum 30	3 hourly
☆ Vertigo; from downward motion; afraid of falling	Borax 30	4 hourly
❑ Vertigo; with sleepiness; worse after rising from seat	Aethusa cy. 30	4 hourly
❑ Vertigo; with eyes out of focus; worse while sitting; better by walking	Alumina 30	4 hourly
❑ Vertigo; with sensation of falling and headache; during epileptic spasms	Calcarea phos. 6X or 30	4 hourly
❑ Vertigo; with pain in liver; inclination to fall forward	Chelidonium 30	4 hourly
☆ Vertigo; with eyes open; motion, on turning head; of old peoples bachelors/maids	Conium mac. 30 or 200	4 hourly
❑ Vertigo; with dimness of vision; worse on walking and seeing objects 'transparently'	Cyclamen 30	4 hourly
❑ Vertigo; with momentary loss of consciousness; after dinner	Nux vomica 30 or 200	4 hourly
❑ Vertigo; on rising from chair, motion; better by lying quietly	Bryonia 30 or 200	4 hourly
❑ Vertigo; on seeing running water; on crossing a bridge	Ferrum phos. 12X or 30	4 hourly
☆ Vertigo; on seeing moving objects, from paresis of accommodation, loss of sleep	Cocculus ind. 30	4 hourly
❑ Feels as if would fall to left side with vertigo; with giddiness in horizontal position	Salicylic acid. 30	4 hourly
☆ Vertigo; in morning; with feeling of falling when standing; in married men, due to excessive semen loss	Phosphoric acid. 30	4 hourly

Symptoms	Remedy	Frequency And Doses
❏ Vertigo; worse on closing eyes, after sleep, suppression of discharges	**Lachesis 30 or 200**	*4 hourly (3)*
☆ Vertigo; worse after rising in the morning, looking upwards	**Pulsatilla 30 or 200**	*4 hourly (3)*
❏ Vertigo, worse in the open air, after eating, in the evening	**Phosphorus 30 or 200**	*4 hourly (3)*
❏ Vertigo; worse on turning over to right side	**Ceanothus Q or 30**	*4 hourly*
Biochemic remedy	**Kali phos. 6X**	*4 hourly*

VISION
Affections Of

Symptoms	Remedy	Frequency And Doses
❏ Diplopia; from excess of sexual activity; from masturbation; loss of vision with nausea	**Sepia 30 or 200**	*4 hourly (3)*
❏ Diplopia; alternating deafness; staring at objects	**Cicuta v. 30**	*4 hourly*
❏ Diplopia after diphtheria; affections of heart; patient feels worse after sleep	**Lachesis 30**	*4 hourly (3)*
❏ Diplopia during pregnancy; drooping of eye-lids	**Gelsemium 30**	*4 hourly*
❏ Disturbed accommodation; myopia, weak feeling in eyes	**Physostigma. 6 or 30**	*4 hourly*
❏ Patient sees rainbow colours; vision foggy; better rubbing eyes; loss of vision due to masturbation	**Acid-phos. 30**	*4 hourly*
❏ See snakes; vision obstructed by mucous	**Argentum nit. 30 or 200**	*4 hourly (3)*
❏ Loss of vision for colours; sudden blind spells with vertigo	**Belladonna 30**	*4 hourly*
❏ Loss of vision from alcoholic drinks	**Terebinth. Q or 30**	*4 hourly*

Symptoms	Remedy	Frequency And Doses
❏ Loss of vision without cause; after looking at white objects steadily	Tabacum 30	4 hourly
❏ Loss of vision with epistaxis	Oxalic ac. 30	4 hourly
❏ Loss of vision due to inflammation in eye	Mancinella 30	4 hourly
❏ Loss of vision from over use of eyes; from grief; due to retinal haemorrhage; Diplopia with nausea	Croton tig. 30 or 200	4 hourly
❏ Loss of vision after sudden fainting	Plumbum met. 30 or 200	4 hourly (3)
❏ Loss of vision with headache; Diplopia while blowing the nose	Causticum 30 or 200	4 hourly (3)
❏ Loss of vision after headache; vision confused, letters run together on reading	Silicea 12X or 30	4 hourly
❏ Loss of vision in hydrocephalus patient	Apocynum Q or 30	4 hourly
❏ Loss of vision while reading; hysterical; from lightning, from tobacco; sees halo around the light; vision misty	Phosphorus 30 or 200	4 hourly (3)
❏ Loss of vision, from optic nerve atrophy; diplopia; one image seen below the other	Syphilinum 200 or 1M	weekly (3)
❏ Loss of vision; periodical; floating black spots before eyes	Merc-sol. 30 or 200	4 hourly
❏ Loss of vision from retro-bulbar neuritis; after malaria fever	Chin-sulph. 30	4 hourly
❏ Loss of vision from lying in sun. Objects look red, striped	Conium mac. 30 or 200	4 hourly (3)
❏ Vision dizzy, confusing; sensitive to light	Theridion 30	4 hourly
❏ Vision dim; Objects flicker; sees countless stars; diplopia	Cyclamen. 30	4 hourly
❏ Objects look black, calls for light; small objects look large	Stramonium. 30 or 200	4 hourly (3)
● Sees fiery spots; intercurrent remedy	Psorinum. 200 or 1M	4 hourly (3)
❏ Sees sparks, fiery and zig-zag appearance around all objects	Natrum mur. 12X or 30	4 hourly
❏ Objects look very yellow; photophobia	Kali bich. 30	4 hourly

Symptoms	Remedy	Frequency And Doses

VOICE, LOSS OF
Aphonia
(See Hoarseness Also)

Symptoms	Remedy	Frequency And Doses
❏ With hoarseness; after debilitating diseases	Carbo veg. 30	4 hourly
❏ From over use of voice; nervous exhaustion	Kali phos. 6X or 30	4 hourly
❏ With laryngitis; constant hawking	Phosphorus 30	4 hourly
❏ Heated, becoming after; due to gastric origin	Antimonium crud. 30	4 hourly
Biochemic remedies	Ferrum phos. 6X and Kali phos. 6X	4 hourly

---

VOMITING

Symptoms	Remedy	Frequency And Doses
☆ With burning pain in the stomach; unquenchable thirst, drinks little water at a time but frequently; retching and fear of death	Arsenic alb. 30	2 hourly
☆ With constant nausea and clean tongue	Ipecac 30	2 hourly
❏ After drinking alcohol; sour vomiting after an hour of eating	Kali bich. 30	2 hourly
☆ Nausea and vomiting; worse after over eating; vomiting during pregnancy	Nux vomica 30 or 200	2 hourly
☆ With face bathed with cold sweat; nausea and vomiting during pregnancy	Lobelia inf. 30	2 hourly
❏ Violent vomiting with deathly nausea	Tabacum 30	2 hourly
❏ Violent, forcible vomiting of slimy acid liquid with food; with painful distortion of face and cold sweat	Verat-alb. 30	2 hourly

WALKING
(See Gait)

WARTS

Symptoms	Remedy	Frequency And Doses
❑ Warts on prepuce	**Cinnabaris 30**	*4 hourly*
❑ Head remedy for warts	**Calc calcinata 3X**	*4 hourly*
❑ Horny; solid, flat or sharp; especially on face, tip of nose, and fingers	**Causticum 200**	*6 hourly*
❑ Small warts around the anus	**Aurum mur. 3X**	*4 hourly*
● Cracky; cauliflower like, moist, in crops; bleeds easily on slightest touch	**Thuja oc. 200**	*6 hourly*
❑ Soft; spongy, horny; bleeds easily; itching and stinging sensation	**Calcarea carb. 200 or 1M**	*6 hourly*
❑ Withered; suppurating; stinging sensation	**Kali silic. 30**	*4 hourly*
● Hard; painful; patient feels hungry at 9-10 a.m.; dread of bathing	**Sulphur 200 or 1M**	*10 min. (3)*
❑ On back of hands; large, smooth, or fleshy on face and hands	**Dulcamara 200 or 1M**	*10 min. (3)*
❑ Covering whole face; pimples all over the body	**Magnesia sulph. 30**	*4 hourly*
❑ Corns with yellowish discoloration and warts; especially hands; epithelial growths	**Natrum carb. 30 or 200**	*4 hourly*
❑ Warts sore, on palms; corns with yellowish colour	**Ferrum pic. 30**	*4 hourly*
❑ Fig-warts, pedunculated; dry, cauliflower like; syphilitic origin	**Staphysagria 200 or 1M**	*6 hourly*
❑ Large, jagged, condylomatous, pedunculated; bleeds easily; painful	**Acid-nit. 200 or 1M**	*6 hourly*

Symptoms	Remedy	Frequency And Doses
● In chronic cases where there is history of malignancy in patient or his family	**Carcinocin 200 or 1M**	*1 dose*

Biochemic remedies

On palms	**Natrum mur. 6X or 12X**	*4 hourly*
On hands	**Kali mur. 6X or 12X**	*4 hourly*

For External Use:

Thuja oc. Q.

WAX
In Ears

Symptoms	Remedy	Frequency And Doses
❑ Wax in ears; hard, yellowish in colour, difficult hearing; loss of thirst	**Pulsatilla 30 o 200**	*4 hourly*
❑ Wax; yellowish white, hard, dry; tearing pain in ears	**Lachesis 30 or 200**	*4 hourly*
❑ Wax reddish, blood colored; defective hearing	**Conium mac. 200 or 1M**	*10 min. (3)*
● Wax reddish; foul smelling; sore pain behind ears	**Psorinum 200 or 1M**	*10 min. (3)*
❑ Excessive ear wax; deafness and re-echo of words	**Causticum 200**	*10 min. (3)*
Biochemic remedy	**Calc-sulph. 2X and Silicea 2X**	*4 hourly*

WEAKNESS
(See Emaciation Also)

Symptoms	Remedy	Frequency And Doses
❑ Due to loss of sleep; nervous tension	**Phosphorus 200**	*10 min. (3)*
❑ Weakness of legs; after diarrhoea	**Bovista 30**	*4 hourly*
❑ Due to nervous exhaustion; chilly patient	**Calcarea carb. 200**	*4 hourly (3)*
❑ General tonic for nervous exhaustion	**Kali phos. 6X or 30**	*4 hourly*
☆ Without any apparent cause; after acute disease	**Alfa alfa tonic**	*before meals*
● Intercurrent remedy, for psoric patients	**Psorinum 200 or 1M**	*weekly (3)*

Symptoms	Remedy	Frequency And Doses

WEEPING

Symptoms	Remedy	Frequency And Doses
❑ Weeps day and night; hard to please	**Apis mel. 30 or 200**	*4 hourly (3)*
❑ Weeps at 11 a.m.; morning	**Sulphur 30 or 200**	*4 hourly (3)*
❑ Weeps in sleep; from contradiction	**Nux vomica 30 or 200**	*4 hourly (3)*
❑ Weeps all night; laughs all day; alternating with cheerfulness; in dark	**Stramonium. 30 or 200**	*4 hourly (3)*
❑ Weeps when alone; worse by consolation; remember unpleasant past events and weeps	**Natrum mur. 30 or 200**	*4 hourly (3)*
❑ Weeps aloud; sobbing; 4 to 8 p.m.; when thanked	**Lycopodium 30 or 200**	*4 hourly (3)*
❑ Weeps on every occasion; when telling her sickness; while nursing; when interrupted, during coryza, answering a question; consolation ameliorates	**Pulsatilla 30 or 200**	*4 hourly (3)*
❑ Weeps after anxiety; from music	**Graphites 30 or 200**	*4 hourly (3)*
❑ Stop weeping only when carried; obstinate	**Chamomilla 30 or 200**	*4 hourly (3)*
❑ Weeps without knowing why; without reason; restlessness	**Rhus tox. 30 or 200**	*4 hourly (3)*
❑ Weeps when demands are not fulfilled; when touched	**Cina 30 or 200**	*4 hourly (3)*
❑ Weeps at trifles; old people for no reason; when sentiments are touched	**Causticum 30 or 200**	*4 hourly (3)*
❑ Weeps before coughing; oversensitive to touch, cold, etc.	**Hepar sulph. 30 or 200**	*4 hourly (3)*
❑ Weeps from joy; superiority complex	**Platinum 30 or 200**	*4 hourly (3)*
❑ Weeps when meeting people; suicidal thoughts	**Aurum mur. 30 or 200**	*4 hourly (3)*
❑ Weeping periodical; every four weeks	**Conium mac. 30 or 200**	*4 hourly (3)*
❑ Weeps after pollutions (masturbation)	**Ustilago 30 or 200**	*4 hourly (3)*
❑ Weeps during pregnancy	**Magnesia carb. 30 or 200**	*4 hourly (3)*

Symptoms	Remedy	Frequency And Doses
❏ Weeps while speaking; day time	**Medorrhinum. 30 or 200**	*4 hourly (3)*
❏ Weeps when spoken to; violent out bursts of passion; due to indignation	**Staphysagria 30 or 200**	*4 hourly (3)*
❏ Weeps when walking in open air	**Sepia 30 or 200**	*4 hourly (3)*

WHEEZING
(See Asthma And Bronchitis Also)

Symptoms	Remedy	Frequency And Doses
☆ With coated tongue; much rattling due to mucous, shortness of breath, dyspnoea	**Antimonium tart. 30 or 200**	*1 dose*
☆ With clean tongue; nausea and vomiting. Wheezing cough; chest full of phlegm	**Ipecac 30**	*4 hourly*
☆ Accumulation of mucous, loose cough; difficult respiration; worse by cold and in cold air	**Hepar sulph. 30**	*4 hourly*
❏ Wheezing, rattling, with rattling in the larynx	**Bromium 30**	*4 hourly*
❏ Inspiration difficult; wheezy, croupy cough; cold extends downwards from head to throat and bronchi	**Iodium 30**	*4 hourly*
❏ With copious purulent expectoration; cough worse in the evening, with efforts to vomit with pain in chest	**Kreosote 30 or 200**	*4 hourly*
❏ Wheezing; worse after lying down, after first sleep with spasmodic cough	**Aralia r. 30**	*4 hourly*
● Intercurrent remedy; for chronic cases	**Bacillinum 200 or 1M**	*fortnightly (3)*
❏ Wheezing and oppression in chest in acute bronchitis; tenacious, profuse, whitish expectoration; sibilant rales	**Grindelia 30**	*4 hourly*
❏ Wheezing; difficulty in raising of tough, profuse mucous (specially for the aged)	**Senega Q or 30**	*4 hourly*

Symptoms	Remedy	Frequency And Doses
❑ Wheezing; cough with rattling chest; spasmodic constriction in chest; worse after eating or drinking	**Nux vomica 30 or 200**	*4 hourly*
❑ Wheezing; cough with relaxed vulva; better by warmth; worse cold and 3 - 4 a.m.	**Kali carb. 30 or 30**	*4 hourly (3)*
❑ Wheezing; paroxysmal cough, with suffocative obstruction of respiration and sneezing	**Justicea Q or 30**	*4 hourly*
❑ Rales, loud, as if lungs were full of mucous; specially in bronchial catarrh of infants	**Lycopodium 30 or 200**	*4 hourly (3)*
❑ From tickling in throat; glairy, greenish, copious, purulent expectoration; worse in damp weather	**Nat-sulph. 30 or 200**	*4 hourly (3)*
● Racking, spasmodic cough; intercurrent remedy; puts warm clothes even in summer	**Psorinum 200 or 1M**	*10 min. (3)*
❑ Rales; until something is expectorated	**Carbo ani. 30 or 200**	*4 hourly (3)*
❑ With copious expectoration of mucous; worse exposure from warmth to cold	**Dulcamara 30 or 200**	*4 hourly (3)*
● Sorenss and pressure in chest; catarrh of pharynx; worse in the morning	**Sulphur 30 or 200**	*4 hourly (3)*
❑ With muco-purulent expectoration; restlessness and unquenchable thirst	**Arsenic alb. 30 or 200**	*4 hourly (3)*
❑ Accumulation of mucous in the throat; tickling in the throat pit	**Causticum 30 or 200**	*4 hourly (3)*
❑ Accumulation of mucous in larynx; whistling, nausea, and rattling in chest	**Kali bich. 30 or 200**	*4 hourly*
❑ Phlegm loose, but can not get it up; cough worse in the evening and after lying down	**Sepia 30 or 200**	*4 hourly (3)*
❑ With greenish, offensive, sweetish sputum	**Stannum met. 30**	*4 hourly*
Biochemic remedies	**Ferrum phos. 6X** and **Kali mur. 6X**	*4 hourly*

Symptoms	Remedy	Frequency And Doses

WHITLOW
(See Abscess And Boils Also)

Deep seated abscess near the end of the finger, often under the nail with pain and swelling is called whitlow. The beginning may be in the shape of a hard tumour like growth which very soon becomes hot and painful.

Symptoms	Remedy	Frequency And Doses
❑ In acute cases; to abort abscess	Myristica seb. Q or 3X	2 hourly
❑ Before suppurative stage; worse from warmth	Mercurius sol. 30	3 hourly
☆ Intense throbbing pain; to promote suppuration	Hepar sulph. 3X	2 hourly
❑ When abscess is deep seated; excruciating pain; to promote suppuration	Silicea 30	3 hourly
❑ Dark red or bluish lesion with intense pain	Lachesis 30 or 200	4 hourly (3)
❑ Blackish; painful, burning pain; better by heat and by warmth	Arsenic alb. 30 and Carbo veg. 30	alternate 2 hourly
☆ When fungoid granulation forms in the effected flesh; with intense pain	Acid-nit. 30 or 200	4 hourly
❑ When the pain is intolerable after exposure of nerves	Allium cepa. 30	3 hourly
❑ When due to injury of nails; effected lesion cold; better by cold compresses	Ledum pal. 30 or 200	3 hourly
❑ Cold applications ameliorates; worse by warmth, feels as if burning vapours were emitted from the effected lesion	Acid-fluor. 30 or 200	3 hourly (3)
Biochemic remedy	Silicea 12X	4 hourly

WHOOPING COUGH
(See Cough Also)

Symptoms	Remedy	Frequency And Doses
● To start the treatment; intercurrent remedy	Syphilinum 1M	1 dose

Symptoms	Remedy	Frequency And Doses
☆ Preventive remedy (give one dose after *Syphilinum 1M* in acute cases)	**Pertussin 200 or 1M**	*1 dose*
❏ Whooping cough with vomiting of tough, ropy mucous; worse by warmth and night; better taking cold drinks and in cold room	**Coccus cact. 30**	*4 hourly*
❏ While starts eating; coughs and vomits after few mouthfuls only	**Bryonia alb. 30 or 200**	*4 hourly*
☆ Head remedy (sudden violent attacks)	**Drosera Q or 6**	*4 hourly (3)*
❏ In young children; worse by least breath, air or fog	**Mentha pip. 30**	*3 hourly*
❏ With cold and clammy perspiration of intermittent nature; spasmodic	**Cuprum ars. 30**	*3 hourly*
☆ With dryness of throat; pain stomach and tears precede the fit of cough; worse by cold	**Belladonna 30**	*4 hourly*
Biochemic remedies	**Magnesia phos. 6X** and **Calcarea phos. 6X**	*4 hourly*

WORMS

Symptoms	Remedy	Frequency And Doses
☆ Head remedy: to start the treatment	**Cina 1M,** *15 min. (3) from 2nd. day -* **Santonine 3X and Natrum phos. 6X,** *twice each for one week or more, as required*	
❏ For tape worms; with morbid hunger	**Anantherum 30**	*4 hourly*
❏ When worms travel over the perineum and get into the vagina and excite masturbation	**Caladium s. 30**	*4 hourly*
❏ Grinding of teeth; distension of abdomen with pain; worse after meal; itching around anus; nocturnal enuresis; desire for sweets	**Embelia ribes Q or 30**	*4 hourly*
❏ For pin worms	**Teucriumm-v. 30**	*4 hourly*
❏ For Ascarides	**Abrotanum 30**	*4 hourly*

Symptoms	Remedy	Frequency And Doses
❑ For hook worms	Chenopodium Q or 6	4 hourly
● Intercurrent remedy	Sulphur 200 or 1M	weekly (3)
Biochemic remedies	Natrum phos. 6X and Kali mur. 6X	4 hourly

WRITER'S CRAMP
(See Cramps)

YAWNING

Symptoms	Remedy	Frequency And Doses
☐ Even while physically occupied; with marked anxiety	Aconite 30 or 200	2 hourly
☐ After eating; with stretching of the limbs	Nux vomica 30 or 200	3 hourly
☐ Though sleeps well at night; yawns during day with desire to sleep	Lycopodium 30 or 200	4 hourly
☐ Constant theorizing; mind always busy; due to constant flow of ideas sleep is not sound, desires to sleep during day and yawns	Sulphur 200 or 1M	10 min. (3)
☐ Spasmodic yawning	Platina 200 or 1M	10 min. (3)
☐ Yawning with dyspnoea	Bromium 30 or 200	4 hourly
☐ Drowsiness without yawning	Chelidonium 30	4 hourly
☐ For complaints that comes on whenever patient yawns; trembling and shuddering	Cina 30 or 200	4 hourly
☐ Yawning with stretching and extending hands	Ruta g. 30 or 200	4 hourly
☐ Violent and spasmodic yawning	Rhus tox. 200 or 1M	4 hourly

Other Important Remedies:

Arnica, Ignatia, Natrum mur., etc..

PLAGUE

SOS – 1994

We are taking this necessary step of including this chapter as an addendum to this book because of a serious recurrence of plague after more than 50 years.

Naturally this matter is not based on our experience. We have culled it from various books and journals even up to a hundred years old. Readers are advised to consult a good *Materia Medica* for further details.

SYMPTOMS OF PLAGUE

The disease commences suddenly, without prodroma, with a rigor, followed quickly by great prostration, fever, and marked pain at the place where the bubo subsequently appears. After the onset the symptoms are headache, great thirst, vomiting, diarrhoea, marked weakness, and, as a rule, intense mental depression. The skin is hot and dry and occasionally, jaundiced. The countenance is drawn, the conjunctive are injected, and the eyes are sunken. The patient presents a dull, heavy, stupefied look. Sometimes this is replaced by an expression of terror. The tongue is swollen, red and coated with a greyish white fur. Occasionally the disease is ushered in with violent delirium, the patients being sometimes quite maniacal. At other times the patients are quiet and indifferent to their surroundings owing to a deadening of the mental faculties. Then appear the buboes or enlarged lymphatic glands.

VARIETIES OF PLAGUE

The main varieties of the disease are three : the bubonic, the pneumonic and the gastro-intestinal.

1. **Bubonic**: 70 percent of the cases come under this heading. Infection occurs through the skin.

2. **Pneumonic**: Fatal as is the bubonic variety, the pneumonic is still more so. The sputum of patients attacked by this variety presents almost a pure culture of plague bacilli. Infection occurs by means of the air-passages. The onset is marked by a rigor, attended by cough and some dyspnoea with slight fever. The temperature soon rises to 103° F. or higher, and in a few hours the patient commences to spit up a quantity of thin blood-stained sputum. The dyspnoea rapidly becomes more marked, there is much cardiac depression, the pulse is rapid and compressible, and there are signs of extreme restlessness, want of sleep, and early delirium; the ausculatory signs are those of catarrhal pneumonia. The disease in this form runs a very rapid course and is almost invariably fatal within three days.

3. **Gastro-intestinal**: This variety, like the pneumonic, has no external buboes and the cases are, as a rule, rapidly fatal. The glands are swollen and also enlarged and inflamed and the mucous membrane of the intestines is thickly coated with mucus and studded with small haemorrhages.

THE VARIOUS STAGES OF PLAGUE AND HOMOEOPATHIC REMEDIES

1. In the invasion or the first stage of the disease: Aconite, Belladonna, Ignatia, Merc. sol., Rhus tox., Pyrogen., Hyoscyamus, Dulcamara, Verat vir., Ferrum phos., Kali mur. and Phosphorus are required.

(If disease goes on unchecked it has a tendency either to invade the brain, heart or other internal organs of the body.)

2. If brain is affected: Belladonna, Naja, Stramoniun, Opium, Nux mos., Ailanthus, etc., are required.

3. If the heart is affected: Aconite, Calc. ars., Naja, Crotalus h., Kali. phos., Hydrocyan acid, Digitalis, Morphinum., etc., are required.

4. For serious cases: Antim tart., Calc. ars., Carbo veg., Crotalus h., Lachesis, Merc. cyn., Naja, Phosphorus, Secale cor., etc.

5. Other useful remedies: Arg. nit., Anthracinum, Apium, Ars. alb., Badiaga, Buboinum, Echinacea, Kali chlor., Pytolacca, Tarentula c., Hepar sulph., Silicea, Iodium, etc..

THERAPEUTICS OF LEADING HOMOEOPATHIC REMEDIES

Curative and preventive for bubonic plague: External heat with internal coldness. Sudden flushes of heat; fever with headache and glandular swelling under armpits and groins. **Ignatia** 200 weekly (6).

Curative and preventive for bubonic plague especially during the period of invasion. Chills followed by intense burning fever; with great thirst, anxiety, restlessness, headache, delirium, copious sweating and retention of urine. **Tarentula c.** 200, S.O.S.

For pneumonic plague: expectoration frothy, pale red, rust coloured, streaked with blood; cold mucus, tasting sour or sweet; difficult respiration, especially in evening; difficult inspiration. Anxiety about heart with nausea. Bleeding from internal organs – blood ,fluid non-coagulable – bleeding from all cavities. Fever with shiverings; flushes of heat over whole body – perspiration profuse on head, hands, and feet. Craving for cold water/drinks. **Phosphorus** 30 or 200 3 hourly (3).

Pestin 200 or **Plaiguinum** 200 is a nosode (prepared from the bacilli of the disease) and is considered the prophylactic remedy.

To combat high fever **Pyrogenium** 200, 1/2 hourly (3).

To combat fear and anxiety **Aconite** 30 or 200, 1/2 hourly (3).

A FEW TIPS FOR THE PREVENTION OF PLAGUE

1. Keep your house scrupulously clean; special attention should be paid to the flushing of drains and removal of refuse.

2. Personal cleanliness should be of the highest kind. Pay an extra amount to your washerman to clean your clothes, bed linen and other things.

3. Allow plenty of fresh air and sufficient light to come to every corner of your house, especially in the bed rooms and sitting rooms.

4. Don't allow rubbish things to accumulate in the corner of your home. These are the resting places for rats.

5. Place your bedding every day in the bright sun and warm it in the sunlight.

6. Don't take any medicines for fear of plague, because that would weaken your constitution and make you liable to diseases. For preventive medicines consult your homoeopathic physician.

7. Fright and fear of the disease should not disturb your mind, because that will induce susceptibility to an attack of plague. Calmness and composure of mind must be kept in tact by all means. We often find people greatly frightened on hearing the report of plague cases in the neighbourhood and it is not unfrequent that they do get the disease out of fear.

8. Take your meals in proper time and take the best nourishing food, at the same time take easily digestible substances. Food or drink polluted with the touch of plague cases or of those who are attending those patients must be avoided by all means. Fresh food and filtered water for drinking purposes must be ensured. Don't allow rotten things to remain in your food store, or rats to infest your storehouse.